W9-DEU-903

Renal
Physiology

Look for these other *Mosby Physiology Monograph Series* titles:

Blankenship: NEUROPHYSIOLOGY (978-0-323-01899-9)

Blaustein et al: CELLULAR PHYSIOLOGY (978-0-323-01341-3)

Cloutier: RESPIRATORY PHYSIOLOGY (978-0-323-03628-3)

Johnson: GASTROINTESTINAL PHYSIOLOGY, 7th Edition (978-0-323-03391-6)

Levy & Pappano: CARDIOVASCULAR PHYSIOLOGY, 9th Edition (978-0-323-03446-3)

Porterfield & White: ENDOCRINE PHYSIOLOGY, 3rd Edition (978-0-323-03666-5)

Renal Physiology

■ ■ ■ ■ ■ ■ ■ ■ ■ ■ ■

FOURTH EDITION

Edited by

BRUCE M. KOEPPEN, MD, PhD

Dean, Academic Affairs
Albert and Wilda Van Dusen Professor of Academic Medicine
Professor of Medicine and Cell Biology
University of Connecticut Health Center
Farmington, Connecticut

BRUCE A. STANTON, PhD

Professor of Physiology
Darmouth Medical School
Hanover, New Hampshire

MOSBY

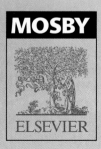

ELSEVIER

1600 John F. Kennedy Blvd.
Ste 1800
Philadelphia, PA 19103-2899

RENAL PHYSIOLOGY

ISBN-13: 978-0-323-03447-0
ISBN-10: 0-323-03447-0

Copyright © 2007 by Mosby, Inc., an affiliate of Elsevier Inc.

All rights reserved. No part of this publication may be reproduced or transmitted in any form or by any means, electronic or mechanical, including photocopying, recording, or any information storage and retrieval system, without permission in writing from the publisher.
Permissions may be sought directly from Elsevier's Health Sciences Rights Department in Philadelphia, PA, USA: phone: (+1) 215 239 3804, fax: (+1) 215 239 3805, e-mail: healthpermissions@elsevier.com. You may also complete your request on-line via the Elsevier homepage (http://www.elsevier.com), by selecting 'Customer Support' and then 'Obtaining Permissions'.

Notice

Knowledge and best practice in this field are constantly changing. As new research and experience broaden our knowledge, changes in practice, treatment and drug therapy may become necessary or appropriate. Readers are advised to check the most current information provided (i) on procedures featured or (ii) by the manufacturer of each product to be administered, to verify the recommended dose or formula, the method and duration of administration, and contraindications. It is the responsibility of the practitioner, relying on their own experience and knowledge of the patient, to make diagnoses, to determine dosages and the best treatment for each individual patient, and to take all appropriate safety precautions. To the fullest extent of the law, neither the Publisher nor the Authors assume any liability for any injury and/or damage to persons or property arising out of or related to any use of the material contained in this book.

The Publisher

Previous editions copyrighted 1992, 1997, 2001

Library of Congress Cataloging-in-Publication Data
Koeppen, Bruce M.
    Renal physiology / Bruce M. Koeppen, Bruce A. Stanton. -- 4th ed.
        p. ; cm. -- (The Mosby physiology monograph series)
    Includes bibliographical references and index.
    ISBN-13: 978-0-323-03447-0 ISBN-10: 0-323-03447-0
    1. Kidneys--Physiology.   I. Stanton, Bruce A. II. Title. III. Series.
    [DNLM: 1. Kidney--physiology.   WJ 301 K78r 2007]
    QP249.K64   2007
    612.4′63--dc22   2006044893

Acquisitions Editor: William Schmitt
Editorial Assistant: Kevin Kochanski
Publishing Services Manager: Linda Van Pelt
Project Manager: Priscilla Crater
Design Direction: Lou Forgione
Cover Designer: Lou Forgione

Printed in China
Last digit is the print number: 9 8 7 6 5 4 3 2

Working together to grow
libraries in developing countries

www.elsevier.com | www.bookaid.org | www.sabre.org

ELSEVIER   BOOK AID International   Sabre Foundation

This book is dedicated to
our family, friends, colleagues, and, most especially, our students.

PREFACE

When we wrote the first edition of *Renal Physiology* in 1992, our goal was to provide a clear and concise overview of the function of the kidneys for health professions students who were studying the topic for the first time. The feedback we have received over the years has affirmed that we met our goal, and that the achievement has been a key element to the book's success. Thus, in this fourth edition we have adhered to our original goal, maintaining all of the proven elements of the last three editions.

Since 1992, much has been learned about kidney function at the cellular and molecular level. Although this new information is exciting and provides new and greater insights into the function of the kidneys in health and disease, it can prove daunting to the first-time student and in some cases may cause them to lose the forest for the trees. In an attempt to balance the needs of the first-time student with our desire to present some of the latest advances in the field of renal physiology, we have added a new feature to this edition. Where appropriate, cellular and molecular details are placed in highlighted text boxes to supplement the main text for those students who wish additional detail. The other features of the book, which include clinical material that illustrates important physiologic principles, multiple-choice questions, self-study problems, and integrated case studies, have been retained and updated. To achieve our goal of keeping the book concise, we have removed some old material as new material was added. Most notable in this regard is the absence of the chapter on the physiologic adaptation to nephron loss—a topic that is well covered, and more appropriately placed, in textbooks focused on renal pathophysiology. We hope that all who use this book find that the changes have made this book an improved learning tool and a valuable source of information.

To the instructor: This book is intended to provide students in the biomedical and health sciences with a basic understanding of the workings of the kidneys. We believe that it is better for the student at this stage to master a few central concepts and ideas rather than to assimilate a large array of facts. Consequently, this book is designed to teach the important aspects and fundamental concepts of normal renal function. We have emphasized clarity and conciseness in presenting the material. To accomplish this goal, we have been selective in the material included. The broader field of nephrology, with its current and future frontiers, is better learned at a later time and only after the "big picture" has been well established. For clarity and simplicity, we have made statements as assertions of fact even though we recognize that not all aspects of a particular problem have been resolved.

To the student: As an aid to learning this material, each chapter includes a listing of objectives that reflect the fundamental concepts to be mastered. At the end of each chapter, we have provided a summary and a listing of key words and concepts that should serve as a checklist while working through the chapter. We have also provided a series of self-study problems, which review the central principles of each chapter. Because these questions are learning tools, answers and explanations are provided in an appendix. A multiple-choice examination and comprehensive clinical cases are included in other appendices. We recommend working through the tests and clinical cases only after completing the book. In this way, they can serve to indicate where additional work or review is required.

We have provided an updated bibliography of selected books, monographs, and papers. This highly selective bibliography is intended to provide the next step in the study of the kidney; it is a place to begin to add details to the subjects presented here and a resource for exploring other aspects of the kidney not treated in this book.

We encourage all who use this book to send us your comments and suggestions. Please let us know what we've done right, as well as what needs improvement.

Bruce M. Koeppen
Bruce A. Stanton

ACKNOWLEDGMENTS

We would like to thank our students at the University of Connecticut School of Medicine and School of Dental Medicine and at Dartmouth Medical School, who continually provide feedback on how to improve this book. We also thank our colleagues and the many individuals from around the world who have contacted us with thoughtful suggestions for this as well as for previous editions. Special thanks go to Drs. Nancy Adams, William Arendhorst, Dennis Brown, Agnieszka Swiatecka-Urban, Jay Bucci, Geza Fejes-Toth, Peter Friedman, Dan Henry, Andre Kaplan, Tom Manger, John Mills, Joseph Palmisano, David Pollack, Brian Remillard, and Cynthia Short, whose insights and suggestions over the many years we have spent writing this monograph have been invaluable.

Finally, we thank William Schmitt, Kevin Kochanski, Priscilla Crater, and the staff at Elsevier for their support and commitment to quality.

CONTENTS

∎ ∎ ∎ ∎ ∎ ∎ ∎ ∎ ∎ ∎

INTRODUCTION TO THE KIDNEY 1

CHAPTER 1

PHYSIOLOGY OF BODY FLUIDS . . .5

Objectives,   5

Physicochemical Properties of Electrolyte
   Solutions,   5

   Molarity and Equivalence,   5

   Osmosis and Osmotic Pressure,   6

   Osmolarity and Osmolality,   7

   Tonicity,   7

   Oncotic Pressure,   8

   Specific Gravity,   8

Volumes of Body Fluid Compartments,   9

Composition of Body Fluid
   Compartments,   10

Fluid Exchange Between Body Fluid
   Compartments,   11

   Capillary Fluid Exchange,   11

   Cellular Fluid Exchange,   13

Summary,   15

Key Words and Concepts,   15

Self-Study Problems,   16

CHAPTER 2

STRUCTURE AND FUNCTION
OF THE KIDNEYS 19

Objectives,   19

Structure of the Kidneys,   19

   Gross Anatomy,   19

   Ultrastructure of the Nephron,   20

   *Ultrastructure of the Renal
      Corpuscle,   24*

   *Ultrastructure of the Juxtaglomerular
      Apparatus,   28*

   Innervation of the Kidneys,   28

Summary,   29

Key Words and Concepts,   29

Self-Study Problems,   30

CHAPTER 3

GLOMERULAR FILTRATION
AND RENAL BLOOD FLOW 31

Objectives,   31

Renal Clearance,   31

   Glomerular Filtration Rate,   32

Glomerular Filtration,   34

   *Determinants of Ultrafiltrate
      Composition,   35*

   Dynamics of Ultrafiltration,   36

Renal Blood Flow, 37

Regulation of Renal Blood Flow and
    Glomerular Filtration Rate, 41

Sympathetic Nerves, 41

Angiotensin II, 42

Prostaglandins, 42

Nitric Oxide, 43

Endothelin, 44

Bradykinin, 44

Adenosine, 44

Natriuretic Peptides, 44

ATP, 44

Glucocorticoids, 44

Histamine, 44

Dopamine, 44

Summary, 45

Key Words and Concepts, 46

Self-Study Problems, 46

CHAPTER 4

RENAL TRANSPORT MECHANISMS: NaCl AND WATER REABSORPTION ALONG THE NEPHRON 47

Objectives, 47

General Principles of Membrane
    Transport, 48

General Principles of Transepithelial Solute
    and Water Transport, 50

NaCl, Solute, and Water Reabsorption Along
    the Nephron, 52

Proximal Tubule, 52

Henle's Loop, 61

Distal Tubule and Collecting
    Duct, 63

Regulation of NaCl and Water
    Reabsorption, 64

Summary, 69

Key Words and Concepts, 70

Self-Study Problems, 70

CHAPTER 5

REGULATION OF BODY FLUID OSMOLALITY: REGULATION OF WATER BALANCE 71

Objectives, 71

Antidiuretic Hormone, 73

Osmotic Control of ADH Secretion, 74

Hemodynamic Control of ADH
    Secretion, 75

ADH Actions on the Kidneys, 76

Thirst, 79

Renal Mechanisms for Dilution and
    Concentration of the Urine, 80

Medullary Interstitium, 85

Vasa Recta Function, 86

Assessment of Renal Diluting
    and Concentrating Ability, 87

Summary, 89

Key Words And Concepts, 89

Self-Study Problems, 90

CHAPTER 6

REGULATION OF EXTRACELLULAR FLUID VOLUME AND NaCl BALANCE 91

Objectives, 91

Concept of Effective Circulating
    Volume, 92

Volume-Sensing Systems, 93

Vascular Low-Pressure Volume
    Sensors, 94

Vascular High-Pressure Volume Sensors,   94

Hepatic Sensors,   95

Central Nervous System Na⁺ Sensors,   95

Volume Sensor Signals,   95

Renal Sympathetic Nerves,   95

Renin-Angiotensin-Aldosterone System,   96

Natriuretic Peptides,   98

Antidiuretic Hormone,   99

Control of Renal NaCl Excretion During Euvolemia,   99

Mechanisms for Maintaining the Delivery of Na⁺ to the Distal Tubule Constant,   101

Regulation of Distal Tubule and Collecting Duct Na⁺ Reabsorption,   101

Control of Na⁺ Excretion with Volume Expansion,   102

Control of Na⁺ Excretion with Volume Contraction,   104

Edema,   106

Alterations in Starling Forces,   106

The Role of the Kidneys,   107

Summary,   108

Key Words and Concepts,   109

Self-Study Problems,   109

CHAPTER 7

REGULATION OF POTASSIUM BALANCE 113

Objectives,   113

Overview of K⁺ Homeostasis,   113

Regulation of Plasma [K⁺],   115

Epinephrine,   116

Insulin,   116

Aldosterone,   117

Alterations of Plasma [K⁺],   117

Acid-Base Balance,   117

Plasma Osmolality,   117

Cell Lysis,   118

Exercise,   118

K⁺ Excretion by the Kidneys,   118

Cellular Mechanisms of K⁺ Secretion by Principal Cells in the Distal Tubule and Collecting Duct,   120

Regulation of K⁺ Secretion by the Distal Tubule and Collecting Duct,   120

Plasma [K⁺],   120

Aldosterone,   122

Antidiuretic Hormone,   123

Factors that Perturb K⁺ Excretion,   124

Flow of Tubular Fluid,   124

Acid-Base Balance,   125

Glucocorticoids,   127

Summary,   128

Key Words and Concepts,   128

Self-Study Problems,   128

CHAPTER 8

REGULATION OF ACID-BASE BALANCE 129

Objectives,   129

The HCO₃⁻ Buffer System,   130

Overview of Acid-Base Balance,   130

Net Acid Excretion by the Kidneys,   131

HCO₃⁻ Reabsorption Along the Nephron,   132

Regulation of H⁺ Secretion,   135

Formation of New HCO₃⁻,   137

Response to Acid-Base Disorders,   141

Extracellular and Intracellular Buffers,   141

Respiratory Compensation,   142

Renal Compensation,   142

Simple Acid-Base Disorders,   143

    Metabolic Acidosis,   143

    Metabolic Alkalosis,   144

    Respiratory Acidosis,   144

    Respiratory Alkalosis,   145

Analysis of Acid-Base Disorders,   145

Summary,   147

Key Words and Concepts,   147

Self-Study Problems,   147

CHAPTER 9

REGULATION OF CALCIUM AND PHOSPHATE HOMEOSTASIS 149

Objectives,   149

Calcium,   150

    Overview of Ca^{++} Homeostasis,   150

    Ca^{++} Transport along the Nephron,   152

    Regulation of Urinary Ca^{++} Excretion,   154

    Calcium-Sensing Receptor,   155

Phosphate,   155

    Overview of Pi Homeostasis,   156

    Pi Transport along the Nephron,   157

    Regulation of Urinary Pi Excretion,   157

Integrative Review of Parathyroid Hormone, Calcitriol, and Calcitonin on Ca^{++} and Pi Homeostasis,   159

Summary,   161

Key Words and Concepts,   161

Self-Study Problems,   161

CHAPTER 10

PHYSIOLOGY OF DIURETIC ACTION,   163

Objectives,   163

General Principles of Diuretic Action,   163

    Sites of Action of Diuretics,   164

    Response of Other Nephron Segments,   164

    Adequate Delivery of Diuretics to Their Site of Action,   164

    Volume of the Extracellular Fluid,   165

Diuretic Braking Phenomenon,   165

Mechanisms of Action of Diuretics,   166

    Osmotic Diuretics,   166

    Carbonic Anhydrase Inhibitors,   167

    Loop Diuretics,   167

    Thiazide Diuretics,   168

    K^{+}-Sparing Diuretics,   168

    Aquaretics,   169

Effect of Diuretics on the Excretion of Water and other Solutes,   169

    Solute-Free Water,   169

    K^{+} Excretion,   170

    HCO$_3^-$ Excretion,   170

    Ca^{++} and Pi Excretion,   171

Summary,   172

Key Words and Concepts,   173

Self-Study Problems,   173

ADDITIONAL READING,   175

APPENDIX **A**

INTEGRATIVE CASE STUDIES . . .179

APPENDIX **B**

NORMAL LABORATORY
VALUES 183

APPENDIX **C**

NEPHRON FUNCTION 185

APPENDIX **D**

ANSWERS TO SELF-STUDY
POBLEMS .189

APPENDIX **E**

ANSWERS TO INTEGRATIVE
CASE STUDIES 203

APPENDIX **F**

REVIEW EXAMINATION 209

INDEX 223

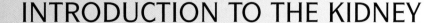

INTRODUCTION TO THE KIDNEY

"The kidney presents in the highest degree the phenomenon of sensibility, the power of reacting to various stimuli in a direction which is appropriate for the survival of the organism; a power of adaptation which almost gives one the idea that its component parts must be endowed with intelligence."

E. Starling—1909

"Certainly, mental integrity is a sine qua non of the free and independent life. But let the composition of our internal environment suffer change, let our kidneys fail for even a short time to fulfill their tasks, and our mental integrity, or personality is destroyed."

Homer W. Smith—1939

As both Starling and Smith recognized, the kidneys are viewed more appropriately as regulatory, rather than excretory, organs. However, it is clear that the excretory function of the kidneys is central to their ability to regulate the composition and volume of the body fluids.

In this book, various aspects of renal physiology are explored. Emphasis is placed on providing insight and understanding into the major functions of the kidneys, which are as follows:

- Regulation of body fluid osmolality and volume
- Regulation of electrolyte balance
- Regulation of acid-base balance
- Excretion of metabolic products and foreign substances
- Production and secretion of hormones

In the chapters that follow, these aspects of renal function are considered in detail. However, in order to provide a broad perspective and overview, they are briefly described here.

Regulation of body fluid osmolality and volume (Chapters 1, 5, and 6): The kidneys are critical components of the systems involved in the control of both the osmolality and volume of the body fluids. The control of body fluid osmolality is important for the maintenance of normal cell volume in virtually all tissues of the body, and control of the volume of body fluids is necessary for normal function of the cardiovascular system. The kidneys, working in an integrated fashion with components of the cardiovascular and central nervous systems, accomplish these tasks by regulating the excretion of water and NaCl.

Regulation of electrolyte balance (Chapters 4, 5, 6, 7, 8, and 9): The kidneys play an essential role in regulating the amounts of several important inorganic ions in the body, including, but not limited to, sodium (Na^+), potassium (K^+), chloride (Cl^-), bicarbonate (HCO_3^-), hydrogen ion (H^+), calcium (Ca^{++}), and phosphate (Pi). The kidneys also contribute to the maintenance of organic ion balance. For example, the excretion of many of the intermediates of the Krebs cycle (e.g., citrate, succinate) is controlled by the kidneys. In order to maintain appropriate balance, the excretion of any one of these electrolytes must be balanced to the daily intake. If intake exceeds excretion, the amount of a particular electrolyte in the body increases. Conversely, if excretion exceeds intake, the amount decreases. For many of these electrolytes

1

the kidneys are the sole or primary route for excretion from the body. Thus, electrolyte balance is achieved by carefully matching daily excretion by the kidneys with daily intake.

Regulation of acid-base balance (Chapter 8): Many of the metabolic functions of the body are exquisitely sensitive to pH. Thus, the pH of the body fluids must be maintained within very narrow limits. This is accomplished by buffers within the body fluids and the coordinated action of the lungs, liver, and kidneys. The importance of the kidneys in acid-base balance is underscored by the fact that acid accumulates in the body fluids of individuals with reduced renal function.

Excretion of metabolic products and foreign substances (Chapters 3 and 4): The kidneys excrete a number of end products of metabolism that are no longer needed by the body. These so-called waste products include urea (from amino acids), uric acid (from nucleic acids), creatinine (from muscle creatine), end products of hemoglobin metabolism, and metabolites of hormones. These substances are eliminated from the body by the kidneys at a rate that matches their production. Thus, their concentrations within the body fluids are maintained at a constant level. The kidneys also represent an important route for elimination of foreign substances from the body, including drugs, pesticides, and other chemicals ingested in the food. When kidney function is compromised, metabolic waste products and foreign substances accumulate in the body because their excretion in the urine decreases.

Production and secretion of hormones (Chapters 6 and 9): The kidneys are important endocrine organs, producing and secreting renin, calcitriol $(1,25\text{-dihydroxyvitamin } D_3)$, and erythropoietin. Although renin is a proteolytic enzyme and not a hormone, it activates the renin-angiotensin-aldosterone system, which is important in regulating blood pressure, as well as Na^+ and K^+ balance. Calcitriol is necessary for normal reabsorption of Ca^{++} by the gastrointestinal tract and for its deposition in bone. With renal disease the ability of the kidneys to produce calcitriol is impaired, and levels of this hormone are reduced. As a result, Ca^{++} reabsorption by the intestine is decreased. This reduced intestinal Ca^{++} reabsorption contributes to the abnormalities in bone formation seen in patients with chronic renal disease.

Erythropoietin stimulates red blood cell formation by the bone marrow. With many kidney diseases, erythropoietin production and secretion are reduced, which by decreasing erythrocyte production is a causal factor in the anemia seen in chronic renal failure. The kidneys also secrete a circulating enzyme (renalase) that metabolizes and inactivates catecholamines. Given the important role of the autonomic nervous system and circulating catecholamines in the regulation of blood pressure, recent studies suggest that the kidneys may play an even more important role in regulating blood pressure than previously thought.

Kidney disease is a major health problem. In the United States:

- Kidney disease affects over 20 million patients and accounts for more than 80,000 deaths per year.
- Each year over 3 million new patients are diagnosed with kidney disease.
- Over 458,000 people are treated for **end-stage renal disease (ESRD)** every year.
- 275,000 patients with ESRD are receiving either hemodialysis or peritoneal dialysis.
- Diabetes, hypertension, glomerulonephritis, and polycystic kidney disease are the leading causes of ESRD.
- ESRD caused by diabetes is increasing at an annual rate of more than 11% per year.
- Health care costs for ESRD are more than $19 billion dollars per year.
- More than 14,000 kidney transplants are performed each year. Unfortunately, more than 54,000 patients are awaiting kidney transplants.
- Urinary tract infections, kidney stones (i.e., urolithiasis), and interstitial cystitis (i.e., inflammation of the urinary bladder) are also major health care problems. Interstitial cystitis (700,000 patients), urinary stones (1.3 million visits annually at a cost of $1.8 billion), urinary tract infections (8.3 million visits annually), and urinary incontinence (13 million adults affected, mostly older than 65, at a cost of $26 billion per year) are serious health concerns.

As noted in the clinical box, a large variety of diseases impair the function of the kidneys, resulting in renal failure. In some instances the impairment of renal function is transient, but in many cases renal function progressively declines. Patients in whom the glomerular filtration rate is less than 10% of normal are said to have end-stage renal disease (ESRD) and must undergo renal replacement therapy in order to survive. Renal replacement therapies include peritoneal dialysis, hemodialysis, and renal transplantation. Both peritoneal dialysis and hemodialysis, as their names indicate, are based on the process of dialysis, whereby small molecules are removed from the blood by diffusion across a selectively permeable membrane into a solution that lacks these small molecules. In peritoneal dialysis, the peritoneal membrane acts as a dialyzing membrane. Several liters of a solution are introduced into the abdominal cavity and small molecules in blood diffuse across the peritoneal membrane into the solution, which is then removed from the abdominal cavity. In hemodialysis, a patient's blood is pumped through an artificial kidney machine. In the kidney machine blood is separated from an artificial solution by a dialysis membrane, which allows small molecules to diffuse from blood into the dialysis solution, thereby removing the small molecules from the blood. Patients who are candidates for renal transplantation are treated with dialysis until an appropriate donor kidney can be obtained. Although anemia also used to be a significant problem because of reduced erythropoietin production in ESRD, patients on chronic dialysis now receive recombinant human erythropoietin.

To understand the mechanisms that contribute to renal disease, it is first necessary to understand the normal physiology of renal function. Thus, in the following chapters of this book various aspects of renal function are considered. Where information is available, these functions are considered at several levels of organization: whole kidney, single nephron, individual tubular cell, cell membrane, and transport protein.

1

PHYSIOLOGY OF BODY FLUIDS

OBJECTIVES

Upon completion of this chapter, the student should be able to answer the following questions:

1. How do the body fluid compartments differ with respect to their volumes and their ionic compositions?

2. What are the driving forces responsible for movement of water across cell membranes and the capillary wall?

3. How do the volumes of the intracellular and extracellular fluid compartments change under various pathophysiologic conditions?

In addition, the student should be able to define, and understand, the following properties of physiologically important solutions and fluids:

1. Molarity and equivalence

2. Osmotic pressure

3. Osmolarity and osmolality

4. Oncotic pressure

5. Tonicity

One of the major functions of the kidneys is to maintain the volume and composition of the body fluids constant despite wide variation in the daily intake of water and solutes. In this chapter, the volume and composition of the body fluids are discussed to provide a background for the study of the kidneys as regulatory organs. Some of the basic principles, terminology, and concepts related to the properties of solutes in solution are also reviewed.

PHYSICOCHEMICAL PROPERTIES OF ELECTROLYTE SOLUTIONS

Molarity and Equivalence

The amount of a substance dissolved in a solution (i.e., its concentration) is expressed in terms of either **molarity** or **equivalence**. Molarity is the amount of a substance relative to its molecular weight. For example, glucose has a molecular weight of 180 g/mole. If 1 L of

water contains 1 g of glucose, the molarity of this glucose solution would be determined as:

$$\frac{1 \text{ g/L}}{180 \text{ g/mole}} = 0.0056 \text{ moles/L or } 5.6 \text{ mmol/L} \qquad (1\text{-}1)$$

For uncharged molecules, such as glucose and urea, concentrations in the body fluids are usually expressed in terms of molarity.[1] Because many of the substances of biologic interest are present at very low concentrations,

---

[1] The units used to express the concentrations of substances in various body fluids differ among laboratories. The system of international units (SI) is used in most countries and in most scientific and medical journals in the United States. Despite this convention, traditional units are still widely used. For urea and glucose the traditional units of concentration are mg/dL (i.e., mg per deciliter or 100 ml), whereas the SI units are mmol/L. Similarly, electrolyte concentrations are traditionally expressed as mEq/L, while the SI units are mmol/L (see Appendix B).

units are more frequently expressed in the millimolar range (mmol/L or mM).

The concentration of solutes, which normally dissociate into more than one particle when dissolved in solution (e.g., NaCl), is usually expressed in terms of equivalence. Equivalence refers to the stoichiometry of the interaction between cation and anion and is determined by the valence of these ions. For example, consider a 1-L solution containing 9 g of NaCl (molecular weight = 58.4 g/mole). The molarity of this solution is 154 mmol/L. Because NaCl dissociates into Na^+ and Cl^- ions, and assuming complete dissociation, this solution contains 154 mmol/L of Na^+ and 154 mmol/L of Cl^-. Because the valence of these ions is 1, these concentrations can also be expressed as milliequivalents (mEq) of the ion per liter (i.e., 154 mEq/L for Na^+ and Cl^-, respectively).

For univalent ions, such as Na^+ and Cl^-, concentrations expressed in terms of molarity and equivalence are identical. However, this is not true for ions having valences greater than 1. Accordingly, the concentration of Ca^{++} (molecular weight = 40.1 g/mole and

valence = 2) in a 1-L solution containing 0.1 g of this ion could be expressed as:

$$\frac{0.1 \text{ g/L}}{40.1 \text{ g/mole}} = 2.5 \text{ mmol/L} \tag{1-2}$$

$$= 2.5 \text{ mmol/L} \times 2 \text{ Eq/mole} = 5 \text{ mEq/L}$$

Although some exceptions exist, it is customary to express concentrations of ions in milliequivalents per liter.

Osmosis and Osmotic Pressure

The movement of water across cell membranes occurs by the process of **osmosis.** The driving force for this movement is the osmotic pressure difference across the cell membrane. Figure 1-1 illustrates the concept of osmosis and the measurement of the osmotic pressure of a solution.

Osmotic pressure is determined solely by the number of solute particles in the solution. It is not dependent upon such factors as the size of the solute particles, their mass, or chemical nature (e.g., valence).

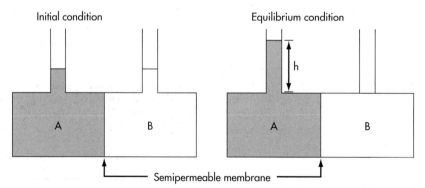

FIGURE 1-1 ■ Schematic representation of osmotic water movement and the generation of an osmotic pressure. Compartment A and compartment B are separated by a semipermeable membrane (i.e., the membrane is highly permeable to water but impermeable to solute). Compartment A contains a solute, and compartment B contains only distilled water. Over time, water moves by osmosis from compartment B to compartment A. (*Note:* This water movement is driven by the concentration gradient for water. Because of the presence of solute particles in compartment A, the concentration of water in compartment A is less than that in compartment B. Consequently, water moves across the semipermeable membrane from compartment B to compartment A down its gradient). This raises the level of fluid in compartment A and decreases the level in compartment B. At equilibrium, the hydrostatic pressure exerted by the column of water (h) stops the movement of water from compartment B to A. This pressure is equal and opposite to the osmotic pressure exerted by the solute particles in compartment A.

Osmotic pressure (π), measured in atmospheres (atm), is calculated by **van't Hoff's law** as:

$$\pi = nCRT \qquad (1\text{-}3)$$

where:

n = Number of dissociable particles per molecule
C = Total solute concentration
R = Gas constant
T = Temperature in degrees Kelvin (°K)

For a molecule that does not dissociate in water, such as glucose or urea, a solution containing 1 mmol/L of these solutes at 37° C can exert an osmotic pressure of 2.54×10^{-2} atm as calculated by equation 1-3 using the following values:

n = 1
C = 0.001 mol/L
R = 0.082 atm L/mol °K
T = 310 °K

Because 1 atmosphere equals 760 mm Hg at sea level, π for this solution can also be expressed as 19.3 mm Hg. Alternatively, osmotic pressure is expressed in terms of osmolarity (see the following). Thus, a solution containing 1 mmol/L of solute particles exerts an osmotic pressure of 1 milliosmole/L (1 mOsm/L).

For substances that dissociate in a solution, n of equation 1-3 has a value other than 1. For example, a 150 mmol/L solution of NaCl has an osmolarity of 300 mOsm/L because each molecule of NaCl dissociates into a Na^+ and a Cl^- ion (i.e., n = 2). If dissociation of a substance into its component ions is not complete, n is not an integer. Accordingly, osmolarity for any solution can be calculated as:

$$\textbf{Osmolarity} = \textbf{concentration} \times \textbf{number of} \qquad (1\text{-}4)$$
$$\textbf{dissociable particles}$$

$$\textbf{mOsm/L} = \textbf{mmol/L} \times \textbf{\# particles/mole}$$

Osmolarity and Osmolality

Osmolarity and **osmolality** are frequently confused and incorrectly interchanged. Osmolarity refers to the number of solute particles per 1 L of solvent, whereas osmolality is the number of solute particles in 1 kg of solvent. For dilute solutions, the difference between osmolarity and osmolality is insignificant. Measurements of osmolarity are temperature dependent

because the volume of solvent varies with temperature (i.e., the volume is larger at higher temperatures). In contrast, osmolality, which is based on the mass of the solvent, is temperature independent. For this reason, osmolality is the preferred term for biologic systems and is used throughout this and subsequent chapters. Osmolality has the units of Osm/kg H_2O. Because of the dilute nature of physiologic solutions and because water is the solvent, osmolalities are expressed as milliosmoles per kilogram water (mOsm/kg H_2O).

Table 1-1 shows the relationship between molecular weight, equivalence, and osmoles for a number of physiologically significant solutes.

Tonicity

The **tonicity** of a solution is related to its effect on the volume of a cell. Solutions that do not change the volume of a cell are said to be **isotonic.** A **hypotonic** solution causes a cell to swell, and a **hypertonic** solution causes a cell to shrink. Although related to osmolality, tonicity also takes into consideration the ability of the solute to cross the cell membrane.

Consider two solutions: a 300 mmol/L solution of sucrose and a 300 mmol/L solution of urea. Both solutions have an osmolality of 300 mOsm/kg H_2O and therefore are said to be **isosmotic** (i.e., they have the

TABLE 1-1			
Units of Measurement for Physiologically Significant Substances			
SUBSTANCE	ATOMIC/ MOLECULAR WEIGHT	EQUIVALENTS/ MOL	OSMOLES/ MOL
Na^+	23.0	1	1
K^+	39.1	1	1
Cl^-	35.4	1	1
HCO_3^-	61.0	1	1
Ca^{++}	40.1	2	1
Phosphate (Pi)	95.0	3	1
NH_4^+	18.0	1	1
NaCl	58.4	2*	2†
$CaCl_2$	111	4‡	3
Glucose	180	—	1
Urea	60	—	1

*One equivalent each from Na^+ and Cl^-.
†NaCl does not dissociate completely in solution. The actual osmoles/mol is 1.88. However, for simplicity, a value of 2 is often used.
‡Ca^{++} contributes two equivalents, as do the Cl^- ions.

same osmolality). When red blood cells, which for the purpose of this illustration also have an intracellular fluid osmolality of 300 mOsm/kg H_2O, are placed in the two solutions, those in the sucrose solution maintain their normal volume but those placed in urea swell and eventually burst. Thus, the sucrose solution is isotonic and the urea solution is hypotonic. The differential effect of these solutions on red cell volume is related to the permeability of the plasma membrane to sucrose and urea. The red cell membrane contains uniporters for urea (see Chapter 4). Thus, urea easily crosses the cell membrane (i.e., the membrane is **permeable** to urea), driven by the concentration gradient (i.e., extracellular [urea] > intracellular [urea]). In contrast, the red cell membrane does not contain sucrose transporters, and sucrose cannot enter the cell (i.e., the membrane is **impermeable** to sucrose).

To exert an osmotic pressure across a membrane, a solute must not permeate that membrane. Because the red cell membrane is impermeable to sucrose, it exerts an osmotic pressure equal and opposite to the osmotic pressure generated by the contents of the red cell (in this case 300 mOsm/kg H_2O). In contrast, urea is readily able to cross the red blood cell membrane, and it cannot exert an osmotic pressure to balance that generated by the intracellular solutes of the red blood cell. Consequently, sucrose is termed an **effective osmole** and urea is an **ineffective osmole.**

To take into account the effect of a solute's membrane permeability on osmotic pressure, it is necessary to rewrite equation 1-3 as:

$$\pi = \sigma(nCRT) \qquad (1\text{-}5)$$

where σ is the **reflection coefficient** or **osmotic coefficient** and is a measure of the relative ability of the solute to cross a cell membrane.

For a solute that can freely cross the cell membrane, such as urea in this example, $\sigma = 0$, and no effective osmotic pressure is exerted. Thus, urea is an ineffective osmole for red blood cells. In contrast, $\sigma = 1$ for a solute that cannot cross the cell membrane (i.e., sucrose). Such a substance is said to be an effective osmole. Many solutes are neither completely able nor completely unable to cross cell membranes (i.e., $0 < \sigma < 1$) and generate an osmotic pressure that is only a fraction of what is expected from the total solute concentration.

Oncotic Pressure

Oncotic pressure is the osmotic pressure generated by large molecules (especially proteins) in solution. As illustrated in Figure 1-2, the magnitude of the osmotic pressure generated by a solution of protein does not conform to van't Hoff's law. The cause of this anomalous relationship between protein concentration and osmotic pressure is not completely understood but appears to be related to the size and shape of the molecule. For example, the correlation to van't Hoff's law is more precise with small, globular proteins than with larger protein molecules.

The oncotic pressure exerted by proteins in human plasma has a normal value of approximately 26 to 28 mm Hg. Although this pressure appears to be small when considered in terms of osmotic pressure (28 mm Hg ≈ 1.4 mOsm/kg H_2O), it is an important force involved in fluid movement across capillaries (details of this topic are presented in the following section on fluid exchange between body fluid compartments).

Specific Gravity

The total solute concentration in a solution can also be measured as **specific gravity.** Specific gravity is defined as the weight of a volume of solution divided by the weight of an equal volume of distilled water. Thus, the specific gravity of distilled water is 1. Because biologic fluids contain a number of different substances, their specific gravities are greater than 1. For example, normal human plasma has a specific gravity in the range of 1.008 to 1.010.

The specific gravity of urine is sometimes measured in clinical settings and used to assess the concentrating ability of the kidney. The specific gravity of urine varies in proportion to its osmolality. However, because specific gravity depends on both the number of solute particles and their weight, the relationship between specific gravity and osmolality is not always predictable. For example, patients who have been injected with radiocontrast dye (molecular weight > 500 g/mole) for x-ray studies can have high values of urine specific gravity (1.040 to 1.050) even though the urine osmolality is similar to that of plasma (e.g., 300 mOsm/kg H_2O).

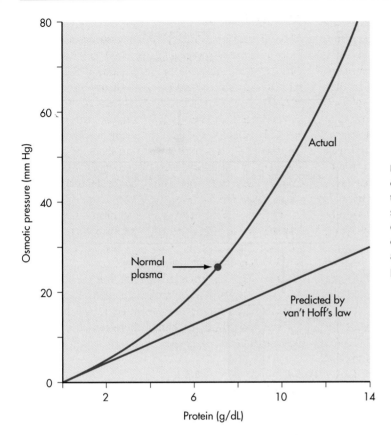

FIGURE 1-2 ■ Relationship between the concentration of plasma proteins in solution and the osmotic pressure (oncotic pressure) they generate. Protein concentration is expressed as g/dL. Normal plasma protein concentration is indicated. Note that the actual pressure generated exceeds that predicted by van't Hoff's law.

VOLUMES OF BODY FLUID COMPARTMENTS

Water makes up approximately 60% of the body's weight, with variability among individuals being a function of the amount of adipose tissue. Because the water content of adipose tissue is lower than that of other tissue, increased amounts of adipose tissue reduce the fraction of total body weight due to water. The percentage of body weight attributed to water also varies with age. In newborns, it is approximately 75%. This decreases to the adult value of 60% by the age of 1 year.

As illustrated in Figure 1-3, **total body water** is distributed between two major compartments, which are divided by the cell membrane.[2] The **intracellular fluid (ICF)** compartment is the larger compartment and contains approximately two thirds of the total body water. The remaining one third is contained in the **extracellular fluid (ECF)** compartment. Expressed as percentages of body weight, the volumes of total body water, ICF, and ECF are:

$$\text{Total body water} = 0.6 \times \text{(body weight)}$$

$$\text{ICF} = 0.4 \times \text{(body weight)}$$

$$\text{ECF} = 0.2 \times \text{(body weight)}$$

The ECF compartment is further subdivided into **interstitial fluid** and **plasma,** which are separated by the capillary wall. The interstitial fluid surrounds the cells in the various tissues of the body and constitutes three fourths of the ECF volume. The ECF includes water contained within the bone and dense connective tissue as well as the cerebrospinal fluid (CSF). Plasma represents the remaining one fourth of the ECF. Under some pathologic conditions, additional fluid

---

[2]In these and all subsequent calculations, it is assumed that 1 L of fluid (e.g., ICF and ECF) has a mass of 1 kg. This allows conversion from measurements of body weight to volume of body fluids.

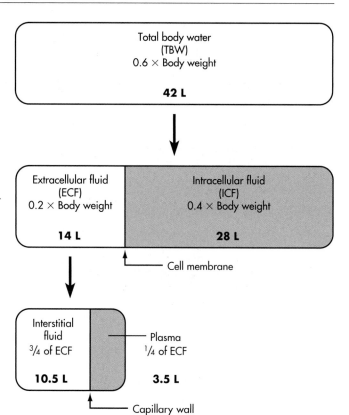

FIGURE 1-3 ■ Relationship between the volumes of the major body fluid compartments. The actual values shown are calculated for a 70-kg individual.

may accumulate in what is referred to as a "third space." Third space collections of fluid are part of the ECF and include, for example, the accumulation of fluid in the peritoneal cavity (**ascites**) of individuals with liver disease.

COMPOSITION OF BODY FLUID COMPARTMENTS

Sodium is the major cation of the ECF, and Cl^- and HCO_3^- are the major anions. The ionic composition of the plasma and interstitial fluid compartments of the ECF is similar because they are separated only by the capillary endothelium, a barrier that is freely permeable to small ions. The major difference between the interstitial fluid and plasma is that the latter contains significantly more protein. This differential concentration of protein can affect the distribution of cations and anions between these two compartments (i.e., Donnan effect) because plasma proteins have a net negative charge that tends to increase the cation concentrations and reduce the anion concentrations in the plasma compartment. However, this effect is small, and the ionic compositions of the interstitial fluid and plasma can be considered to be identical. Because of its abundance, Na^+ (and its attendant anions, primarily Cl^- and HCO_3^-) is the major determinant of ECF osmolality. Accordingly, a rough estimate of the ECF osmolality can be obtained by simply doubling the sodium concentration [Na^+]. For example, if the plasma [Na^+] is 145 mEq/L, the osmolality of plasma and ECF can be estimated as:

$$\text{Plasma osmolality} = 2(\text{plasma } [Na^+]) \quad (1\text{-}6)$$
$$= 290 \text{ mOsm/kg } H_2O$$

Because water is in osmotic equilibrium across the capillary endothelium and the plasma membrane of cells, measurement of the plasma osmolality also provides a measure of the osmolality of the ECF and ICF.

In clinical situations a more accurate estimate of the plasma osmolality is obtained by also considering the contribution of glucose and urea to the plasma osmolality. Accordingly, plasma osmolality can be estimated as:

$$\text{Plasma osmolality} = \qquad\qquad (1\text{-}7)$$

$$2(\text{plasma [Na}^+]) + \frac{[\text{glucose}]}{18} + \frac{[\text{urea}]}{2.8}$$

The glucose and urea concentrations are expressed in units of mg/dL (dividing by 18 for glucose and 2.8 for urea[5] allows conversion from the units of mg/dL to mmol/L and thus to mOsm/kg H_2O). This estimation of plasma osmolality is especially useful when dealing with patients who have an elevated plasma [glucose] secondary to diabetes mellitus and patients with chronic renal failure, whose plasma [urea] is elevated.

In contrast to the ECF, where the [Na$^+$] is approximately 145 mEq/L, the [Na$^+$] of the ICF is only 10 to 15 mEq/L. K$^+$ is the predominant cation of the ICF, and its concentration is approximately 150 mEq/L. This asymmetric distribution of Na$^+$ and K$^+$ across the plasma membrane is maintained by the activity of the ubiquitous sodium-potassium adenosine triphosphatase (Na$^+$, K$^+$-ATPase). By its action, Na$^+$ is extruded from the cell in exchange for K$^+$. The anion composition of the ICF also differs from that of the ECF. For example, Cl$^-$ and HCO$_3^-$ are the predominant anions of the ECF, and organic molecules and the negatively charged groups on proteins are the major anions of the ICF.

FLUID EXCHANGE BETWEEN BODY FLUID COMPARTMENTS

Water moves freely and rapidly between the various body fluid compartments. Two forces determine this movement: hydrostatic pressure and osmotic pressure. Hydrostatic pressure from the pumping of the heart (and the effect of gravity on the column of blood in the vessel) and osmotic pressure exerted by plasma

proteins (oncotic pressure) are important determinants of fluid movement across the capillary wall. By contrast, because hydrostatic pressure gradients are not present across the cell membrane, only osmotic pressure differences between ICF and ECF cause fluid movement into and out of cells.

Capillary Fluid Exchange

The movement of fluid across a capillary wall is determined by the algebraic sum of the hydrostatic and oncotic pressures (the so-called **Starling forces**) as expressed by the following equation:

$$\textbf{Filtration rate} = K_f\,[(P_c - P_i) - \sigma(\pi_c - \pi_i)] \qquad (1\text{-}8)$$

where the filtration rate is the volume of fluid moving across the capillary wall and is expressed in units of either volume/capillary surface area or volume/time and where:

K_f = Filtration coefficient of the capillary wall
P_c = Hydrostatic pressure within the capillary lumen
π_c = Oncotic pressure of the plasma
P_i = Hydrostatic pressure of the interstitial fluid
π_i = Oncotic pressure of the interstitial fluid
σ = Reflection coefficient for proteins across the capillary wall

The Starling forces for capillary fluid exchange vary between tissues and organs. They can also change in a given capillary bed under physiologic (e.g., exercising muscle) and pathophysiologic (e.g., congestive heart failure) conditions. Figure 1-4 illustrates these forces for a capillary bed located in skeletal muscle at rest.

The capillary filtration coefficient (K_f) reflects the intrinsic permeability of the capillary wall to the movement of fluid as well as the surface area available for filtration. The K_f varies among different capillary beds. For example, the K_f of glomerular capillaries in the kidneys is approximately 100 times greater in magnitude than that of skeletal muscle capillaries. This difference in K_f accounts for the large volume of fluid filtered across glomerular capillaries compared with the amount filtered across skeletal muscle capillaries (see Chapter 3).

The hydrostatic pressure within the lumen of a capillary (P_c) is a force promoting the movement of

---

[5]The [urea] in plasma is measured as the nitrogen in the urea molecule, or blood urea nitrogen (BUN).

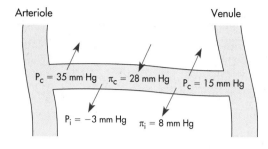

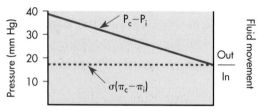

FIGURE 1-4 ■ **Upper panel,** Schematic representation of the Starling forces responsible for the filtration and absorption of fluid across the wall of a typical skeletal muscle capillary. P_c, capillary hydrostatic pressure; P_i, interstitial hydrostatic pressure; π_c, capillary oncotic pressure; π_i, interstitial oncotic pressure. Note that Pc decreases from the arteriole end to the venule end of the capillary, whereas all the other Starling forces are constant along the length of the capillary. Fluid filtered into the interstitium is taken up by lymphatic vessels and returned to the vascular system (not shown). **Lower panel,** Graph of hydrostatic and oncotic pressure differences along the capillary. (In this example, $\sigma = 0.9$.) Net fluid movement across the wall of the capillary is also indicated. Note that fluid is filtered out of the capillary except at the venous end, where the net driving forces are zero.

fluid from the lumen into the interstitium. Its magnitude depends on arterial pressure, venous pressure, and precapillary (arteriolar) and postcapillary (venular and small vein) resistances. An increase in the arterial or venous pressures results in an increase in P_c, and a decrease in these pressures has the opposite effect. P_c increases with either a decrease in precapillary resistance or an increase in postcapillary resistance. Likewise, an increase in precapillary resistance or a decrease in postcapillary resistance decreases P_c. For virtually all capillary beds, precapillary resistance is greater than postcapillary resistance and thus the precapillary resistance plays a greater role in determining P_c. An important exception is the glomerular capillaries,

where both precapillary and postcapillary resistances modulate P_c (see Chapter 3). The magnitude of P_c varies among not only tissues but also capillary beds within a given tissue, and it is also dependent upon the physiologic state of the tissue.

Precapillary sphincters not only control the hydrostatic pressure within an individual capillary but also control the number of perfused capillaries in the tissue. For example, in skeletal muscle at rest, not all capillaries are perfused. During exercise, relaxation of precapillary sphincters allows perfusion of more capillaries. The increased number of perfused capillaries reduces the diffusion distance between the cells and capillaries and thereby facilitates the exchange of O_2 and cellular metabolites (e.g., CO_2 and lactic acid).

The hydrostatic pressure within the interstitium (P_i) is difficult to measure, but in the absence of edema (abnormal accumulation of fluid in the interstitium) its value is near zero or slightly negative. Thus, under normal conditions, it causes fluid to move out of the capillary. However, when edema is present, P_i is positive and it opposes the movement of fluid out of the capillary (see Chapter 6).

The oncotic pressure of plasma proteins (π_c) retards the movement of fluid out of the capillary lumen. At a normal plasma protein concentration, π_c has a value of approximately 26 to 28 mm Hg. The degree to which oncotic pressure influences capillary fluid movement depends on the permeability of the capillary wall to the protein molecules. If the capillary wall is highly permeable to protein, σ is near zero and the oncotic pressure generated by plasma proteins plays little or no role in capillary fluid exchange. This situation is seen in the capillaries of the liver (i.e., hepatic sinusoids), which are highly permeable to proteins. As a result, the protein concentration of the interstitial fluid is essentially the same as that of plasma. In the capillaries of skeletal muscle, σ is approximately 0.9, whereas in the glomeruli of the kidneys, the value is essentially 1. Therefore, plasma protein oncotic pressure plays an important role in fluid movement across these capillary beds.

The protein that leaks across the capillary wall into the interstitium exerts an oncotic pressure (π_i) and promotes the movement of fluid out of the capillary lumen. In skeletal muscle capillaries under normal conditions, π_i is small and has a value of only 8 mm Hg.

As depicted in Figure 1-4, the balance of Starling forces across muscle capillaries causes fluid to leave the lumen (filtration) along its entire length. Some of this filtered fluid reenters the vasculature across the postcapillary venule where the Starling forces are reversed (i.e., the net driving force for fluid movement is into the vessel). The remainder of the filtered fluid is returned to the circulation through the lymphatics. The sinusoids of the liver also filter along their entire length. In contrast, during digestion of a meal, the balance of forces across capillaries of the gastrointestinal tract results in the net uptake of fluid into the capillary.

Normally, 8 to 12 L/day of fluid moves across capillary beds throughout the body and is collected by lymphatic vessels. This lymphatic fluid flows first to lymph nodes, where most of the fluid is returned to the circulation. Fluid not returned to the circulation at the lymph nodes (1 to 4 L/day) reenters the circulation through the thoracic and right lymphatic ducts. However, under conditions of increased capillary filtration, such as occurs in congestive heart failure, thoracic and right lymphatic duct flow can increase 10-fold to 20-fold.

Cellular Fluid Exchange

Osmotic pressure differences between ECF and ICF are responsible for fluid movement between these compartments. Because the plasma membrane of cells contains water channels (aquaporins), water can easily cross the membrane. Thus, a change in the osmolality of either ICF or ECF results in rapid movement (i.e., minutes) of water between these compartments. Thus, except for transient changes, the ICF and ECF compartments are in osmotic equilibrium.

Water movement across the plasma membrane of cells occurs through a class of integral membrane proteins called **aquaporins (AQPs).** Although water can cross the membrane through other transporters (e.g., Na^+-glucose symporter), aquaporins are the main route of water movement into and out of the cell. To date, 11 aquaporins have been identified. These can be divided into two subgroups. One group, which includes the aquaporin (AQP-2) involved in the regulation of water movement across the apical membrane of renal collecting duct cells by antidiuretic hormone (see Chapter 5), is permeable only to water. The second group is permeable not only to water but also to small molecular weight substances. Because glycerol can cross the membrane via this group of aquaporins, they are termed aquaglyceroporins. Aquaporins exist in the plasma membrane as a tetramer, with each monomer functioning as a water channel (see also Chapter 4).

In contrast to that of water, the movement of ions across cell membranes is more variable from cell to cell and depends on the presence of specific membrane transport proteins. Consequently, as a first approximation, fluid exchange between the ICF and ECF under pathophysiologic conditions can be analyzed by assuming that appreciable shifts of ions between the compartments do not occur.

A useful approach for understanding the movement of fluids between the ICF and the ECF is outlined in Box 1-1. To illustrate this approach, consider what happens when solutions containing various amounts of NaCl are added to the ECF.[3]

Example 1: Addition of Isotonic NaCl to ECF Addition of an isotonic NaCl solution (e.g., intravenous infusion of 0.9% NaCl: osmolality ≈ 290 mOsm/kg H_2O to a patient)[4] to the ECF increases the volume of this compartment by the volume of fluid administered. Because this fluid has the same osmolality as ECF and therefore also ICF, there is no driving force for fluid movement between these compartments, and the volume of ICF is unchanged. Although Na^+ can cross cell membranes, it is effectively restricted to the ECF by the activity of the Na^+, K^+-ATPase, which is present in the plasma membrane of all cells. Therefore, there is no net movement of the infused NaCl into the cells.

---

[3]Fluids are usually administered intravenously. When electrolyte solutions are infused by this route, there is rapid (i.e., minutes) equilibration between plasma and interstitial fluid because of the high permeability of the capillary wall to water and electrolytes. Thus, these fluids are essentially added to the entire ECF.
[4]A 0.9% NaCl solution (0.9 g NaCl/100 ml) contains 154 mmoles/L of NaCl. Because NaCl does not dissociate completely in solution (i.e., 1.88 osmoles/mole) the osmolality of this solution is 290 mOsm/kg H_2O, which is very similar to that of normal ECF.

BOX 1-1
PRINCIPLES FOR ANALYSIS OF FLUID SHIFTS BETWEEN THE ICF AND THE ECF

■ The volumes of the various body fluid compartments can be estimated in the normal adult by the following:

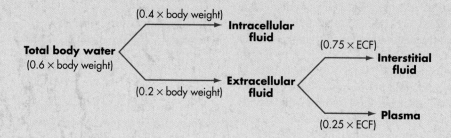

■ All exchanges of water and solutes with the external environment occur through the ECF (e.g., intravenous infusion and intake or loss via the gastrointestinal tract). Changes in the ICF are secondary to fluid shifts between the ECF and the ICF. Fluid shifts occur only if the perturbation of the ECF alters its osmolality.
■ Except for brief periods of seconds to minutes, the ICF and the ECF are in osmotic equilibrium. A measurement of plasma osmolality will provide a measure of both the ECF and the ICF osmolality.
■ For the sake of simplification, it can be assumed that equilibration between the ICF and the ECF occurs only by movement of water and not by movement of osmotically active solutes.
■ Conservation of mass must be maintained, especially when considering either addition or removal of water and/or solutes from the body.

Neurosurgical procedures and cerebrovascular accidents (strokes) often result in the accumulation of interstitial fluid in the brain (i.e., edema) and swelling of the neurons. Because the brain is enclosed within the skull, edema can raise intracranial pressure and thereby disrupt neuronal function, leading to coma and death. The blood-brain barrier, which separates the cerebrospinal fluid and brain interstitial fluid from blood, is freely permeable to water but not to most other substances. As a result, excess fluid in brain tissue can be removed by imposing an osmotic gradient across the blood-brain barrier. Mannitol can be used for this purpose. Mannitol is a sugar (molecular weight = 182 g/mol) that does not readily cross the blood-brain barrier and membranes of cells (neurons as well as other cells in the body). Therefore, mannitol is an effective osmole, and intravenous infusion results in the movement of fluid from the brain tissue by osmosis.

Example 2: Addition of Hypotonic NaCl to ECF
Addition of a hypotonic NaCl solution to the ECF (e.g., intravenous infusion of 0.45% NaCl: osmolality < 145 mOsm/kg H_2O to a patient) decreases the osmolality of this fluid compartment, resulting in the movement of water into the ICF. After osmotic equilibration, the osmolalities of ICF and ECF are equal but lower than before the infusion, and the volume of each compartment is increased. The increase in ECF volume is greater than the increase in ICF volume.

Example 3: Addition of Hypertonic NaCl to ECF
Addition of a hypertonic NaCl solution to the ECF (e.g., intravenous infusion of 3% NaCl: osmolality ≈ 1000 mOsm/kg H_2O to a patient) increases the osmolality of this compartment, resulting in the movement of water out of cells. After osmotic equilibration, the osmolalities of ECF and ICF are equal but higher than before the infusion. The volume of the ECF is increased, whereas that of the ICF is decreased.

Fluid and electrolyte disorders are seen commonly in clinical practice (e.g., in patients with vomiting and/or diarrhea). In most instances these disorders are self-limited and correction of the disorder occurs without need for intervention. However, more severe or prolonged disorders may require fluid replacement therapy. Such therapy may be administered orally with special electrolyte solutions, or intravenous fluid may be administered.

Intravenous solutions are available in many formulations. The type of fluid administered to a particular patient is dictated by the patient's need. For example, if an increase in the patient's vascular volume is necessary, a solution containing substances that do not readily cross the capillary wall is infused (e.g., 5% albumin solution). The oncotic pressure generated by the albumin molecules retains fluid in the vascular compartment, expanding its volume. Expansion of ECF is accomplished most often by using isotonic saline solutions (e.g., 0.9% NaCl).

As already noted, administration of an isotonic NaCl solution does not result in the development of an osmotic pressure gradient across the plasma membrane of cells. Therefore, the entire volume of the infused solution remains in the ECF. Patients whose body fluids are hyperosmotic need hypotonic solutions. These solutions may be hypotonic NaCl (e.g., 0.45% NaCl or 5% dextrose in water, called D5W). Administration of the D5W solution is equivalent to infusion of distilled water because the dextrose is metabolized to CO_2 and water. Administration of these fluids increases the volumes of both the ICF and ECF. Finally, patients whose body fluids are hypotonic need hypertonic solutions. These are typically NaCl-containing solutions (e.g., 3% and 5% NaCl). These solutions expand the volume of the ECF but decrease the volume of the ICF. Other constituents, such as electrolytes (e.g., K^+) or drugs, can be added to intravenous solutions to tailor the therapy to the patient's fluid, electrolyte, and metabolic needs.

SUMMARY

1. Water is a major constituent of the human body, accounting for 60% of the body weight. Body water is divided between two major compartments: intracellular fluid (ICF) and extracellular fluid (ECF). Two thirds of the water is in the ICF, and one third is in the ECF. Osmotic pressure gradients between ICF and ECF drive water movement between these compartments. Because the plasma membrane of most cells is highly permeable to water, ICF and ECF are in osmotic equilibrium.

2. The ECF is divided into a vascular compartment (plasma) and an interstitial fluid compartment. Starling forces across capillaries determine the exchange of fluid between these compartments.

3. Sodium is the major cation of ECF. Potassium is the major cation of the ICF. This asymmetric distribution of Na^+ and K^+ is maintained by the activity of the Na^+, K^+-ATPase.

KEY WORDS AND CONCEPTS

- Molarity
- Equivalence
- Osmosis
- Osmotic pressure
- van't Hoff's law
- Osmolarity
- Osmolality
- Tonicity (isotonic, hypotonic, and hypertonic)
- Effective osmole
- Ineffective osmole
- Reflection coefficient
- Osmotic coefficient
- Oncotic pressure
- Specific gravity
- Total body water
- Intracellular fluid (ICF)

- Extracellular fluid (ECF)
- Interstitial fluid
- Plasma
- Capillary wall
- Starling forces
- Capillary filtration coefficient (K_f)
- Aquaporin (AQP)

SELF-STUDY PROBLEMS

1. Calculate the molarity and osmolality of a 1-L solution containing the following solutes. Assume complete dissociation of all electrolytes.

		Molarity (mmol/L)	Osmolality (mOsm/kg H_2O)
9 g	NaCl	*155*	
72 g	Glucose		
22.2 g	CaCl$_2$		
3 g	Urea		
8.4 g	NaHCO$_3$		

2. The intracellular contents of a cell generate an osmotic pressure of 300 mOsm/kg H_2O. The cell is placed in a solution containing 300 mmol/L of a solute (x). If solute x remains as a single particle in solution and has a reflection coefficient of 0.5, what happens to the volume of the cell in this solution? What would be the composition of an isotonic solution (i.e., a solution that does not cause a change in the volume of the cell) containing substance x ?

3. An individual's plasma [Na$^+$] is measured and found to be 130 mEq/L (normal = 145 mEq/L). What is the individual's estimated plasma osmolality? What effect does the lower than normal plasma [Na$^+$] have on water movement across cell plasma membranes? Across the capillary endothelium?

4. Figure 1-4 illustrates the normal values for the Starling forces involved in fluid movement across a typical skeletal muscle capillary. Draw the new hydrostatic ($P_c - P_i$) and oncotic $\sigma(\pi_c - \pi_i)$ pressure curves if P_c at the venous end of the capillary was increased to 20 mm Hg. What effect would this have on fluid exchange across the capillary wall?

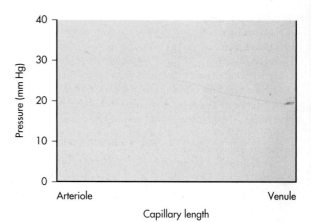

5. A healthy volunteer (body weight = 50 kg) is infused with 1 L of a 5% dextrose and water solution (D5W: osmolality ~ 290 mOsm/kg H_2O). What would be the immediate and long-term (several hours) effects of this infusion on the following parameters? Assume an initial plasma [Na$^+$] of 145 mEq/L and, for simplicity, no urine output.

Immediate effect:
ECF volume: ___*11*___ L
ICF volume: ___*20*___ L
Plasma [Na$^+$]: ___*132*___ mEq/L

$$\frac{145\ mEq}{L} \times 10\ L = 1450$$

Long-term effect:
ECF volume: ___*10.3*___ L
ICF volume: ___*20.67*___ L
Plasma [Na$^+$]: _____ mEq/L

$$\frac{1450\ mEq}{11\ L} = 132\ \frac{mEq}{L}$$

Based on these effects of the 5% dextrose solution on the volumes and compositions of the body fluids, how would this solution be used clinically?

6. A second healthy volunteer (body weight = 50 kg) is infused with 1 L of a 0.9% NaCl solution (isotonic saline: osmolality ~ 290 mOsm/kg H_2O). What would be the immediate and long-term (several hours) effects of this infusion on the following parameters? Assume an initial plasma [Na$^+$] of 145 mEq/L and, for simplicity, no urine output.

Immediate effect:
ECF volume: ___*11*___ L
ICF volume: ___*20*___ L
Plasma [Na$^+$]: _____ mEq/L

Long-term effect:

ECF volume: _____ L
ICF volume: _____ L
Plasma [Na$^+$]: _____ mEq/L

Based on these effects of the NaCl solution on the volumes and compositions of the body fluids, how would this solution be used clinically?

7. A 60-kg individual has an episode of gastroenteritis with vomiting and diarrhea. Over a 2-day period this individual loses 4 kg of body weight. Before becoming ill, this individual had a plasma [Na$^+$] of 140 mEq/L, which was unchanged by the illness. Assuming the entire loss of body weight represents the loss of fluid (a reasonable assumption), estimate the following:

Initial conditions (before gastroenteritis):

Total body water:	36	L
ICF volume:	24	L
ECF volume:	12	L
Total body osmoles:	10080	mOsm
ICF osmoles:		mOsm
ECF osmoles:		mOsm

New equilibrium conditions (after gastroenteritis):

Total body water:	32	L
ICF volume:	24	L
ECF volume:	8	L
Total body osmoles:	8960	mOsm
ICF osmoles:	6720	mOsm
ECF osmoles:	2240	mOsm

8. A 50-kg individual with a plasma [Na$^+$] of 145 mEq/L is infused with 5 g/kg of mannitol (molecular weight of mannitol = 182 g/mol) to reduce brain swelling after a stroke. After equilibration, estimate the following, assuming mannitol is restricted to the ECF compartment, no excretion occurs, and the infusion volume of the mannitol solution is negligible (i.e., total body water unchanged):

Initial conditions (before mannitol infusion):

Total body water:	30	L
ICF volume:	20	L
ECF volume:	10	L
Total body osmoles:	8700	mOsm
ICF osmoles:	5800	mOsm
ECF osmoles:	2900	mOsm

New equilibrium conditions (after mannitol infusion):

Total body water:	30	L
ICF volume:	20	L
ECF volume:	10	L
Total body osmoles:	10074	mOsm
ICF osmoles:	5800	mOsm
ECF osmoles:	4274	mOsm
Plasma osmolality:	335.8	mOsm/kg H$_2$O
Plasma [Na$^+$]:		mEq/L

9. Two normal individuals (body weight = 60 kg) excrete the following urine over the same time period.

Subject A: 1 L of urine with an osmolality of 1000 mOsm/kg H$_2$O
Subject B: 4 L of urine with an osmolality of 400 mOsm/kg H$_2$O

If both individuals have no fluid intake, what is their plasma osmolality? *Hint*: Assume both individuals have an initial plasma [Na$^+$] of 145 mEq/L and thus a plasma osmolality of approximately 290 mOsm/kg H$_2$O.

Subject A: _____ 270 _____
Subject B: _____ 276. _____

2

STRUCTURE AND FUNCTION OF THE KIDNEYS

OBJECTIVES

Upon completion of this chapter, the student should be able to answer the following questions:

1. Which structures in the renal corpuscle are filtration barriers to plasma proteins?

2. What is the physiologic significance of the juxta-glomerular apparatus?

3. What blood vessels supply the kidneys?

4. What nerves innervate the kidneys?

In addition, the student should be able to describe the following:

1. The location of the kidneys and their gross anatomic features

2. The different parts of the nephron and their locations within the cortex and medulla

3. The components of the renal corpuscle and the cell types located in each component

STRUCTURE OF THE KIDNEYS

Structure and function are closely linked in the kidneys. Consequently, an appreciation of the gross anatomic and histologic features of the kidneys is a prerequisite for an understanding of their function.

Gross Anatomy

The kidneys are paired organs that lie on the posterior wall of the abdomen behind the peritoneum on either side of the vertebral column. In the adult human, each kidney weighs between 115 and 170 g and is approximately 11 cm long, 6 cm wide, and 3 cm thick.

The gross anatomic features of the human kidney are illustrated in Figure 2-1. The medial side of each kidney contains an indentation through which pass the renal artery and vein, nerves, and pelvis. If a kidney were cut in half, two regions would be evident: an outer region called the **cortex** and an inner region

called the **medulla.** The cortex and medulla are composed of **nephrons** (the functional units of the kidney), blood vessels, lymphatics, and nerves. The medulla in the human kidney is divided into conical masses called **renal pyramids.** The base of each pyramid originates at the corticomedullary border, and the apex terminates in a **papilla,** which lies within a **minor calyx.** Minor calyces collect urine from each papilla. The numerous minor calyces expand into two or three open-ended pouches, the **major calyces.** The major calyces in turn feed into the **pelvis.** The pelvis represents the upper, expanded region of the **ureter,** which carries urine from the pelvis to the urinary bladder. The walls of the calyces, pelvis, and ureters contain smooth muscle that contracts to propel the urine toward the **urinary bladder.**

The blood flow to the two kidneys is equal to about 25% (1.25 L/min) of the cardiac output in resting individuals. However, the kidneys constitute less than

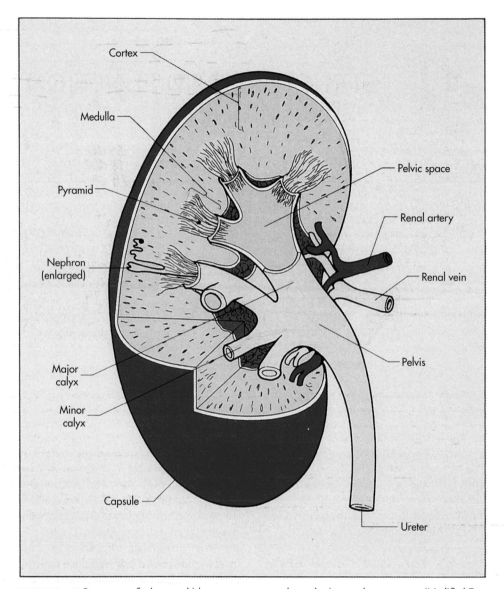

FIGURE 2-1 ■ Structure of a human kidney, cut open to show the internal structures. *(Modified From Marsh DJ: Renal physiology. New York, 1983, Raven.)*

0.5% of total body weight. As illustrated in Figure 2-2 (left), the **renal artery** branches progressively to form the **interlobar artery,** the **arcuate artery,** the **interlobular artery,** and the **afferent arteriole,** which leads into the **glomerular capillaries** (i.e., **glomerulus**). The glomerular capillaries come together to form the **efferent arteriole,** which leads into a second capillary network, the **peritubular capillaries,** which supply blood to the nephron. The vessels of the venous system

run parallel to the arterial vessels and progressively form the **interlobular vein, arcuate vein, interlobar vein,** and **renal vein,** which courses beside the ureter.

Ultrastructure of the Nephron

The functional unit of the kidneys is the nephron. Each human kidney contains approximately 1.2 million nephrons, which are hollow tubes composed of a single

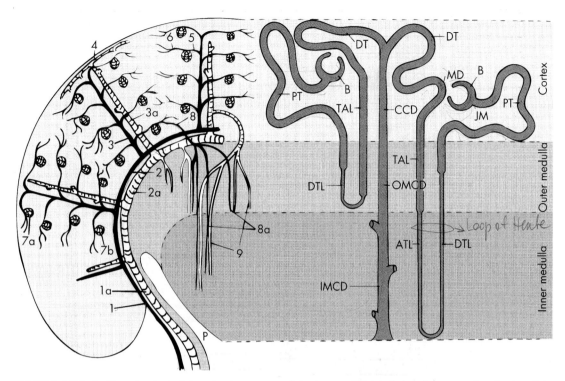

FIGURE 2-2 ■ **Left,** Organization of the vascular system of the human kidney. 1, Interlobar arteries; 1a, interlobar veins; 2, arcuate arteries; 2a, arcuate veins; 3, interlobular arteries; 3a, interlobular veins; 4, stellate vein; 5, afferent arterioles; 6, efferent arterioles; 7a, 7b, glomerular capillary networks; 8, descending vasa recta; 9, ascending vasa recta. **Right,** Organization of the human nephron. A superficial nephron is illustrated on the left and a juxtamedullary (JM) nephron is illustrated on the right. The loop of Henle includes the straight portion of the proximal tubule (PT), descending thin limb (DTL), ascending thin limb (ATL), and thick ascending limb (TAL). B, Bowman's capsule; CCD, cortical collecting duct; DT, distal tubule; IMCD, inner medullary collecting duct; MD, macula dense; OMCD, outer medullary collecting duct; P, pelvis. *(Modified from Kriz W, Bankir LA: A standard nomenclature for structures of the kidney. Am J Physiol 254:F1, 1988; and Koushanpour E, Kriz W: Renal physiology: principles, structure, and function, ed 2. New York, 1986, Springer-Verlag.)*

cell layer. The nephron consists of a **renal corpuscle, proximal tubule, loop of Henle, distal tubule,** and **collecting duct system**[1] (Figure 2-3; see Figure 2-2). The renal corpuscle consists of glomerular capillaries and **Bowman's capsule.** The proximal tubule initially

forms several coils, followed by a straight piece that descends toward the medulla. The next segment is the loop of Henle, which is composed of the straight part of the proximal tubule, descending thin limb (which ends in a hairpin turn), ascending thin limb (only in nephrons with long loops of Henle), and thick ascending limb. Near the end of the thick ascending limb, the nephron passes between the afferent and efferent arterioles of the same nephron. This short segment of the thick ascending limb is called the **macula densa.** The distal tubule begins a short distance beyond the macula densa and extends to the point in the cortex where two or more nephrons join to form a cortical collecting duct. The **cortical collecting duct** enters

---

[1]The organization of the nephron is actually more complicated than presented here. However, for simplicity and clarity of presentation in subsequent chapters, the nephron is divided into five segments. For details on the subdivisions of the five nephron segments consult the references by Kriz and Bankir, Kriz and Kaissling, and Madsen and Tisher (see Additional Reading). The collecting duct system is not actually part of the nephron. However, for simplicity, we consider the collecting duct system part of the nephron.

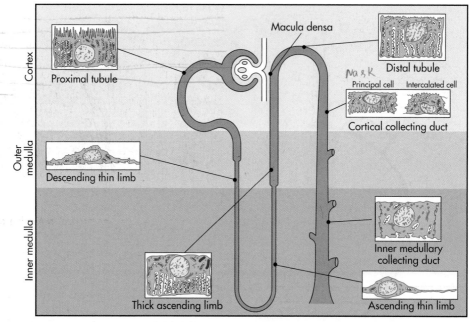

FIGURE 2-3 ■ Diagram of a nephron, including the cellular ultrastructure.

the medulla and becomes the outer **medullary collecting duct** and then the **inner medullary collecting duct.**

Each nephron segment is made up of cells that are uniquely suited to perform specific transport functions (see Figure 2-3). Proximal tubule cells have an extensively amplified apical membrane (the urine side of the cell) called the **brush border,** which is present only in the proximal tubule. The basolateral membrane (the blood side of the cell) is highly invaginated. These invaginations contain many mitochondria. In contrast, the descending and ascending thin limbs of Henle's loop have poorly developed apical and basolateral surfaces and few mitochondria. The cells of the thick ascending limb and the distal tubule have abundant mitochondria and extensive infoldings of the basolateral membrane.

The collecting duct is composed of two cell types: principal cells and intercalated cells. **Principal cells** have a moderately invaginated basolateral membrane and contain few mitochondria. Principal cells play an important role in NaCl reabsorption (see Chapters 4 and 6)

and K^+ secretion (see Chapter 7). **Intercalated cells,** which play an important role in regulating acid-base balance, have a high density of mitochondria. One population of intercalated cells secretes H^+ (i.e., reabsorbs HCO_3^-) and a second population of intercalated cells secretes HCO_3^- (see Chapter 8). The final segment of the nephron, the inner medullary collecting duct, is composed of inner medullary collecting duct cells. Cells of the inner medullary collecting duct have poorly developed apical and basolateral surfaces and few mitochondria.

All cells in the nephron, except intercalated cells, have in the apical plasma membrane a single nonmotile primary cilium, which protrudes into tubule fluid (Figure 2-4). Primary cilia are mechanosensors (i.e., they sense changes in the flow rate of tubule fluid) and chemosensors (i.e., they sense or respond to compounds in the surrounding fluid), and they initiate Ca^{++}-dependent signaling pathways including those that control kidney cell function, proliferation, differentiation, and apoptosis (i.e., programmed cell death).

Polycystin 1 (encoded by the *PKD1* gene) and polycystin 2 (encoded by the *PKD2* gene) are expressed in the membrane of primary cilia and mediate Ca^{++} entry into cells. PKD1 and PKD2 are thought to play an important role in flow-dependent K$^+$ secretion by principal cells of the collecting duct (see Chapter 7). As described in more detail in Chapter 7, increased flow of tubule fluid in the collecting duct is a strong stimulus for K$^+$ secretion. Increased flow bends the primary cilium in principal cells, which activates the PKD1/PKD2 Ca^{++} conducting channel complex allowing Ca^{++} to enter the cell and increase intracellular [Ca^{++}]. The increase in [Ca^{++}] activates K$^+$ channels in the apical plasma membrane, which enhances K$^+$ secretion from the cell into the tubule fluid.

Polycystic kidney disease (PKD) is a genetic disease occurring in about 1 in 800 people. Approximately 4 million to 6 million people worldwide have PKD, which is caused primarily by mutations in *PKD1* (85% to 90% of cases) and *PKD2* (10% to 15% of cases). The major phenotype of PKD is enlargement of the kidneys related to the presence of hundreds to thousands of renal cysts that can be as large as 20 cm in diameter. Cysts are also seen in the liver and other organs. PKD causes renal failure, usually in the fifth decade of life, and accounts for 10% of patients with end-stage renal failure. Although it is not clear how mutations in *PKD1* and *PKD2* cause polycystic kidney disease, renal cyst formation may result from defects in Ca^{++} uptake that lead to alterations in Ca^{++}-dependent signaling pathways including those that control kidney cell proliferation, differentiation, and apoptosis.

Nephrons may be subdivided into superficial and juxtamedullary types (see Figure 2-2). The renal corpuscle of each superficial nephron is located in the outer region of the cortex. Its loop of Henle is short, and its efferent arteriole branches into peritubular capillaries that surround the nephron segments of its own and adjacent nephrons. This capillary network conveys oxygen and important nutrients to the nephron segments in the cortex, delivers substances to the nephron for secretion (i.e., the movement of a substance from the blood into the tubular fluid),

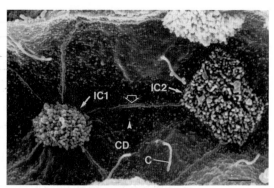

FIGURE 2-4 ■ Scanning electron micrograph illustrating primary cilia (labeled C) in the apical plasma membrane of principal cells within the cortical collecting duct. Note that intercalated cells (IC) do not have cilia. Primary cilia are approximately 2 to 30 μm long and 0.5 μm in diameter. CD, collecting duct principal cells with short microvilli *(arrowhead)*. The straight ridges *(open arrow)* represent the cell borders between principal cells. C, cilia; IC1 and IC2, intercalated cells with numerous long microvilli in the apical membrane. *(From Kriz W, Kaissling B: Structural organization of the mammalian kidney. In Seldin DW, Giebisch G, editors: The kidney: physiology and pathophysiology, ed 3, Philadelphia, 2000, Lippincott Williams & Wilkins.)*

and serves as a pathway for the return of reabsorbed water and solutes to the circulatory system. A few species, including humans, also possess very short superficial nephrons whose Henle's loops never enter the medulla.

The renal corpuscle of each **juxtamedullary nephron** is located in the region of the cortex adjacent to the medulla (see Figure 2-2, right). In comparison with the superficial nephrons, the juxtamedullary nephrons differ anatomically in two important ways: the loop of Henle is longer and extends deeper into the medulla, and the efferent arteriole forms not only a network of peritubular capillaries but also a series of vascular loops called the **vasa recta.**

As shown in Figure 2-2, the vasa recta descend into the medulla, where they form capillary networks that surround the collecting ducts and ascending limbs of the loop of Henle. The blood returns to the cortex in the ascending vasa recta. Although less than 0.7% of the blood enters the vasa recta, these vessels subserve important functions in the renal medulla, including

(1) conveying oxygen and important nutrients to nephron segments, (2) delivering substances to the nephron for secretion, (3) serving as a pathway for the return of reabsorbed water and solutes to the circulatory system, and (4) concentrating and diluting the urine (urine concentration and dilution are discussed in more detail in Chapter 5).

Ultrastructure of the Renal Corpuscle

The first step in urine formation begins with the passive movement of a plasma ultrafiltrate from the glomerular capillaries (i.e., glomerulus) into **Bowman's space.** The term ultrafiltration refers to the passive movement of an essentially protein-free fluid from the glomerular capillaries into Bowman's space. To appreciate the process of ultrafiltration, one must understand the anatomy of the renal corpuscle. The glomerulus consists of a network of capillaries supplied by the afferent arteriole and drained by the efferent arteriole (Figures 2-5 and 2-6). During embryologic development, the glomerular capillaries press into the closed end of the proximal tubule, forming **Bowman's capsule** of a renal corpuscle. The capillaries are covered by epithelial cells, called **podocytes,** which form the **visceral layer** of Bowman's capsule (see Figures 2-7 through 2-9; and Figure 2-5). The visceral cells face outward at the vascular pole (i.e., where the afferent and efferent arterioles enter and exit Bowman's capsule) to form the **parietal layer** of Bowman's capsule. The space between the visceral layer and the parietal layer is Bowman's space, which at the urinary pole (i.e., where the proximal tubule joins Bowman's capsule) of the glomerulus becomes the lumen of the proximal tubule.

The endothelial cells of glomerular capillaries are covered by a basement membrane, which is surrounded by **podocytes** (see Figure 2-10; and Figures 2-5; and 2-7 to 2-9). The capillary endothelium, basement membrane, and foot processes of podocytes form the

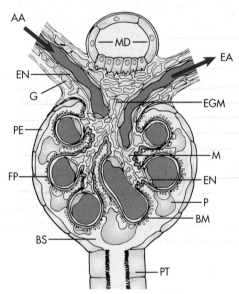

FIGURE 2-5 ■ Anatomy of the renal corpuscle and juxta-glomerular apparatus. The juxtaglomerular apparatus is composed of the macula densa (MD) region of the thick ascending limb, extraglomerular mesangial cells (EGM), and renin- and angiotensin II–producing granular cells (G) of the afferent arterioles (AA). BM, basement membrane; BS, Bowman's space; EA, efferent arteriole; EN, endothelial cell; FP, foot processes of podocyte; M, mesangial cells between capillaries; P, podocyte cell body (visceral cell layer); PE, parietal epithelium; PT, proximal tubule cell. *(Modified from Kriz W, Kaissling B: Structural organization of the mammalian kidney. In Seldin DW, Giebisch G, editors: The kidney: physiology and pathophysiology, ed 2. New York, 1992, Raven.)*

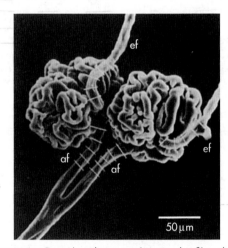

FIGURE 2-6 ■ Scanning electron micrograph of interlobular artery, afferent arteriole (af), efferent arteriole (ef), and glomerulus. The white bars on the afferent and efferent arterioles indicate that they are about 15 to 20 μm wide. *(From Kimura K, Hirata Y, Nanba S, et al: Effects of atrial natriuretic peptide on renal arterioles: morphometric analysis using microvascular casts. Am J Physiol 259:F936, 1990.)*

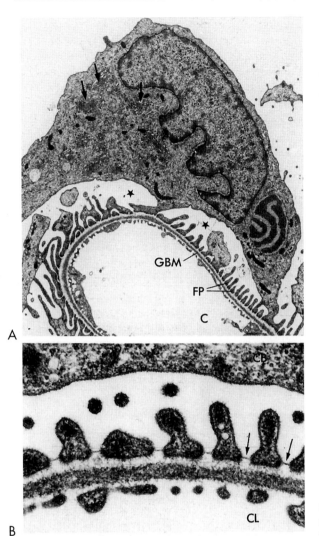

A

B

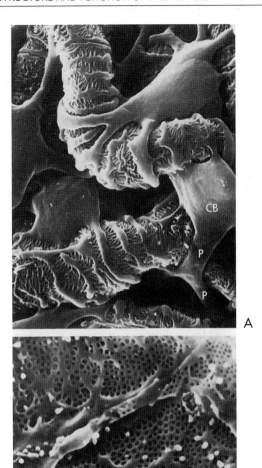

A

B

FIGURE 2-7 ■ A, Electron micrograph of a podocyte surrounding a glomerular capillary. The cell body of the podocyte contains a large nucleus with three indentations. Cell processes of the podocyte form the interdigitating foot processes (FP). The arrows in the cytoplasm of the podocyte indicate the well-developed Golgi apparatus, and the asterisks indicate Bowman's space. C, capillary lumen; GBM, glomerular basement membrane. B, Electron micrograph of the filtration barrier of a glomerular capillary. The filtration barrier is composed of three layers: the endothelium, basement membrane, and foot processes of the podocytes. Note the filtration slit diaphragm bridging the floor of the filtration slits (arrows). CB, cell body of a podocyte; CL, capillary lumen. (From Kriz W, Kaissling B: Structural organization of the mammalian kidney. In Seldin DW, Giebisch G, editors: The kidney: physiology and pathophysiology, ed 2. New York, 1992, Raven.)

FIGURE 2-8 ■ A, Scanning electron micrograph showing the outer surface of glomerular capillaries. This is the view that would be seen from Bowman's space. Processes (P) of podocytes run from the cell body (CB) toward the capillaries, where they ultimately split into foot processes. Interdigitation of the foot processes creates the filtration slits. B, Scanning electron micrograph of the inner surface (blood side) of a glomerular capillary. This view would be seen from the lumen of the capillary. The fenestrations of the endothelial cells are seen as small 700-Å holes. (From Kriz W, Kaissling B: Structural organization of the mammalian kidney. In Seldin DW, Giebisch G, editors: The kidney: physiology and pathophysiology, ed 2. New York, 1992, Raven.)

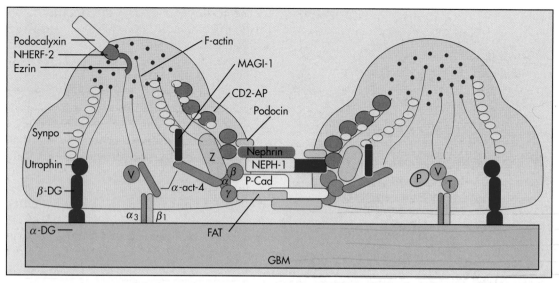

FIGURE 2-9 ■ Anatomy of podocyte foot processes. This figure illustrates the proteins that make up the slit diaphragm between two adjacent foot processes. Nephrin and neph-1 are membrane-spanning proteins that have large extracellular domains that interact. Podocin, also a membrane-spanning protein, organizes nephrin and neph-1 in specific microdomains in the plasma membrane, which is important for signaling events that determine the structural integrity of podocyte foot processes. Many of the proteins that compose the slit diaphragm interact with adapter proteins inside the cell, including CD2-AP, that bind to the filamentous actin (F-actin) cytoskeleton, which in turn binds either directly or indirectly to proteins such as $\alpha3\beta1$ and MAGI-1 that interact with proteins expressed by the glomerular basement membrane (GBM). α-act 4, α-actinin 4; $\alpha3\beta1$, $\alpha3\beta1$ integrin, α-DG, α-dystroglycan; CD2-AP, an adapter protein that links nephrin and podocin to intracellular proteins; FAT, a protocadherin that organizes actin polymerization; MAGI-1, a membrane-associated guanylate kinase protein; NHERF-2, Na^+-H^+ exchanger regulatory factor 2; P, paxillin; p-Cad, p-cadherin; synpo, synaptopodin; T, talin; V, vinculin; ZO-1, zona occludens. *(Adapted from Mundel P, Shankland SJ: Podocyte biology and response to injury. J Am Soc Nephrol 13:3005-3015, 2002.)*

so-called **filtration barrier** (see Figures 2-5 and 2-7 through 2-10). The endothelium is fenestrated (i.e., contains 700-Å holes where $1 Å = 10^{-10}$ m) and is freely permeable to water, small solutes (such as Na^+, urea, and glucose), and most proteins but is not permeable to red blood cells, white blood cells, or platelets. Because endothelial cells express negatively charged glycoproteins on their surface, they may retard the filtration into Bowman's space of very large anionic proteins (see Chapter 3). In addition to their role as a barrier to filtration, the endothelial cells synthesize a number of vasoactive substances (e.g., nitric oxide (NO), a vasodilator, and endothelin-1 (ET-1), a vasoconstrictor) that are important in controlling renal plasma flow (see Chapter 3).

The basement membrane, which is a porous matrix of negatively charged proteins including type IV collagen, laminin, the proteoglycans agrin and perlecan, and fibronectin, is an important filtration barrier to plasma proteins. The basement membrane is thought to function primarily as a charge-selectivity filter, allowing proteins to cross on the basis of charge.[2]

---

[2]Because the basement membrane and filtration slits of podocytes contain negatively charged glycoproteins, some proteins are held back (i.e., not filtered into Bowman's space) on the basis of size and charge. For molecules with an effective molecular radius between 20 and 42 Å, cationic molecules are filtered more readily than anionic molecules (see Chapter 3).

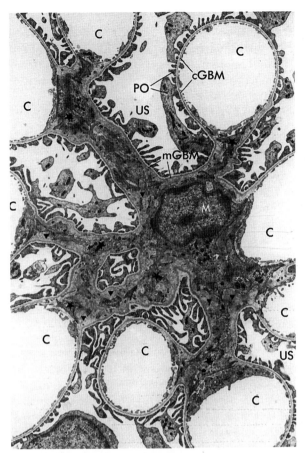

FIGURE 2-10 ■ Electron micrograph of the mesangium, the area between glomerular capillaries containing mesangial cells. C, glomerular capillaries; cGBM, capillary glomerular basement membrane surrounded by foot processes of podocytes (PO) and endothelial cells; mGBM, mesangial glomerular basement membrane surrounded by foot processes of podocytes and mesangial cells; M, mesangial cell that gives rise to several processes, some marked by asterisks; US, urinary space. Note the extensive extracellular matrix surrounded by mesangial cells (marked by arrowheads). (Magnification ~4100.) *(From Kriz W, Kaissling B: Structural organization of the mammalian kidney. In Seldin DW, Giebisch G, editors: The kidney: physiology and pathophysiology, ed 2., New York, 1992, Raven.)*

The podocytes, which are endocytic (i.e., the process of endocytosis allows materials to enter the cell without passing through the plasma membrane), have long finger-like processes that completely encircle the outer surface of the capillaries (see Figure 2-8). The processes of the podocytes interdigitate to cover the basement membrane and are separated by apparent gaps called **filtration slits.** Each filtration slit is bridged by a thin diaphragm, which contains pores with dimensions of 40×140 Å. The **filtration slit diaphragm,** which appears as a continuous structure when viewed by electron microscopy (see Figure 2-7B), is composed of several proteins including **nephrin** (*NPHS1*), **NEPH-1, podocin** (*NPHS2*), α-**actinin 4** *(ACTN4),* and **CD2-AP** (see Figure 2-9). Filtration slits, which function primarily as the size-selective filter, retard the filtration of proteins and macromolecules that cross the basement membrane from entering Bowman's space.

The **nephrotic syndrome** is produced by a variety of disorders and is characterized by an increase in the permeability of the glomerular capillaries to proteins and by a loss of normal podocyte structure including effacement (i.e., thinning) of foot processes. The augmented permeability to proteins results in an increase in urinary protein excretion **(proteinuria).** Thus, the appearance of proteins in the urine can indicate kidney disease. Individuals with this syndrome often develop hypoalbuminemia as a result of the proteinuria. In addition, generalized edema is commonly seen in individuals with the nephrotic syndrome (see Chapter 6). Mutations in several genes that encode slit diaphragm proteins (see Figure 2-9), including **nephrin, NEPH-1, podocin, CD2-AP, and** α**-actinin 4,** or knock out of these genes in mice cause proteinuria and kidney disease. For example, mutations in the nephrin gene (*NPHS1*) lead to abnormal or absent slit diaphragms, causing massive proteinuria and renal failure (i.e., congenital nephrotic syndrome). In addition, mutations in the podocin gene (*NPHS2*) cause autosomal recessive, steroid-resistant nephrotic syndrome. These naturally occurring mutations and knockout studies in mice demonstrate that nephrin, NEPH-1, podocin, CD2-AP, and α-actinin 4 play key roles in podocyte structure and function.

Alport's syndrome is characterized by hematuria (i.e., blood in the urine) and progressive glomerulonephritis (i.e., inflammation of the glomerular capillaries) and accounts for 1% to 2% of all cases of end-stage renal disease (ESRD). Alport's syndrome is caused by defects in type IV collagen (encoded by the *COL4A5* gene), a major component of the glomerular basement membrane. In about 85% of patients with Alport's syndrome, the disease is X-linked with mutations in the *COL4A5* gene. The remaining 15% of patients also have mutations in type IV collagen genes; six have been identified, but the mode of inheritance is autosomal recessive. In Alport's syndrome, the glomerular basement membrane becomes irregular in thickness and fails to serve as an effective filtration barrier to blood cells and protein.

Another important component of the renal corpuscle is the **mesangium**, which consists of **mesangial cells** and the **mesangial matrix** (see Figure 2-10). Mesangial cells, which possess many properties of smooth muscles cells, surround the glomerular capillaries, provide structural support for the glomerular capillaries, secrete the extracellular matrix, exhibit phagocytic activity that removes macromolecules from the mesangium, and secrete prostaglandins and proinflammatory cytokines. Because they also contract and are adjacent to glomerular capillaries, mesangial cells may influence the glomerular filtration rate (GFR) by regulating blood flow through the glomerular capillaries or by altering the capillary surface area (see Chapter 3). Mesangial cells located outside the glomerulus (between the afferent and efferent arterioles) are called **extraglomerular mesangial cells.**

Mesangial cells are involved in the development of **immune complex–mediated glomerular disease.** Because the glomerular basement membrane does not completely surround all glomerular capillaries (see Figure 2-10), some immune complexes can enter the mesangial area without crossing the glomerular basement membrane. Accumulation of immune complexes induces the infiltration of inflammatory cells into the mesangium and promotes the production of proinflammatory cytokines and autacoids by cells in the mesangium. These cytokines and autacoids enhance the inflammatory response. This inflammatory response can lead to cell death, scarring and eventually obliterates the glomerulus.

Ultrastructure of the Juxtaglomerular Apparatus

The **juxtaglomerular apparatus** is one component of an important feedback mechanism, the tubuloglomerular feedback mechanism, that is described in Chapter 3. The structures that make up the juxtaglomerular apparatus (JGA) include (see Figure 2-5):

1. The **macula densa** of the thick ascending limb
2. The extraglomerular mesangial cells
3. The renin- and angiotensin II–producing **granular cells** of the afferent arteriole

The cells of the macula densa represent a morphologically distinct region of the thick ascending limb. This region passes through the angle formed by the afferent and efferent arterioles of the same nephron. The cells of the macula densa are in contact with the extraglomerular mesangial cells and the granular cells of the afferent arterioles. Granular cells of the afferent arterioles are derived from metanephric mesenchymal cells. They contain smooth muscle myofilaments and they manufacture, store, and release **renin.** Renin is involved in the formation of **angiotensin II** and ultimately in the secretion of **aldosterone** (see Chapters 4 and 6). The juxtaglomerular apparatus is one component of the tubuloglomerular feedback mechanism that is involved in the autoregulation of renal blood flow (RBF) and the glomerular filtration rate (GFR) (see Chapter 3).

Innervation of the Kidneys

Renal nerves regulate renal blood flow, glomerular filtration rate, and salt and water reabsorption by the nephron. The nerve supply to the kidneys consists of sympathetic nerve fibers that originate in the celiac plexus. There is no parasympathetic innervation. Adrenergic fibers that innervate the kidneys release norepinephrine and dopamine. The adrenergic fibers lie adjacent to the smooth muscle cells of the major branches of the renal artery (interlobar, arcuate, and interlobular arteries) and the afferent and efferent arterioles. Moreover, sympathetic nerves innervate the renin-producing granular cells of the afferent arterioles. Renin secretion is stimulated by increased sympathetic activity. Nerve fibers also innervate the proximal tubule, loop of Henle, distal tubule, and collecting duct; activation of these nerves enhances Na^+ reabsorption by these nephron segments.

SUMMARY

1. The functional unit of the kidneys is the nephron, which consists of a renal corpuscle, proximal tubule, Henle's loop, distal tubule, and collecting duct.

2. Cilia play an important role in mechanosensation and chemosensation in nephron cells. Mutations in *PKD1* and *PKD2*, which encode proteins that associate with the central cilium and mediate Ca^{++} entry into cells, cause polycystic kidney disease.

3. The renal corpuscle consists of glomerular capillaries and Bowman's capsule.

4. The first step in urine formation begins with the passive movement of a plasma ultrafiltrate from the glomerular capillaries into Bowman's space. The term ultrafiltration refers to the passive movement of an essentially protein-free fluid from the glomerular capillaries into Bowman's space. The endothelial cells of glomerular capillaries are covered by a basement membrane, which is surrounded by podocytes. The capillary endothelium, basement membrane, and foot processes of podocytes form the so-called filtration barrier.

5. The filtration slit diaphragm is composed of several proteins including nephrin, NEPH-1, podocin, CD2-AP, and α-actinin 4. Mutations in these genes cause the nephrotic syndrome, which is associated with proteinuria and ultimately renal failure.

6. The juxtaglomerular apparatus is one component of an important feedback mechanism (i.e., tubuloglomerular feedback) that regulates renal blood flow and the glomerular filtration rate. The structures that make up the juxtaglomerular apparatus include the macula densa, extraglomerular mesangial cells, and renin—producing granular cells.

7. The kidneys are innervated by sympathetic nerves that regulate renal blood flow, glomerular filtration rate, and salt and water reabsorption by the nephron.

KEY WORDS AND CONCEPTS

- Cortex
- Medulla
- Nephrons
- Renal pyramids
- Calyx
- Pelvis
- Major calyces
- Minor calyces
- Urinary bladder
- Interlobar artery
- Arcuate artery
- Interlobular artery
- Afferent arteriole
- Glomerulus
- Efferent arteriole
- Renal corpuscle
- Bowman's capsule
- Proximal tubule
- Henle's loop
- Descending thin limb (of Henle)
- Ascending thin limb (of Henle)
- Thick ascending limb (of Henle)
- Macula densa
- Distal tubule
- Cortical collecting duct
- Outer medullary collecting duct
- Inner medullary collecting duct
- Brush border
- Principal cells
- Intercalated cells
- Superficial nephrons
- Juxtamedullary nephrons
- Vasa recta
- Collecting ducts
- Podocytes
- Visceral layer
- Parietal layer
- Bowman's space
- Filtration barrier
- Filtration slits
- Filtration slit diaphragm
- Nephrin
- NEPH-1
- Podocin
- CD2-AP
- α-actinin 4
- Mesangium
- Mesangial cells
- Mesangial matrix
- Extraglomerular mesangial cells (lacis cells)

- Juxtaglomerular apparatus
- Proteinuria
- Nephrotic syndrome

SELF-STUDY PROBLEMS

1. Describe the gross anatomic features of the kidney.
2. Identify the five segments of the nephron.
3. Describe the blood supply to the kidneys.
4. What is the renal corpuscle?
5. Describe the structures that form the filtration barriers to plasma proteins in the glomerulus.
6. What structures are parts of the juxtaglomerular apparatus?
7. What is the functional significance of the juxtaglomerular apparatus?
8. What is the mesangium, and what is its functional significance?
9. What nerves innervate the kidneys, and what functions are regulated by renal nerves?

GLOMERULAR FILTRATION AND RENAL BLOOD FLOW

■ ■ ■ ■ ■ ■ ■ ■ ■ ■ ■

OBJECTIVES

Upon completion of this chapter, the student should be able to answer the following questions:

1. How can the concepts of mass balance be used to measure the glomerular filtration rate?

2. Why can inulin clearance and creatinine clearance be used to measure the glomerular filtration rate?

3. What are the factors that determine which molecules cross the glomerular filtration barrier and enter Bowman's space?

4. Why does a loss of negative charge on the glomerular filtration barrier result in proteinuria (loss of protein in the urine)?

5. What Starling forces are involved in the formation of the glomerular ultrafiltrate and how do changes in each force affect the glomerular filtration rate?

6. What is autoregulation of renal blood flow and glomerular filtration rate, and which factors and hormones are responsible for autoregulation?

7. Which hormones regulate renal blood flow?

8. Why do hormones influence renal blood flow despite autoregulation?

The first step in the formation of urine by the kidneys is the production of an ultrafiltrate of plasma across the filtration barrier. The process of glomerular filtration and the regulation of glomerular filtration rate and renal blood flow are discussed in this chapter. The concept of renal clearance, which is the theoretical basis for the measurements of glomerular filtration rate and renal blood flow, is also presented.

RENAL CLEARANCE

The concept of renal **clearance** is based on the Fick principle (i.e., mass balance or conservation of mass). Figure 3-1 illustrates the various factors required to describe the mass balance relationships of a kidney. The renal artery is the single input source to the kidney, whereas the renal vein and ureter constitute the two output routes. The following equation defines the mass balance relationship:

$$P^a_x \times RPF^a = (P^v_x \times RPF^v) + (U_x \times \dot{V}) \qquad (3\text{-}1)$$

where:

P^a_x and P^v_x = Concentrations of substance x in the renal artery and renal vein plasma, respectively

RPF^a and RPF^v = **Renal plasma flow** (RPF) rates in the artery and vein, respectively

U_x = Concentration of x in the urine

$\dot{V}$ = Urine flow rate

This relationship permits the quantification of the amount of x excreted in the urine versus the amount returned to the systemic circulation in the renal venous blood. Thus, for any substance that is neither synthesized nor metabolized, the amount that enters

31

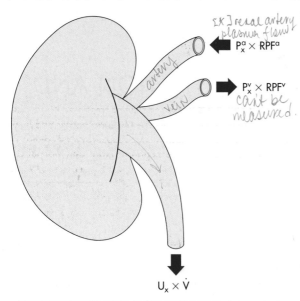

[x] renal artery
plasma flow↑
$P_x^a \times RPF^a$

$P_x^v \times RPF^v$
can't be
measured.

arterial

vein

$U_x \times \dot{V}$

Input		Output
Renal artery	=	Renal vein + ureter
$P_x^a \times RPF^a$		$P_x^v \times RPF^v + U_x \times \dot{V}$

FIGURE 3-1 ■ Mass balance relationships for the kidney. See text for definition of symbols.

the kidneys is equal to the amount that leaves the kidneys in the urine plus the amount that leaves the kidneys in the renal venous blood.

The principle of renal clearance emphasizes the excretory function of the kidneys; it considers only the rate at which a substance is excreted into the urine and not its rate of return to the systemic circulation in the renal vein. Therefore, in terms of mass balance (equation 3-1), the urinary excretion rate of x ($U_x \times \dot{V}$) is proportional to the plasma concentration of x (P_x^a):

$$P_x^a \propto U_x \times \dot{V} \qquad (3\text{-}2)$$

To equate the urinary excretion rate of x to its renal arterial plasma concentration, it is necessary to determine the rate at which x is removed from the plasma by the kidneys. This removal rate is the clearance (C_x).

$$P_x^a \times C_x = U_x \times \dot{V} \qquad (3\text{-}3)$$

If equation 3-3 is rearranged and the concentration of x in the renal artery plasma (P_x^a) is assumed to be identical to its concentration in a plasma sample from

any peripheral blood vessel, the following relationship is obtained:

$$C_x = \frac{U_x \times \dot{V}}{P_x^a} \quad \left(\frac{volume}{time}\right) \qquad (3\text{-}4)$$

Clearance has the dimensions of volume/time, and it represents a volume of plasma from which all the substance has been removed and excreted into the urine per unit time. The last point is best illustrated by considering the following example. If a substance is present in the urine at a concentration of 100 mg/ml and the urine flow rate is 1 ml/min, the excretion rate for this substance is calculated as follows:

$$\text{Excretion rate} = U_x \times \dot{V} = 100\ \text{mg/ml} \times (1\ \text{ml/min}) \quad (3\text{-}5)$$
$$= 100\ \text{mg/min}$$

If this substance is present in the plasma at a concentration of 1 mg/ml, its clearance according to equation 3-4 is as follows:

$$C_x = \frac{U_x \times \dot{V}}{P_x^a} = \frac{100\ \text{mg/min}}{1\ \text{mg/ml}} = 100\ \text{ml/min} \qquad (3\text{-}6)$$

In other words, 100 ml of plasma are completely cleared of substance x each minute. The definition of clearance as a volume of plasma from which all the substance has been removed and excreted into the urine per unit time is somewhat misleading because it is not a real volume of plasma; rather, it is an idealized volume.[1] The concept of clearance is important because it can be used to measure the glomerular filtration rate and RPF and determine whether a substance is reabsorbed or secreted along the nephron.

Glomerular Filtration Rate

The glomerular filtration rate (GFR) is equal to the sum of the filtration rates of all functioning nephrons. Thus, it is an index of kidney function. A fall in GFR generally means that kidney disease is progressing, whereas a recovery generally suggests recuperation. Thus, knowledge of the patient's GFR is essential in evaluating the severity and course of kidney disease.

---

[1]For most substances cleared from the plasma by the kidneys, only a portion is actually removed and excreted in a single pass through the kidneys.

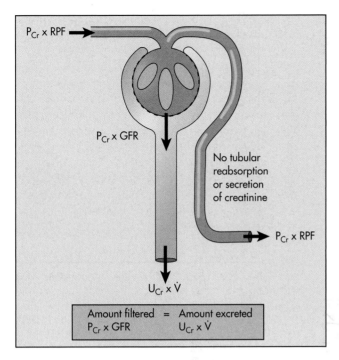

$P_{Cr} \times RPF$

$P_{Cr} \times GFR$

No tubular
reabsorption
or secretion
of creatinine

$P_{Cr} \times RPF$

$U_{Cr} \times \dot{V}$

Amount filtered	=	Amount excreted
$P_{Cr} \times GFR$		$U_{Cr} \times \dot{V}$

FIGURE 3-2 ■ Renal handling of creatinine. Creatinine is freely filtered across the filtration barrier and is, to a first approximation, not reabsorbed, secreted, or metabolized by the nephron. Note that not all the creatinine coming to the kidney in the renal artery is filtered (normally, 15% to 20% of plasma creatinine is filtered). The portion that is not filtered is returned to the systemic circulation in the renal vein. P_{Cr}, plasma creatinine concentration; RPF, renal plasma flow; U_{Cr}, urinary concentration of creatinine; $\dot{V}$, urine flow rate.

Creatinine is a by-product of skeletal muscle creatine metabolism, and it can be used to measure the GFR.[2] Creatinine is freely filtered across the filtration barrier into Bowman's space, and to a first approximation it is not reabsorbed, secreted, or metabolized by the cells of the nephron. Accordingly, the amount of creatinine excreted in the urine per minute equals the amount of creatinine filtered across the filtration barrier each minute (Figure 3-2):

Amount filtered = amount excreted

$$GFR \times P_{Cr} = U_{Cr} \times \dot{V} \qquad (3\text{-}7)$$

where:

P_{Cr} = Plasma concentration of creatinine
U_{Cr} = Urine concentration of creatinine
$\dot{V}$ = Urine flow

---

[2] Under experimental conditions GFR is usually measured using inulin, a polyfructose molecule (molecular weight ≈ 5000). However, inulin is not produced by the body and must be infused. Therefore, it is not used in most clinical situations.

If equation 3-7 is solved for the GFR:

$$GFR = \frac{C_{cr} \times \dot{V}}{P_{cr}} \qquad (3\text{-}8)$$

This equation is the same form as that for clearance (equation 3-4). Thus, the clearance of creatinine provides a means for determining the GFR. Clearance has the dimensions of volume/time, and it represents a volume of plasma from which all the substance has been removed and excreted into the urine per unit time.

Creatinine is not the only substance that can be used to measure the GFR. Any substance that meets the following criteria can serve as an appropriate marker for the measurement of GFR. The substance must:

1. Be freely filtered across the filtration barrier into Bowman's space
2. Not be reabsorbed or secreted by the nephron
3. Not be metabolized or produced by the kidney
4. Not alter the GFR

Creatinine is used to estimate the GFR in clinical practice. It is synthesized at a relatively constant rate, and the amount produced is proportional to the muscle mass. However, creatinine is not a perfect substance for measuring GFR because it is secreted to a small extent by the organic cation secretory system in the proximal tubule (see Chapter 4). The error introduced by this secretory component is approximately 10%. Thus, the amount of creatinine excreted in the urine exceeds the amount expected from filtration alone by 10%. However, the method used to measure the plasma creatinine concentration (P_{Cr}) overestimates the true value by 10%. Consequently, the two errors cancel, and in most clinical situations creatinine clearance provides a reasonably accurate measure of the GFR.

Not all of the creatinine (or other substances used to measure the GFR) that enters the kidney in the renal arterial plasma is filtered at the glomerulus (see Figure 3-2). Likewise, not all of the plasma coming into the kidneys is filtered. Although nearly all of the plasma that enters the kidneys in the renal artery passes through the glomerulus, approximately 10% does not. The portion of filtered plasma is termed the **filtration fraction** and is determined as:

$$\text{Filtration fraction} = \text{GFR/RPF} \qquad (3\text{-}9)$$

Under normal conditions, the filtration fraction averages 0.15 to 0.20. This means that only 15% to 20% of the plasma that enters the glomerulus is actually filtered. The remaining 80% to 85% continues on through the glomerular capillaries and into the efferent arterioles and peritubular capillaries. It is finally returned to the systemic circulation in the renal vein.

A fall in the GFR may be the first and only clinical sign of kidney disease. Thus, measuring the GFR is important when kidney disease is suspected. A 50% loss of functioning nephrons reduces the GFR by only about 25%. The decline in GFR is not 50% because the remaining nephrons compensate. Because measurements of GFR are cumbersome, kidney function is usually assessed in the clinical setting by measuring the P_{Cr}, which is inversely related to the GFR (Figure 3-3). However, as Figure 3-3 shows, the GFR must decline substantially before an increase in the

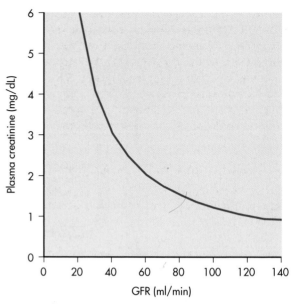

FIGURE 3-3 ■ Relationship between GFR and plasma [creatinine] (P_{Cr}). The amount of creatinine filtered is equal to the amount excreted; thus, GFR × P_{Cr} = U_{Cr} × V̇. Because the production of creatinine is constant, excretion must be constant to maintain creatinine balance. Therefore, if the GFR falls from 120 to 60 ml/min, the P_{Cr} must increase from 1 to 2 mg/dL to keep the filtration of creatinine and its excretion equal to the production rate.

P_{Cr} can be detected in a clinical setting. For example, a fall in GFR from 120 to 100 ml/min is accompanied by an increase in the P_{Cr} from 1.0 to 1.2 mg/dL. This does not appear to be a significant change in the P_{Cr}, but the GFR has actually fallen by almost 20%.

GLOMERULAR FILTRATION

The first step in the formation of urine is ultrafiltration of the plasma by the glomerulus. In normal adults, the GFR ranges from 90 to 140 ml/min for males and from 80 to 125 ml/min for females. Thus, in 24 hours as much as 180 L of plasma is filtered by the glomeruli. The plasma ultrafiltrate is devoid of cellular elements (i.e., red and white blood cells and platelets) and is essentially protein free. The concentrations of salts and of organic molecules, such as glucose and amino acids, are similar in the plasma and ultrafiltrate. Starling forces drive ultrafiltration across the glomerular capillaries, and changes in these forces alter the GFR. The GFR and RPF are normally held within very narrow ranges by a phenomenon called autoregulation. The next sections of this chapter review the composition of the glomerular filtrate, the dynamics of its formation, and the relationship between RPF and GFR. In addition, the factors that contribute to the autoregulation, and regulation, of GFR and RBF are discussed.

Determinants of Ultrafiltrate Composition

The glomerular filtration barrier determines the composition of the plasma ultrafiltrate. It restricts the filtration of molecules on the basis of both size and electrical charge (Figure 3-4). In general, neutral molecules with a radius smaller than 20 Å are filtered freely, molecules larger than 42 Å are not filtered, and molecules between 20 and 42 Å are filtered to various degrees. For example, serum albumin, an anionic protein that has an effective molecular radius of 35.5 Å, is filtered poorly. Because, normally, the filtered albumin is reabsorbed avidly by the proximal tubule, almost no albumin appears in the urine.

Figure 3-4 shows how electrical charge affects the filtration of macromolecules (e.g., dextrans) by the glomerulus. Dextrans are a family of exogenous polysaccharides manufactured in various molecular weights. They can be electrically neutral or have either negative charges (polyanionic) or positive charges

(polycationic). As the size (i.e., effective molecular radius) of a dextran molecule increases, the rate at which it is filtered decreases. For any given molecular radius, cationic molecules are more readily filtered than anionic molecules. The reduced filtration rate for anionic molecules is explained by the presence of negatively charged glycoproteins on the surfaces of all components of the glomerular filtration barrier. These charged glycoproteins repel similarly charged molecules. Because most plasma proteins are negatively charged, the negative charge on the filtration barrier restricts the filtration of proteins that have a molecular radius of 20 to 42 Å or more.

The importance of the negative charges on the filtration barrier in restricting the filtration of plasma proteins is shown in Figure 3-5. The removal of negative charges from the filtration barrier causes proteins to be filtered solely on the basis of their effective molecular radius. Hence, at any molecular radius between approximately 20 and 42 Å, the filtration of polyanionic proteins exceeds the filtration that prevails in the normal state (in which the filtration barrier has anionic charges). In a number of glomerular diseases, the negative charges on the filtration barrier are reduced because of immunologic damage and inflammation. As a result, the filtration of proteins is increased, and proteins appear in the urine **(proteinuria).**

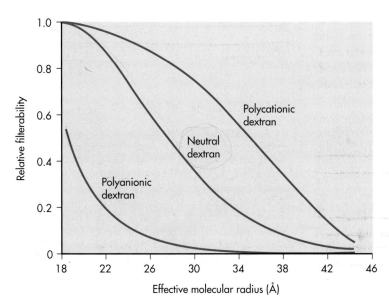

FIGURE 3-4 ■ Influence of size and electrical charge of dextran on its filterability. A value of one indicates that it is filtered freely, whereas a value of zero indicates that it is not filtered. The filterability of dextrans between approximately 20 and 42 Å depends on charge. Dextrans larger than 42 Å are not filtered regardless of charge, and polycationic dextrans and neutral dextrans smaller than 20 Å are freely filtered. The major proteins in plasma are albumin and immunoglobulins. Because the effective molecular radii of immunoglobulin G (IgG) (53 Å) and IgM (>100 Å) are greater than 42 Å, they are not filtered. Although the effective molecular radius of albumin is 35 Å, it is a polyanionic protein; thus, it does not cross the filtration barrier to a significant degree.

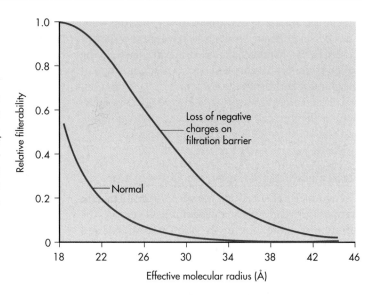

FIGURE 3-5 ■ Reduction of the negative charges on the glomerular wall results in the filtration of proteins on the basis of size only. In this situation the relative filterability of proteins depends only on the molecular radius. Accordingly, the excretion of polyanionic proteins (20 to 42 Å) in the urine increases because more proteins of this size are filtered.

Dynamics of Ultrafiltration

The forces responsible for the glomerular filtration of plasma are the same as those in all capillary beds (see Chapter 1). Ultrafiltration occurs because the Starling forces (i.e., hydrostatic and oncotic pressures) drive fluid from the lumen of glomerular capillaries, across the filtration barrier, and into Bowman's space (Figure 3-6). The hydrostatic pressure in the glomerular capillary (P_{GC}) is oriented to promote the movement of fluid from the glomerular capillary into Bowman's space. Because the reflection coefficient (σ) for proteins across the glomerular capillary is essentially one, the glomerular ultrafiltrate is protein free, and the oncotic pressure in Bowman's space (π_{BS}) is near zero. Therefore, P_{GC} is the only force that favors filtration. The hydrostatic pressure in Bowman's space (P_{BS}) and the oncotic pressure in the glomerular capillary (π_{GC}) oppose filtration.

As shown in Figure 3-6, a net ultrafiltration pressure (P_{UF}) of 17 mm Hg exists at the afferent end of the glomerulus, whereas at the efferent end, it is 8 mm Hg (where $P_{UF} = P_{GC} - P_{BS} - \pi_{GC}$). Two additional points concerning Starling forces and this pressure change are important. First, P_{GC} decreases slightly along the length of the capillary because of the resistance to flow along the length of the capillary. Second, π_{GC} increases along the length of the glomerular capillary. Because water is filtered and protein is retained in the

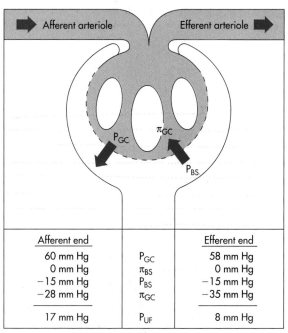

Afferent end		Efferent end
60 mm Hg	P_{GC}	58 mm Hg
0 mm Hg	π_{BS}	0 mm Hg
−15 mm Hg	P_{BS}	−15 mm Hg
−28 mm Hg	π_{GC}	−35 mm Hg
17 mm Hg	P_{UF}	8 mm Hg

FIGURE 3-6 ■ Idealized glomerular capillary and the Starling forces across it. The reflection coefficient (σ) for protein across the glomerular capillary is one. P_{BS}, hydrostatic pressure in Bowman's space; P_{GC}, hydrostatic pressure in the glomerular capillary; P_{UF}, net ultrafiltration pressure; π_{GC}, oncotic pressure in the glomerular capillary; π_{BS}, oncotic pressure in Bowman's space. The negative signs for P_{BS} and π_{GC} indicate that these forces oppose the formation of the glomerular filtrate.

glomerular capillary, the protein concentration in the capillary rises, and π_{GC} increases.

The GFR is proportional to the sum of the Starling forces that exist across the capillaries $[(P_{GC} - P_{BS}) - \sigma(\pi_{GC} - \pi_{BS})]$ multiplied by the ultrafiltration coefficient (K_f). That is:

$$GFR = K_f[(P_{GC} - P_{BS}) - \sigma(\pi_{GC} - \pi_{BS})] \quad (3\text{-}10)$$

K_f is the product of the intrinsic permeability of the glomerular capillary and the glomerular surface area available for filtration. The rate of glomerular filtration is considerably greater in glomerular capillaries than in systemic capillaries, mainly because K_f is approximately 100 times greater in glomerular capillaries. Furthermore, the P_{GC} is approximately twice as great as the hydrostatic pressure in systemic capillaries.

The GFR can be altered by changing K_f or by changing any of the Starling forces. In normal individuals, the GFR is regulated by alterations in the P_{GC} that are mediated mainly by changes in afferent or efferent arteriolar resistance. P_{GC} is affected in three ways:

1. *Changes in afferent arteriolar resistance:* a decrease in resistance increases the P_{GC} and GFR, whereas an increase in resistance decreases them.
2. *Changes in efferent arteriolar resistance:* a decrease in resistance reduces the P_{GC} and GFR, whereas an increase in resistance elevates them.
3. *Changes in renal arteriolar pressure:* an increase in blood pressure transiently increases the P_{GC} (which enhances the GFR), whereas a decrease in blood pressure transiently decreases the P_{GC} (which reduces the GFR).

A reduction in the GFR in disease states is most often due to decreases in K_f because of the loss of filtration surface area. The GFR also changes in pathophysiologic conditions because of changes in P_{GC}, π_{GC}, and P_{BS}.

1. Changes in K_f: an increased K_f enhances the GFR, whereas a decreased K_f reduces the GFR. Some kidney diseases reduce the K_f by decreasing the number of filtering glomeruli (i.e., diminished surface area). Some drugs and hormones that dilate the glomerular arterioles also increase the K_f. Similarly, drugs and hormones that constrict the glomerular arterioles also decrease the K_f.

2. Changes in P_{GC}: with decreased renal perfusion, the GFR declines because the P_{GC} falls. As previously discussed, a reduction in the P_{GC} is caused by a decline in renal arterial pressure, an increase in afferent arteriolar resistance, or a decrease in efferent arteriolar resistance.
3. Changes in π_{GC}: an inverse relationship exists between the π_{GC} and the GFR. Alterations in the π_{GC} result from changes in protein synthesis outside the kidneys. In addition, protein loss in the urine caused by some renal diseases can lead to a decrease in the plasma protein concentration and thus in the π_{GC}.
4. Changes in P_{BS}: an increased P_{BS} reduces the GFR, whereas a decreased P_{BS} enhances the GFR. Acute obstruction of the urinary tract (e.g., a kidney stone occluding the ureter) increases the P_{BS}.

RENAL BLOOD FLOW

Blood flow through the kidneys serves several important functions including the following:

1. Indirectly determines the GFR
2. Modifies the rate of solute and water reabsorption by the proximal tubule
3. Participates in the concentration and dilution of urine
4. Delivers O_2, nutrients, and hormones to the cells of the nephron and returns CO_2 and reabsorbed fluid and solutes to the general circulation
5. Delivers substrates for excretion in the urine

Blood flow through any organ may be represented by the following equation:

$$Q = \frac{\Delta P}{R} \quad (3\text{-}11)$$

where:

Q = Blood flow
ΔP = Mean arterial pressure minus venous pressure for that organ
R = Resistance to flow through that organ

Accordingly, RBF is equal to the pressure difference between the renal artery and the renal vein divided by the renal vascular resistance:

$$RBF = \frac{\text{Aortic Pressure} - \text{Renal Venous Pressure}}{\text{Renal Vascular Resistance}} \qquad (3\text{-}12)$$

The afferent arteriole, efferent arteriole, and interlobular artery are the major resistance vessels in the kidneys and thereby determine renal vascular resistance. Like most other organs, the kidneys regulate their blood flow by adjusting the vascular resistance in response to changes in arterial pressure. As shown in Figure 3-7, these adjustments are so precise that blood flow remains relatively constant as arterial blood pressure fluctuates between 90 and 180 mm Hg. The GFR is also regulated over the same range of arterial pressures. The phenomenon whereby RBF and GFR are maintained relatively constant, namely **autoregulation,** is achieved by changes in vascular resistance, mainly through the afferent arterioles of the kidneys. Because both the GFR and RBF are regulated over the same range of pressures and because RBF is an important determinant of GFR, it is

not surprising that the same mechanisms regulate both flows.

Two mechanisms are responsible for the autoregulation of RBF and GFR: one mechanism that responds to changes in arterial pressure and another that responds to changes in the NaCl concentration of tubular fluid. Both regulate the tone of the afferent arteriole. The pressure-sensitive mechanism, the so-called **myogenic mechanism,** is related to an intrinsic property of vascular smooth muscle: the tendency to contract when it is stretched. Accordingly, when the arterial pressure rises and the renal afferent arteriole is stretched, the smooth muscle contracts. Because the increase in the resistance of the arteriole offsets the increase in pressure, RBF and therefore GFR remain constant (that is, RBF is constant if $\Delta P/R$ is kept constant [see equation 3-11]).

The second mechanism responsible for the autoregulation of GFR and RBF is the NaCl concentration-dependent mechanism known as **tubuloglomerular feedback** (Figure 3-8). This mechanism involves a feedback loop in which the NaCl concentration of tubular fluid is sensed by the macula densa of the **juxtaglomerular apparatus** (JGA; see Figure 2-5 in Chapter 2) and converted into a signal or signals that affect afferent arteriolar resistance and, thus, the GFR. When the GFR increases and causes the NaCl concentration of tubular fluid at the macula densa to rise, more NaCl enters macula densa cells. This leads to an increase in the formation and release of ATP and adenosine, a metabolite of ATP, by macula densa cells, which cause vasoconstriction of the afferent arteriole. Vasoconstriction of the afferent arteriole returns the GFR to normal levels. In contrast, when the GFR and NaCl concentration of tubule fluid decrease, less NaCl enters macula densa cells, and ATP, and adenosine, production and release decline. The fall in ATP and adenosine causes vasodilation of the afferent arteriole, which returns the GFR to normal. Nitric oxide (NO), a vasodilator produced by the macula densa, attenuates tubuloglomerular feedback, whereas angiotensin II enhances tubuloglomerular feedback. Thus, the macula densa may release both vasoconstrictors (e.g., ATP and adenosine) and a vasodilator (e.g., NO), which oppose each other's action at the level of the afferent arteriole. Production and release of vasoconstrictors and vasodilators assure exquisite control over tubuloglomerular feedback.

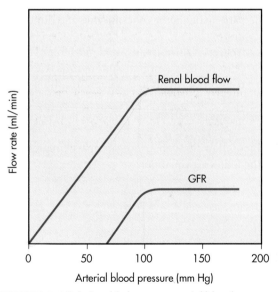

FIGURE 3-7 ■ Relationship between arterial blood pressure and RBF and between arterial blood pressure and GFR. Autoregulation maintains the GFR and RBF relatively constant as blood pressure fluctuates between 90 and 180 mm Hg.

Figure 3-8B also illustrates the role of the macula densa in controlling the secretion of renin by the granular cells of the afferent arteriole. This aspect of JGA function is considered in detail in Chapter 6.

Tubuloglomerular feedback is absent in mice that do not express the adenosine receptor (A1). This underscores the importance of adenosine signaling in tubuloglomerular feedback. Studies have shown that when the GFR increases and causes the NaCl concentration of tubular fluid at the macula densa to rise, more NaCl enters cells through the Na^+-K^+-$2Cl^-$ cotransporter

(*NKCC2*) located in the apical plasma membrane (see Chapter 4). Increased intracellular [NaCl] in turn stimulates the release of ATP through ATP-conducting ion channels located in the basolateral membrane of macula densa cells. In addition, adenosine production is enhanced. Adenosine binds to A1 receptors and ATP binds to P2X receptors located on the plasma membrane of smooth muscle cells in the afferent arteriole. Both hormones increase intracellular [Ca^{++}], which causes vasoconstriction of the afferent artery and therefore a fall in GFR. Although adenosine is a vasodilator in most other vascular beds, it constricts the afferent arteriole in the kidney.

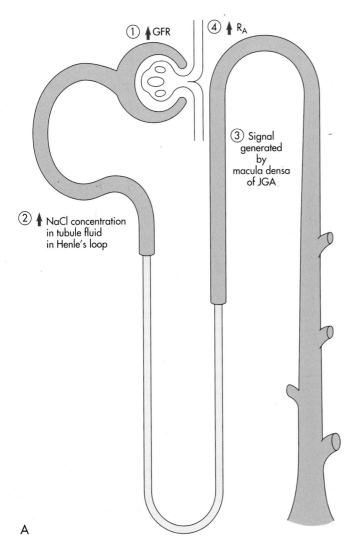

① ↑GFR

④ ↑R_A

③ Signal generated by macula densa of JGA

② ↑ NaCl concentration in tubule fluid in Henle's loop

FIGURE 3-8 ■ A, Tubuloglomerular feedback. An increase in the GFR (1) increases NaCl concentration in tubule fluid in the loop of Henle (2), which is sensed by the macula densa and converted into a signal (3) that increases the resistance of the afferent arteriole (R_A) (4), which decreases the GFR. (**A,** *Modified from Cogan MG: Fluid and electrolytes: physiology and pathophysiology. Norwalk, Conn, 1991, Appleton & Lange.*)

Continued

A

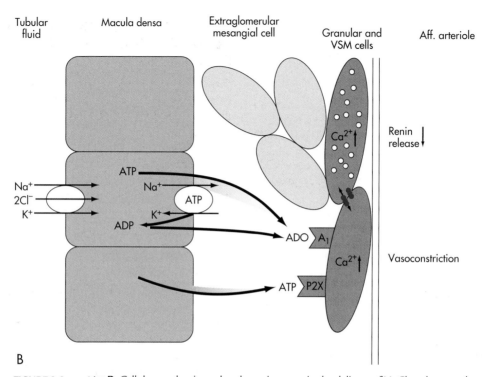

FIGURE 3-8, cont'd ■ **B,** Cellular mechanism whereby an increase in the delivery of NaCl to the macula densa causes vasoconstriction of the afferent arteriole of the same nephron (i.e., tubuloglomerular feedback). An increase in GFR elevates the [NaCl] in tubule fluid at the macula densa. This in turn enhances NaCl uptake across the apical cell membrane of macula densa cells through the $Na^+/K^+/2Cl^-$ (*NKCC2*) symporter, which leads to an increase in [ATP] and [adenosine] (ADO). ATP binds to P2X receptors and adenosine binds to adenosine A1 receptors in the plasma membrane of smooth muscle cells surrounding the afferent arteriole, both of which increase intracellular $[Ca^{++}]$. The rise in $[Ca^{++}]$ induces vasoconstriction of the afferent arteriole, returning GFR to normal levels. Note that ATP and adenosine also inhibit renin release by granular cells in the afferent arteriole. This too results from an increase in intracellular $[Ca^{++}]$ reflecting electrical coupling of the granular and vascular smooth muscle cells. When GFR is reduced, [NaCl] in tubule fluid falls, as does NaCl uptake into macula densa cells. This in turn decreases ATP and adenosine release, which decreases intracellular $[Ca^{++}]$ and thereby increases GFR and stimulates renin release by granular cells. In addition, a decrease in NaCl entry into macula densa cells enhances the production of PGE_2, which also stimulates renin secretion by granular cells. As discussed in detail in Chapters 4 and 6, renin increases plasma angiotensin II, a hormone that enhances NaCl and water retention by the kidneys. (**B,** *Modified from Persson AEG, Ollerstam R, Liu R, Brown R: Mechanisms for macula densa cell release of renin. Acta Physiol Scand 181:471-474, 2004.*)

Because animals engage in many activities that can change arterial blood pressure, mechanisms that maintain RBF and GFR relatively constant despite changes in arterial pressure are highly desirable. If the GFR and RBF were to rise or fall suddenly in proportion to changes in blood pressure, urinary excretion of fluid and solute would also change suddenly. Such changes in water and solute excretion without comparable changes in intake would alter the fluid and electrolyte balance (the reason for which is discussed in Chapter 6).

Accordingly, autoregulation of the GFR and RBF provides an effective means for uncoupling renal function from arterial pressure, and it ensures that fluid and solute excretion remain constant.

Three points concerning autoregulation should be noted:

1. Autoregulation is absent when arterial pressure is less than 90 mm Hg.
2. Autoregulation is not perfect; the RBF and GFR do change slightly as the arterial blood pressure varies.
3. Despite autoregulation, the RBF and GFR can be changed by certain hormones and by changes in sympathetic nerve activity (Table 3-1).

Individuals with **renal artery stenosis** (narrowing of the artery lumen) caused by atherosclerosis, for example, can have an elevated systemic arterial blood pressure mediated by stimulation of the renin-angiotensin system (see Chapter 6). Pressure in the renal artery proximal to the stenosis is increased, but pressure distal to the stenosis is normal or reduced. Autoregulation is important in maintaining RBF, P_{GC}, and GFR in the presence of this stenosis. The administration of drugs to lower the systemic blood pressure also lowers the pressure distal to the stenosis; accordingly, the RBF, P_{GC}, and GFR fall.

REGULATION OF RENAL BLOOD FLOW AND GLOMERULAR FILTRATION RATE

Several factors and hormones affect the GFR and RBF (see Table 3-1). As discussed, the myogenic mechanism and tubuloglomerular feedback play key roles in maintaining GFR and RBF constant. In addition, sympathetic nerves, angiotensin II, prostaglandins, NO, endothelin, bradykinin, ATP, and adenosine exert major control over RBF and GFR. Figure 3-9 shows how changes in afferent and efferent arteriolar resistance, mediated by changes in the hormones listed in Table 3-1, modulate the GFR and RBF.

Sympathetic Nerves

The afferent and efferent arterioles are innervated by sympathetic neurons; however, sympathetic tone is minimal when the volume of extracellular fluid is normal (see Chapter 6). Sympathetic nerves release norepinephrine and dopamine, and circulating epinephrine (a catecholamine like norepinephrine and dopamine) is secreted by the adrenal medulla. Norepinephrine and epinephrine cause vasoconstriction by binding to α_1-adrenoceptors, which are located mainly on the afferent arterioles. Activation of α_1-adrenoceptors decreases the GFR and RBF. Dehydration or strong emotional stimuli, such as fear

TABLE 3-1			
Major Hormones that Influence GFR and RBF			
	STIMULUS	EFFECT ON GFR	EFFECT ON RBF
Vasoconstrictors			
Sympathetic nerves	↓ ECFV	↓	↓
Angiotensin II	↓ ECFV	↓	↓
Endothelin	↑ Stretch, AII, bradykinin, epinephrine, ↓ ECFV	↓	↓
Vasodilators			
Prostaglandins (PGE1, PGE2, PGI2)	↓ ECFV, ↑ shear stress, AII	No change/↑	↑
Nitric oxide (NO)	↑ shear stress, acetylcholine, histamine, bradykinin, ATP	↑	↑
Bradykinin	Prostaglandins, ↓ ACE	↑	↑
Natriuretic peptides (ANP, BNP)	↑ ECFV	↑	No change

ACE, angiotensin-converting enzyme; AII, angiotensin II; ECFV, extracellular fluid volume; GFR, glomerular filtration rate; RBF, renal blood flow.

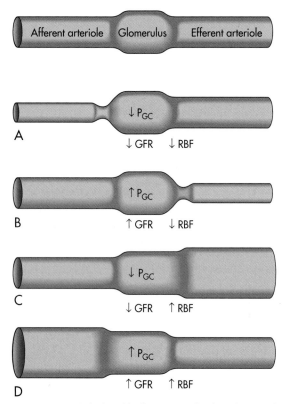

FIGURE 3-9 ■ Relationship between selective changes in the resistance of either the afferent arteriole or the efferent arteriole on RBF and GFR. Constriction of either the afferent or efferent arteriole increases resistance, and according to equation 3-11 ($Q = \Delta P/R$), an increase in resistance (R) decreases flow (Q) (i.e., RBF). Dilation of either the afferent or efferent arteriole increases flow (i.e., RBF). **(A)** Constriction of the afferent arteriole decreases the P_{GC} because less of the arterial pressure is transmitted to the glomerulus, thereby reducing the GFR. **(B)** In contrast, constriction of the efferent arteriole elevates the P_{GC} and thus increases the GFR. **(C)** Dilation of the efferent arteriole decreases the P_{GC} and thus decreases the GFR. **(D)** Dilation of the afferent arteriole increases the P_{GC} because more of the arterial pressure is transmitted to the glomerulus, thereby increasing the GFR. (*Modified from Rose BD, Rennke KG: Renal pathophysiology: the essentials. Baltimore, 1994, Williams & Wilkins.*)

and pain, activate sympathetic nerves and reduce the GFR and RBF.

Renalase, a catecholamine-metabolizing hormone produced by kidneys, facilitates the degradation of catecholamines.

Angiotensin II

Angiotensin II is produced systemically and locally within the kidneys. It constricts the afferent and efferent arterioles[3] and decreases the RBF and GFR. Figure 3-10 shows how norepinephrine, epinephrine, and angiotensin II act together to decrease the RBF and GFR and thereby increase blood pressure and extracellular fluid (ECF) volume, as would occur, for example, with hemorrhage.

> **Hemorrhage** decreases arterial blood pressure and therefore activates the sympathetic nerves to the kidneys by the baroreceptor reflex (Figure 3-10). Norepinephrine causes intense vasoconstriction of the afferent and efferent arterioles and thereby decreases the GFR and RBF. The rise in sympathetic activity also increases the release of epinephrine and angiotensin II, which cause further vasoconstriction and a fall in RBF. The rise in the vascular resistance of the kidneys and other vascular beds increases the total peripheral resistance. The resulting tendency for blood pressure to increase (blood pressure = cardiac output × total peripheral resistance) offsets the tendency of blood pressure to decrease in response to hemorrhage. Hence, this system works to preserve the arterial pressure at the expense of maintaining a normal GFR and RBF.

Prostaglandins

Prostaglandins do not play a major role in regulating RBF in healthy, resting people. However, during pathophysiologic conditions such as hemorrhage,

---

[3]The efferent arteriole is more sensitive to angiotensin II than the afferent arteriole. Therefore, with low concentrations of angiotensin II, constriction of the efferent arteriole predominates, and GFR increases and RBF decreases. However, with high concentrations of angiotensin II, constriction of both afferent and efferent arterioles occurs and both GFR and RBF fall (see Figure 3-9).

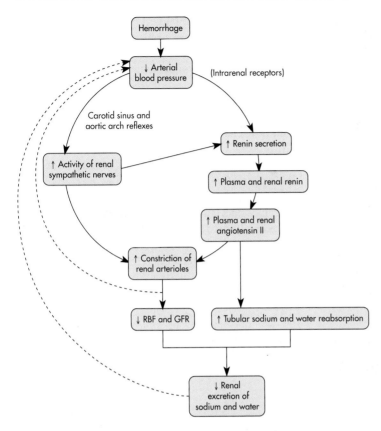

FIGURE 3-10 ■ Pathway by which hemorrhage activates renal sympathetic nerve activity and stimulates the production of angiotensin II. GFR, glomerular filtration rate; RBF, renal blood flow. *(Modified from Vander AJ: Renal physiology, ed 2. New York, 1980, McGraw-Hill.)*

prostaglandins (PGI_2, PGE_1, and PGE_2) are produced locally within the kidneys, and they increase RBF without changing the GFR. Prostaglandins increase RBF by dampening the vasoconstrictor effects of sympathetic nerves and angiotensin II. This effect is important because it prevents severe and potentially harmful vasoconstriction and renal ischemia. Prostaglandin synthesis is stimulated by dehydration and stress (e.g., surgery, anesthesia), angiotensin II, and sympathetic nerves. Nonsteroidal anti-inflammatory drugs (NSAIDs), such as aspirin and ibuprofen, inhibit the synthesis of prostaglandins. Thus, administration of these drugs during renal ischemia and hemorrhagic shock is contraindicated because, by blocking the production of prostaglandins, they decrease RBF and increase renal ischemia. Prostaglandins play an increasingly important role in maintaining RBF and

GFR as individuals age. Accordingly, NSAIDs can significantly reduce RBF and GFR in elderly people.

Nitric Oxide

NO, an endothelium-derived relaxing factor, is an important vasodilator under basal conditions, and it counteracts the vasoconstriction produced by angiotensin II and catecholamines. When blood flow increases, a greater shear force acts on the endothelial cells in the arterioles and increases the production of NO. Also, a number of vasoactive hormones, including acetylcholine, histamine, bradykinin, and ATP, cause the release of NO from endothelial cells. Increased production of NO causes dilation of the afferent and efferent arterioles in the kidneys. Whereas increased levels of NO decrease the total peripheral resistance, inhibition of NO production increases the total peripheral resistance.

Abnormal production of NO is observed in individuals with **diabetes mellitus** and **hypertension.** Excess renal NO production in diabetes may be responsible for glomerular hyperfiltration (i.e., increased GFR) and damage of the glomerulus, problems characteristic of this disease. Elevated NO levels increase the glomerular capillary pressure secondary to a fall in the resistance of the afferent arteriole. The ensuing hyperfiltration is thought to cause glomerular damage. The normal response to an increase in dietary salt intake includes the stimulation of renal NO production, which prevents an increase in blood pressure. In some individuals, however, NO production may not increase appropriately in response to an elevation in salt intake, and blood pressure rises.

Endothelin

Endothelin is a potent vasoconstrictor secreted by endothelial cells of the renal vessels, mesangial cells, and distal tubular cells in response to angiotensin II, bradykinin, epinephrine, and endothelial shear stress. Endothelin causes profound vasoconstriction of the afferent and efferent arterioles and decreases the GFR and RBF. Although this potent vasoconstrictor may not influence the GFR and RBF in resting subjects, endothelin production is elevated in a number of glomerular disease states (e.g., renal disease associated with diabetes mellitus).

Bradykinin

Kallikrein is a proteolytic enzyme produced in the kidneys. Kallikrein cleaves circulating kininogen to bradykinin, which is a vasodilator that acts by stimulating the release of NO and prostaglandins. Bradykinin increases the GFR and RBF.

Adenosine

Adenosine is produced within the kidneys and causes vasoconstriction of the afferent arteriole, thereby reducing the GFR and RBF. As previously mentioned, adenosine may play a role in tubuloglomerular feedback.

Natriuretic Peptides

Secretion of atrial natriuretic peptide (ANP) by the cardiac atria and brain natriuretic peptide (BNP) from the cardiac ventricle increases when the ECF volume is expanded. Both ANP and BNP dilate the afferent arteriole and constrict the efferent arteriole. Therefore, ANP and BNP produce a modest increase in the GFR with little change in RBF.

ATP

Cells release ATP into the renal interstitial fluid. ATP has dual effects on the GFR and RBF. Under some conditions, ATP constricts the afferent arteriole, reduces RBF and GFR, and may play a role in tubuloglomerular feedback. In contrast, ATP may stimulate NO production and increase the GFR and RBF.

Glucocorticoids

Administration of therapeutic doses of glucocorticoids increases the GFR and RBF.

Histamine

The local release of histamine modulates RBF in the resting state and during inflammation and injury. Histamine decreases the resistance of the afferent and efferent arterioles and thereby increases RBF without elevating the GFR.

Dopamine

The proximal tubule produces the vasodilator substance dopamine. Dopamine has several actions within the kidney, such as increasing RBF and inhibiting renin secretion.

Finally, as illustrated in Figure 3-11, endothelial cells play an important role in regulating the resistance of the renal afferent and efferent arterioles by producing a number of paracrine hormones, including NO, prostacyclin (PGI_2), endothelin, and angiotensin II. These hormones regulate contraction or relaxation of smooth muscle cells in afferent and efferent arterioles and mesangial cells. Shear stress, acetylcholine, histamine, bradykinin, and ATP stimulate the production of NO, which increases the GFR and RBF.

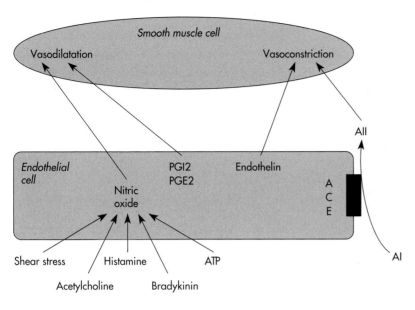

FIGURE 3-11 ■ Examples of the interactions of endothelial cells with smooth muscle and mesangial cells. ACE, angiotensin converting enzyme; AI, angiotensin I; AII, angiotensin II; ATP, adenosine triphosphate. (Modified from Navar LG, Inscho EW, Majid SA, et al: Paracrine regulation of the renal microcirculation. Physiol Rev 76:425, 1996.)

Angiotensin-converting enzyme (ACE), located on the surface of endothelial cells lining the afferent arteriole and glomerular capillaries, converts angiotensin I to angiotensin II, which decreases the GFR and RBF. Angiotensin II is also produced locally in the granular cells in the afferent arteriole and proximal tubular cells. PGI_2 and PGE_2 secretion by endothelial cells, stimulated by sympathetic nerve activity and angiotensin II, increases the GFR and RBF. Finally, the release of endothelin from endothelial cells decreases the GFR and RBF.

Angiotensin-converting enzyme **(ACE)** degrades and thereby inactivates bradykinin, and it converts angiotensin I, an inactive hormone, to angiotensin II, an active hormone. Thus, ACE increases angiotensin II levels and decreases bradykinin levels. Drugs called **ACE inhibitors** (e.g., enalapril, captopril), which reduce systemic blood pressure in patients with hypertension, decrease angiotensin II levels and elevate bradykinin levels. Both effects lower systemic vascular resistance, reduce blood pressure, and decrease renal vascular resistance, thereby increasing the GFR and RBF. **Angiotensin II receptor antagonists** (e.g., losartan) are also used to treat high blood pressure. As their name suggests, they block the binding of angiotensin II to the angiotensin II receptor (AT1). These antagonists block the vasoconstrictor effects of angiotensin II on the afferent arteriole; thus, they increase GFR and RBF. In contrast to ACE inhibitors, angiotensin II receptor antagonists do not inhibit kinin metabolism (e.g., bradykinin).

S U M M A R Y

1. Creatinine and inulin clearance can be used to measure the glomerular filtration rate.
2. Clinically, the GFR is evaluated by measuring plasma [creatinine].
3. Starling forces across the glomerular capillaries provide the driving force for the ultrafiltration of plasma from the glomerular capillaries into Bowman's space.
4. The glomerular ultrafiltrate is devoid of cellular elements, including red and white blood cells and platelets, and contains very little protein but is otherwise identical to plasma.

5. RBF (1.25 L/min) is about 25% of the cardiac output. RBF determines the GFR; modifies solute and water reabsorption by the proximal tubule; participates in the concentration and dilution of the urine; delivers O_2, nutrients, and hormones to the cells of the nephron; returns CO_2 and reabsorbed fluid and solutes to the general circulation; and delivers substrates for excretion in the urine.

6. Autoregulation allows the GFR and RBF to remain constant despite fluctuations in arterial blood pressure between 90 and 180 mm Hg.

7. Hemorrhage activates renal sympathetic nerves and stimulates angiotensin II production and thereby reduces renal perfusion and urinary excretion of NaCl and water.

8. Sympathetic nerves, catecholamines, angiotensin II, prostaglandins, NO, endothelin, natriuretic peptides, prostaglandins, bradykinin, and adenosine exert substantial control over the GFR and RBF.

KEY WORDS AND CONCEPTS

- Clearance
- Mass balance
- Renal plasma flow
- Inulin
- Glomerular filtration rate
- Creatinine
- Creatinine clearance
- Filtration fraction
- Autoregulation
- Myogenic mechanism
- Tubuloglomerular feedback
- Juxtaglomerular apparatus
- Sympathetic nerves, angiotensin II, prostaglandins, nitric oxide (NO), endothelin, bradykinin, and adenosine
- Renalase

SELF-STUDY PROBLEMS

1. Phlorhizin is a drug that completely inhibits the reabsorption of glucose by the kidneys. The following data are obtained to assess the effect of phlorhizin on the clearance of glucose. Fill in the missing data.

Before phlorhizin administration

Plasma (inulin):	1 mg/ml
Plasma (glucose):	1 mg/ml
GFR Inulin excretion rate:	100 mg/min
Glucose excretion rate:	0 mg/min
Inulin clearance:	_100_ ml/min
Glucose clearance:	_0_ ml/min

After phlorhizin administration

Plasma (inulin):	1 mg/ml
Plasma (glucose):	1 mg/ml
Inulin excretion rate:	100 mg/min
Glucose excretion rate:	_____ mg/min
Inulin clearance:	_100_ ml/min
Glucose clearance:	_____ ml/min

How do you explain the change in glucose excretion and clearance seen with phlorhizin?

2. Finding which of the following substances in the urine would indicate damage to the glomerular ultrafiltration barrier?
   a. Red blood cells
   b. Glucose
   c. Sodium
   d. Proteins

3. Explain how hormones (e.g., sympathetic agonists, angiotensin II, and prostaglandins) change RBF.

4. Explain why the use of nonsteroidal anti-inflammatory drugs (e.g., indomethacin for arthritis) does not affect GFR or RBF in patients with normal renal function and why administration of nonsteroidal anti-inflammatory agents is not recommended for patients with severe reductions in GFR and RBF.

RENAL TRANSPORT MECHANISMS: NaCl AND WATER REABSORPTION ALONG THE NEPHRON

OBJECTIVES

Upon completion of this chapter, the student should be able to answer the following questions:

1. What three processes are involved in the production of urine?

2. What is the composition of "normal" urine?

3. What transport mechanisms are responsible for NaCl reabsorption by the nephron? Where are they located along the nephron?

4. How is water reabsorption "coupled" to NaCl reabsorption in the proximal tubule?

5. Why are solutes, but not water, reabsorbed by the thick ascending limb of Henle's loop?

6. What transport mechanisms are involved in the secretion of organic anions and cations? What is the physiologic relevance of these transport processes?

7. What is glomerulotubular balance, and what is its physiologic importance?

8. What are the major hormones that regulate NaCl and water reabsorption in the kidneys? What is the nephron site of action of each hormone?

The formation of urine involves three basic processes: (1) **ultrafiltration** of plasma by the glomerulus, (2) **reabsorption** of water and solutes from the ultrafiltrate, and (3) **secretion** of select solutes into the tubular fluid. Although an average of 115 to 180 L/day for women and 130 to 200 L/day for men of essentially protein-free fluid is filtered by the human glomeruli each day,[1] less than 1% of the filtered water and sodium chloride (NaCl) and variable amounts

of other solutes are excreted in the urine (Table 4-1). By the processes of reabsorption and secretion, the renal tubules modulate the volume and composition of urine (Table 4-2). Consequently, the tubules precisely control the volume, osmolality, composition, and pH of the intracellular and extracellular fluid compartments. Transport proteins in cell membranes of the nephron mediate the reabsorption and secretion of solutes and water in the kidneys. Approximately 5% to 10% of all human genes code for transport proteins, and genetic and acquired defects in transport proteins are the cause of many kidney diseases (Table 4-3). In addition, numerous transport proteins are important drug targets. This chapter discusses NaCl and water reabsorption, organic anion and cation transport, the transport proteins involved in solute and water

---

[1]The normal glomerular filtration rate (GFR) averages 115 to 180 L/day in women and 130 to 200 L/day in men. Thus, the volume of the ultrafiltrate represents a volume that is approximately 10 times the extracellular fluid volume. For simplicity, we assume throughout the remainder of this book that the GFR is 180 L/day.

TABLE 4-1

Filtration, Excretion, and Reabsorption of Water, Electrolytes, and Solutes by the Kidneys

SUBSTANCE	MEASURE	FILTERED*	EXCRETED	REABSORBED	% FILTERED LOAD REABSORBED
Water	L/day	180	1.5	178.5	99.2
Na^+	mEq/day	25,200	150	25,050	99.4
K^+	mEq/day	720	100	620	86.1
Ca^{++}	mEq/day	540	10	530	98.2
Bicarbonate (HCO_3^-)	mEq/day	4,320	2	4,318	99.9+
Cl^-	mEq/day	18,000	150	17,850	99.2
Glucose	mmol/day	800	0	800	100.0
Urea	g/day	56	28	28	50.0

*The filtered amount of any substance is calculated by multiplying the concentration of that substance in the ultrafiltrate by the glomerular filtration rate (GFR); for example, the filtered load of Na^+ is calculated as $[Na^+]_{ultrafiltrate}$ (140 mEq/L) × GFR (180 L/day) = 25,200 mEq/day.

transport, and some of the factors and hormones that regulate NaCl transport. Details on acid-base transport and on K^+, Ca^{++}, and inorganic phosphate (Pi) transport and their regulation are provided in Chapters 7 through 9.

TABLE 4-2

Composition of Urine*

SUBSTANCE	CONCENTRATION
Na^+	50-130 mEq/L
K^+	20-70 mEq/L
Ammonium	30-50 mEq/L
Ca^{++}	5-12 mEq/L
Mg^{++}	2-18 mEq/L
Cl^-	50-130 mEq/L
Inorganic phosphate	20-40 mEq/L
Urea	200-400 mM
Creatinine	6-20 mM
pH	5.0-7.0
Osmolality	500-800 mOsm/kg H_2O
Glucose	0
Amino acids	0
Protein	0
Blood	0
Ketones	0
Leukocytes	0
Bilirubin	0

*The composition and volume of the urine can vary widely in the healthy state. These values represent average ranges. Water excretion ranges between 0.5 and 1.5 L/day.
Modified from Valtin HV: *Renal physiology,* ed 2, Boston, 1983, Little, Brown.

GENERAL PRINCIPLES OF MEMBRANE TRANSPORT

Solutes may be transported across cell membranes by passive mechanisms, active transport mechanisms, or endocytosis. In mammals, solute movement occurs by both passive and active mechanisms, whereas all water movement is passive. The movement of a solute across a membrane is passive if it develops spontaneously and does not require direct expenditure of metabolic energy. **Passive transport** (diffusion) of uncharged solutes occurs from an area of higher concentration to one of lower concentration (i.e., down its chemical concentration gradient). In addition to concentration gradients, the passive diffusion of ions (but not uncharged solutes, such as glucose and urea) is affected by the electrical potential difference (i.e., electrical gradient) across cell membranes and the renal tubules. Cations (e.g., Na^+, K^+) move to the negative side of the membrane, whereas anions (e.g., Cl^-, HCO_3^-) move to the positive side of the membrane. Diffusion of gases (e.g., O_2, CO_2, NH_3) may occur across the lipid bilayer, or through aquaporin channels. Diffusion of water (**osmosis**) occurs through channels in the cell membrane and is driven by osmotic pressure gradients. When water is reabsorbed across tubule segments, the solutes dissolved in the water are also carried along with the water. This process is called **solvent drag** and can account for a substantial amount of solute reabsorption across the proximal tubule.

TABLE 4-3

Some Monogenic Renal Diseases Involving Transport Proteins

DISEASES	MODE OF INHERITANCE	GENE	TRANSPORT PROTEIN	NEPHRON SEGMENT	PHENOTYPE
Cystinuria, type I	AR	SLC3A1, also known as D2/rBAT	Basic amino acid transporter	Proximal tubule	Increased excretion of basic amino acids, nephrolithiasis (kidney stones)
Cystinuria, types I and III	IAR	SLC7A9, also known as b°, $^+$AT	B°, $^+$AT	Proximal tubule	Increased excretion of basic amino acids, nephrolithiasis
Proximal renal tubular acidosis	AR	SLC4A4, also known as NBCe1	Na^+-HCO_3^- cotransporter	Proximal tubule	Hyperchloremic metabolic acidosis
X-linked nephrolithiasis (Dent's disease)	XLR	CLC5, also known as ClC-5	Chloride channel	Distal tubule	Hypercalciuria, nephrolithiasis
Bartter's syndrome	AR-type I	SLC12A1, also known as NKCC2	Na^+/K^+/$2Cl^-$ transporter (furosemide sensitive)	TAL	Hypokalemia, metabolic alkalosis, hyperaldosteronism
	AR-type II	KCNJ1, also known as ROMK	Potassium channel	TAL	Hypokalemia, metabolic alkalosis, hyperaldosteronism
	AR-type III	CLCNKB	Chloride channel (basolateral membrane)	TAL	Hypokalemia, metabolic alkalosis, hyperaldosteronism
	AR-type IV	BSND, also known as Barttin	Chloride channel (Barttin recruits CLCNKB to the basolateral membrane)	TAL	Hypokalemia, metabolic alkalosis, hyperaldosteronism
Hypomagnesemia-hypercalciuria syndrome	AR	CLDN16	Claudin-16, also known as paracellin 1	TAL	Hypomagnesemia-hypercalciuria, nephrolithiasis
Gitelman syndrome	AR	SLC12A3, also known as NCC/TSC	Thiazide-sensitive cotransporter	Distal tubule	Hypomagnesemia, hypokalemic metabolic alkalosis, hypocalciuria, hypotension
Pseudohypoaldosteronism	AR	SCNN1A, SCNN1B, and SCNN1G, also known as α-ENaC, β-ENaC and γ-ENaC	α, β, and γ subunit of amiloride-sensitive Na^+ channel	Collecting duct	Increased excretion of Na^+, hyperkalemia, hypotension
Pseudohypoaldosteronism	AD	MR	Mineralocorticoid receptor	Collecting duct	Increased excretion of Na^+, hyperkalemia, hypotension
Liddle's syndrome	AD	SCNN1B, SCNN1G, also known as β-ENaC and γ-ENaC	β and γ subunit of amiloride-sensitive Na^+ channel	Collecting duct	Decreased excretion of Na^+, hypertension
Nephrogenic diabetes insipidus (NDI)	AR	AQP-2	Aquaporin 2 water channel	Collecting duct	Polyuria, polydipsia, plasma hyperosmolality
Distal renal tubular acidosis	AD/AR	SLC4A1, also known as AE1	Cl^-/HCO_3^- exchanger	Collecting duct	Metabolic acidosis, hypokalemia, hypercalciuria, nephrolithiasis
Distal renal tubular acidosis	AR	ATP6V1B1	Subunit of H^+-ATPase	Collecting duct	Metabolic acidosis, hypokalemia, hypercalciuria, nephrolithiasis
Distal renal tubular acidosis	AR	ATP6V0A4	Accessory subunit of H^+-ATPase	Collecting duct	Metabolic acidosis, hypokalemia, hypercalciuria, nephrolithiasis

AD, autosomal dominant; AR, autosomal recessive; IAR, incomplete autosomal recessive; TAL, thick ascending limb of Henle's loop; XLR, X-linked recessive; nephrolithiasis = kidney stones. There are 40 different solute transporter families, which form the so-called SLC (solute carrier) series.
Modified from Guay-Woodford LM: Overview: the genetics of renal disease. *Semin Nephrol* 19:312-318, 1999.

In **facilitated diffusion,** transport depends on the interaction of the solute with a specific protein in the membrane that facilitates its movement across the membrane. If defined broadly, the term facilitated diffusion can be used to describe several different types of membrane transporters. For example, one form of facilitated diffusion is the diffusion of ions, such as Na^+ and K^+, through aqueous-filled channels created by proteins that span the plasma membrane. Also, the movement of a single molecule across the membrane by means of a transport protein (**uniport**), as occurs with urea and glucose, is a form of facilitated diffusion.[2]

Another form of facilitated diffusion is coupled transport, in which the movement of two or more solutes across a membrane depends on their interaction with a specific transport protein. Coupled transport of two or more solutes in the same direction is mediated by a **symport** mechanism. Examples of symport mechanisms in the kidneys include Na^+-glucose, Na^+–amino acid, and Na^+-Pi symporters in the proximal tubule and the $1Na^+$-$1K^+$-$2Cl^-$ symporter in the thick ascending limb of Henle's loop. Coupled transport of two or more solutes in opposite directions is mediated by an **antiport** mechanism. An Na^+-H^+ antiporter in the proximal tubule mediates Na^+ reabsorption and H^+ secretion. With coupled transporters, at least one of the solutes is usually transported against its electrochemical gradient. The energy for this uphill movement is derived from the passive downhill movement of at least one of the other solutes into the cell. For example, in the proximal tubule, operation of the Na^+-H^+ antiporter in the apical membrane of the cell results in the movement of H^+ against its electrochemical gradient out of the cell into the tubular lumen. The movement of Na^+ from the tubular lumen into the cell, down its electrochemical gradient, drives this uphill movement of H^+. The uphill movement of H^+ is termed **secondary active transport** to reflect the fact that the movement of H^+ is not directly coupled to the hydrolysis of

adenosine triphosphate (ATP) (see the following). Instead, the energy is derived from the gradient of the other coupled ion (in this example, Na^+).

Transport is **active** if it is coupled directly to energy derived from metabolic processes (i.e., it consumes ATP). Active transport of solutes usually takes place from an area of lower concentration to an area of higher concentration. In the kidneys, the most prevalent active transport mechanism is the Na^+,K^+-ATPase (or sodium pump), which is located in the basolateral membrane. The Na^+,K^+-ATPase is made up of several proteins that together actively move Na^+ out of the cell and K^+ into the cell. Other active transport mechanisms in the kidneys include the H^+-ATPase and H^+,K^+-ATPase, which are responsible for H^+ secretion in the collecting duct system (see Chapter 8), and the Ca^{++}-ATPase, which is responsible for Ca^{++} movement from the cytoplasm into the blood (see Chapter 9).

Endocytosis is the movement of a substance across the plasma membrane by a process involving the invagination of a piece of membrane until it completely pinches off and forms a vesicle in the cytoplasm. This is an important mechanism for the reabsorption of small proteins and macromolecules by the proximal tubule. Because endocytosis requires ATP, it is a form of active transport.

GENERAL PRINCIPLES OF TRANSEPITHELIAL SOLUTE AND WATER TRANSPORT

As illustrated in Figure 4-1, tight junctions hold renal cells together. Below the tight junctions, the cells are separated by **lateral intercellular spaces.** The tight junctions separate the apical membranes from the basolateral membranes. An epithelium can be compared with a six-pack of soda, wherein the cans are the cells and the plastic holder represents the tight junctions.

In the nephron, a substance can be reabsorbed or secreted through cells, the so-called **transcellular pathway,** or between cells, the so-called **paracellular pathway** (see Figure 4-1). Na^+ reabsorption by the proximal tubule is a good example of transport by the transcellular pathway. Na^+ reabsorption in this

---

[2]Some authors restrict the term facilitated diffusion to this type of transport and use as the classic example the glucose uniporter that brings glucose into many cells (e.g., skeletal muscle).

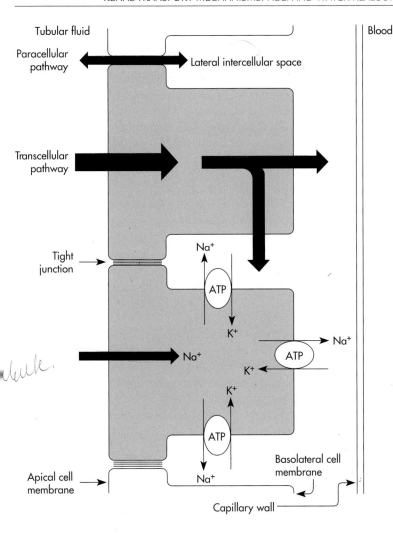

Tubular fluid

Blood

Paracellular pathway

Lateral intercellular space

Transcellular pathway

Tight junction

Na^+

ATP

K^+

Na^+

ATP

Na^+

K^+

K^+

ATP

Basolateral cell membrane

Apical cell membrane

Na^+

Capillary wall

FIGURE 4-1 ■ Paracellular and transcellular transport pathways in the proximal tubule. See text for details.

nephron segment depends on the operation of the Na^+,K^+-ATPase pump (see Figure 4-1). The Na^+, K^+-ATPase pump, which is located exclusively in the basolateral membrane, moves Na^+ out of the cell into the blood and K^+ into the cell. Thus, the operation of the Na^+,K^+-ATPase pump lowers intracellular [Na^+] and increases intracellular [K^+]. Because intracellular [Na^+] is low (12 mEq/L) and the [Na^+] in tubular fluid is high (140 mEq/L), Na^+ moves across the apical cell membrane, down a chemical concentration gradient from the tubular lumen into the cell. The Na^+, K^+-ATPase pump senses the addition of Na^+ to the cell and is stimulated to increase its rate of Na^+ extrusion into the blood, thereby returning intracellular Na^+ to normal levels. Thus, transcellular Na^+ reabsorption by

the proximal tubule is a two-step process:

1. Movement across the apical membrane into the cell, down an electrochemical gradient established by the Na^+,K^+-ATPase pump
2. Movement across the basolateral membrane against an electrochemical gradient through the Na^+,K^+-ATPase pump

The reabsorption of Ca^{++} and K^+ across the proximal tubule is a good example of paracellular transport. Some of the water reabsorbed across the proximal tubule traverses the paracellular pathway. Some solutes dissolved in this water, particularly Ca^{++} and K^+, are entrained in the reabsorbed fluid and thereby reabsorbed by the process of **solvent drag.**

The tight junction in renal epithelial cells is a specialized membrane domain that creates a barrier that regulates the paracellular diffusion of solutes across the epithelia. Tight junctions are composed of linear arrays of several integral membrane proteins including occludins (20 related proteins), claudins (three isoforms), and several members of the immunoglobulin superfamily. The tight junction complex of proteins has biophysical properties of ion channels including the ability to allow ions to diffuse selectively across the complex based on size and charge (see later).

NaCl, SOLUTE, AND WATER REABSORPTION ALONG THE NEPHRON

Quantitatively, the reabsorption of NaCl and water represents the major function of nephrons. Approximately 25,000 mEq/day of Na^+ and 179 L/day of water are reabsorbed by the renal tubules (see Table 4-1). In addition, renal transport of many other important solutes is linked either directly or indirectly to Na^+ reabsorption. In the following sections, the NaCl and water transport processes of each nephron segment and its regulation by hormones, and other factors, are presented.

Proximal Tubule

The proximal tubule reabsorbs approximately 67% of filtered water, Na^+, Cl^-, K^+, and other solutes. In addition, the proximal tubule reabsorbs virtually all the glucose and amino acids filtered by the glomerulus. The key element in proximal tubule reabsorption is the Na^+,K^+-ATPase in the basolateral membrane. The reabsorption of every substance, including water, is linked in some manner to the operation of the Na^+,K^+-ATPase.

Na+ Reabsorption Na^+ is reabsorbed by different mechanisms in the first and the second halves of the proximal tubule. In the first half of the proximal tubule, Na^+ is reabsorbed primarily with bicarbonate (HCO_3^-) and a number of other solutes (e.g., glucose, amino acids, Pi, lactate). In contrast, in the second half, Na^+ is reabsorbed mainly with Cl^-. This disparity is mediated by differences in the Na^+ transport systems in the first

and second halves of the proximal tubule and by differences in the composition of tubular fluid at these sites.

In the first half of the proximal tubule, Na^+ uptake into the cell is coupled with either H^+ or organic solutes (Figure 4-2). Specific transport proteins mediate Na^+ entry into the cell across the apical membrane. For example, the Na^+-H^+ antiporter (see Figure 4-2A) couples Na^+ entry with H^+ extrusion from the cell. H^+ secretion results in sodium bicarbonate ($NaHCO_3$) reabsorption (see Chapter 8). Na^+ also enters proximal cells by several symporter mechanisms, including Na^+-glucose, Na^+–amino acid, Na^+-Pi, and Na^+-lactate (see Figure 4-2B). The glucose and other organic solutes that enter the cell with Na^+ leave the cell across the basolateral membrane by passive transport mechanisms. Any Na^+ that enters the cell across the apical membrane leaves the cell and enters the blood by the Na^+,K^+-ATPase. In brief, the reabsorption of Na^+ in the first half of the proximal tubule is coupled to that of HCO_3^- and a number of organic molecules. The reabsorption of many organic molecules is so avid that they are almost completely removed from the tubular fluid in the first half of the proximal tubule (Figure 4-3). The reabsorption of $NaHCO_3$ and Na^+–organic solutes across the proximal tubule establishes a transtubular osmotic gradient (i.e., the osmolality of the interstitial fluid bathing the basolateral side of the cells is higher than the osmolality of tubule fluid) that provides the driving force for the passive reabsorption of water by osmosis. Because more water than Cl^- is reabsorbed in the first half of the proximal tubule, the Cl^- concentration in tubular fluid rises along the length of the proximal tubule (see Figure 4-3).

In the second half of the proximal tubule, Na^+ is mainly reabsorbed with Cl^- across both the transcellular and paracellular pathways (Figure 4-4). Na^+ is primarily reabsorbed with Cl^- rather than organic solutes or HCO_3^- as the accompanying anion because the Na^+ transport mechanisms in the second half of the proximal tubule differ from those in the first half. Furthermore, the tubular fluid that enters the second half contains very little glucose and amino acids, but the high concentration of Cl^- (140 mEq/L) in tubule fluid exceeds that in the first half (105 mEq/L). The high Cl^- concentration is due to the preferential reabsorption of Na^+ with HCO_3^- and organic solutes in the first half of the proximal tubule.

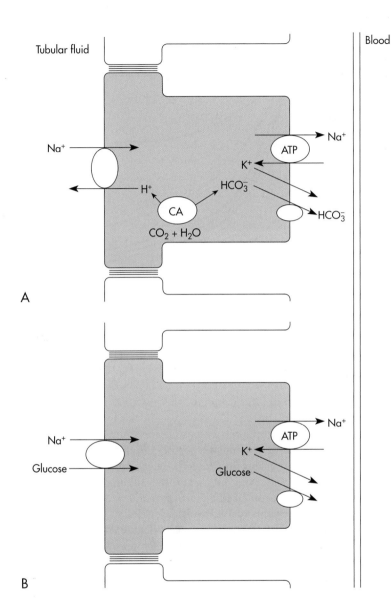

FIGURE 4-2 ■ Na⁺ transport processes in the first half of the proximal tubule. These transport mechanisms are present in all cells in the first half of the proximal tubule but are separated into different cells to simplify the discussion. **A,** Operation of the Na^+-H^+ antiporter (NHE3) in the apical membrane and the Na^+,K^+-ATPase and bicarbonate transporters, including the Cl^--HCO_3^- antiporter (AE2) and the $1Na^+$-$3 HCO_3^-$ cotransporter (NBC1; see also Chapter 8), in the basolateral membrane mediates $NaHCO_3$ reabsorption. Note that a single HCO_3^- transporter is illustrated for simplicity. Carbon dioxide and water combine inside the cells to form H^+ and HCO_3^- in a reaction facilitated by the enzyme carbonic anhydrase (CA). **B,** Operation of the Na^+-glucose transporter (SGLT-2) in the apical membrane, in conjunction with the Na^+,K^+-ATPase and glucose transporter (GLUT-2) in the basolateral membrane, mediates Na^+-glucose reabsorption. Inactivating mutations in the GLUT-2 gene lead to decreased glucose reabsorption in the proximal tubule and glucosuria (i.e., glucose in the urine). Although not shown, Na^+ reabsorption is also coupled with other solutes, including amino acids, Pi, and lactate. Reabsorption of these solutes is mediated by the Na^+-amino acid, Na^+-Pi, and Na^+-lactate symporters located in the apical membrane and the Na^+, K^+-ATPase, amino acid, Pi, and lactate transporters located in the basolateral membrane. Three classes of amino acid transporters have been identified in the proximal tubule: two that transport Na^+ in conjunction with either acidic or basic amino acids and one that does not require Na^+ and transports basic amino acids.

The mechanism of transcellular Na^+ reabsorption in the second half of the proximal tubule is shown in Figure 4-4. Na^+ enters the cell across the luminal membrane primarily through the parallel operation of a Na^+-H^+ antiporter and one or more Cl^--anion antiporters. Because the secreted H^+ and anion combine in the tubular fluid and reenter the cell, the operation of the Na^+-H^+ and Cl^--anion antiporters is equivalent to NaCl uptake from tubular fluid into the cell. Na^+ leaves the cell through Na^+,K^+-ATPase, and Cl^- leaves the cell and enters the blood through a K^+-Cl^- symporter in the basolateral membrane.

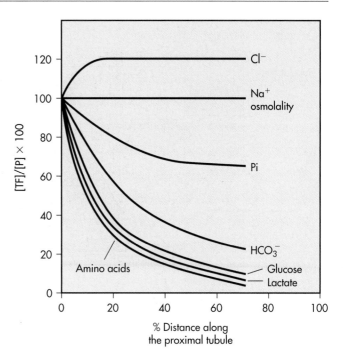

FIGURE 4-3 ■ Concentration of solutes in tubule fluid as a function of length along the proximal tubule. [TF] is the concentration of the substance in tubular fluid; [P] is the concentration of the substance in plasma. Values above 100 indicate that relatively less of the solute than water was reabsorbed, and values below 100 indicate that relatively more of the substance than water was reabsorbed. *(Modified from Vander AJ: Renal physiology, ed 4. New York, 1991, McGraw-Hill.)*

NaCl is also reabsorbed across the second half of the proximal tubule by a **paracellular route.** Paracellular NaCl reabsorption occurs because the rise in the Cl^- concentration in the tubule fluid in the first half of the proximal tubule creates a Cl^- concentration gradient (140 mEq/L in the tubule lumen and 105 mEq/L in the interstitium). This concentration gradient favors the diffusion of Cl^- from the tubular lumen across the tight junctions into the lateral intercellular space. Movement of the negatively charged Cl^- causes the tubular fluid to become positively charged relative to the blood. This positive transepithelial voltage causes the diffusion of positively charged Na^+ out of the tubular fluid across the tight junction into the blood. Thus, in the second half of the proximal tubule, some Na^+ and Cl^- are reabsorbed across the tight junctions by passive diffusion. The reabsorption of NaCl establishes a transtubular osmotic gradient that provides the driving force for the passive reabsorption of water by osmosis.

In summary, the reabsorption of Na^+ and Cl^- in the proximal tubule occurs across paracellular and transcellular pathways. Approximately 67% of the NaCl filtered each day is reabsorbed in the proximal tubule. Of this, two thirds moves across the transcellular pathway, whereas the remaining one third moves across the paracellular pathway (see Table 4-4).

Water Reabsorption The proximal tubule reabsorbs 67% of the filtered water. The driving force for water reabsorption is a transtubular osmotic gradient established by solute reabsorption (e.g., NaCl, Na^+-glucose). The reabsorption of Na^+ along with organic solutes, HCO_3^-, and Cl^- from the tubular fluid into the lateral intercellular spaces reduces the osmolality of the tubular fluid and increases the osmolality of the lateral intercellular space (Figure 4-5). Because the apical and basolateral membranes of the proximal

Fanconi's syndrome, a renal disease that is either hereditary or acquired, is often associated with glucosuria, osteomalacia, acidosis, and hypokalemia. It results from an impaired ability of the proximal tubule to reabsorb HCO_3^-, amino acids, glucose, and low-molecular-weight proteins. Because other segments of the nephron cannot reabsorb these solutes and protein, Fanconi's syndrome results in increased urinary excretion of HCO_3^-, amino acids, glucose, Pi, and low-molecular-weight proteins.

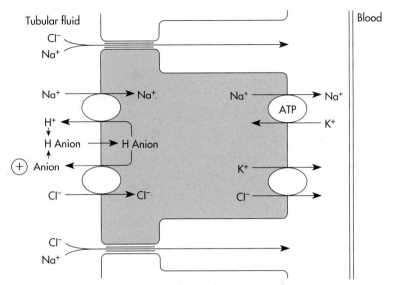

FIGURE 4-4 ■ Na^+ transport processes in the second half of the proximal tubule. Na^+ and Cl^- enter the cell across the apical membrane through the operation of parallel Na^+-H^+ and Cl^--anion antiporters. More than one Cl^- anion antiporter may be involved in this process, but only one is depicted. The secreted H^+ and anion combine in the tubular fluid to form an H^+-anion complex that can recycle across the plasma membrane. Accumulation of the H^+-anion complex in tubular fluid establishes an H^+-anion concentration gradient that favors H^+-anion recycling across the apical plasma membrane into the cell. Inside the cell, H^+ and the anion dissociate and recycle back across the apical plasma membrane. The net result is NaCl uptake across the apical membrane. The anion may be hydroxde ions (OH^-), formate (HCO_2^-), oxalate$^-$, HCO_3^-, or sulfate. The lumen-positive transepithelial voltage, indicated by the plus sign inside the circle in the tubular lumen, is generated by the diffusion of Cl^- (lumen to blood) across the tight junction. The high Cl^- concentration of tubular fluid provides the driving force for Cl^- diffusion. Some glucose is also reabsorbed in the second half of the proximal tubule by a mechanism similar to that described in the first half of the proximal tubule, except that the Na^+-glucose symporter (SGLT-1 gene) transports $2Na^+$ with one glucose and has a higher affinity and lower capacity than the Na^+-glucose symporter in the first part of the proximal tubule (i.e., SGLT-2). Also, glucose exits the cell across the basolateral membrane through GLUT-1 rather than GLUT-2 as in the first part of the proximal tubule.

tubule express aquaporin water channels, the proximal tubule is highly permeable to water, and water is reabsorbed by osmosis primarily through the cells. However, some water is also reabsorbed across the tight junction. The accumulation of fluid and solutes within the lateral intercellular space increases the hydrostatic pressure in this compartment. This increased hydrostatic pressure forces fluid and solutes into the capillaries.[3] Thus, water reabsorption follows solute reabsorption in the proximal tubule. The reabsorbed fluid is slightly hyperosmotic to plasma.

---

[3]In addition, the protein oncotic pressure in the peritubular capillaries (π_{pc}) is elevated because of the process of glomerular filtration (see Chapter 3). The elevated π_{pc} also facilitates fluid and solute uptake into the capillary.

However, this difference in osmolality is so small that it is commonly said that proximal tubule reabsorption is isosmotic (i.e., 67% of the filtered load of solute and water is reabsorbed). Indeed, there is little difference in the osmolality of tubular fluid at the start and end of the proximal tubule. An important consequence of osmotic water flow across the proximal tubule is that some solutes, especially K^+ and Ca^{++}, are entrained in the reabsorbed fluid and are thereby reabsorbed by the process of solvent drag (see Figure 4-5). The reabsorption of virtually all organic solutes, Cl^- and other ions, and water is coupled to Na^+ reabsorption. Therefore, changes in Na^+ reabsorption influence the reabsorption of water and other solutes by the proximal tubule.

Water channels called **aquaporins (AQPs)** mediate the transcellular reabsorption of water across many nephron segments. In 2003, Dr. Peter Agre received the Nobel Prize in Chemistry for his discovery that AQPs regulate and facilitate water transport across cell membranes, a process essential to all living organisms. To date, 11 aquaporins have been identified. The AQP family is divided into two groups on the basis of their permeability characteristics. One group (aquaporins) is permeable to water (AQP-0, AQP-1, AQP-2, AQP-4, AQP-5, AQP-6, and AQP-8). The other group (aquaglyceroporins) is permeable to water and small solutes, especially glycerol (AQP-3, AQP-5, AQP-7, AQP-9, and AQP-10). Aquaporins form tetramers in the plasma membrane of cells, with each subunit forming a water channel. In the kidneys, AQP-1 is expressed in the apical and basolateral membranes of the proximal tubule and descending thin limb of Henle's loop. The importance of AQP-1 in renal water reabsorption is underscored by studies in which AQP-1 was "knocked out" in mice. These mice had increased urine output (polyuria) and a reduced ability to concentrate the urine. In addition, the rate of water reabsorption by the proximal tubule was 50% less in mice lacking APQ-1 than in normal mice. AQP-7 and AQP-8 are also expressed in the proximal tubule. AQP-2 is expressed in the apical plasma membrane of principal cells in the collecting duct, and its expression in the membrane is regulated by ADH (see Chapter 5). AQP-3 and AQP-4 are expressed in the basolateral membrane of principal cells in the collecting duct. Mice deficient in AQP-3 or AQP-4

(i.e., knockout mice) have defects in the ability to concentrate urine (see Chapter 5). AQPs are also expressed in many other organs in the body including the lung, eye, skin, secretory glands, and brain, where they play key physiologic roles. For example, AQP-4 is expressed in cells that form the blood-brain barrier. Knockout of AQP-4 in mice affects the water permeability of the blood-brain barrier such that brain edema is reduced in AQP-4 knockout mice following acute water loading and hyponatremia (see Chapter 5).

Protein Reabsorption Proteins filtered by the glomerulus are reabsorbed in the proximal tubule. As mentioned previously, peptide hormones, small proteins, and small amounts of large proteins such as albumin are filtered by the glomerulus. Overall, only a small percentage of proteins cross the glomerulus and enter Bowman's space (i.e., the concentration of proteins in the glomerular ultrafiltrate is only 40 mg/L). However, the amount of protein filtered per day is significant because the glomerular filtration rate (GFR) is so high:

$$\text{Filtered protein} = \text{GFR} \times [\text{protein}] \text{ in the ultrafiltrate}$$
$$\text{Filtered protein} = 180 \text{ L/day} \times 40 \text{ mg/L} \quad (4\text{-}1)$$
$$= 7200 \text{ mg/day, or } 7.2 \text{ g/day}$$

The endocytosis of protein by the proximal tubule is mediated by apical membrane proteins that specifically bind luminal proteins and peptides. These peptides, called **multiligand endocytic receptors,** can bind a wide range of peptides and proteins and thereby mediate their endocytosis. **Megalin** and **cubilin** mediate protein and peptide endocytosis in the proximal tubule. Both are glycoproteins, with megalin being a member of the low-density lipoprotein receptor gene family.

Proteins are either endocytosed intact or endocytosed after being partially degraded by enzymes on the surface of the proximal tubule cells. Once the proteins and peptides are inside the cell, enzymes digest them into their constituent amino acids, which then leave the cell across the basolateral membrane by transport

	TABLE 4-4		
	NaCl Transport Along the Nephron		
SEGMENT	PERCENTAGE OF FILTERED LOAD REABSORBED	MECHANISM OF Na$^+$ ENTRY ACROSS APICAL MEMBRANE	MAJOR REGULATORY HORMONES
Proximal tubule	67	Na$^+$-H$^+$ exchange, Na$^+$ cotransport with amino acids and organic solutes, Na$^+$/H$^+$-Cl$^-$/anion exchange, paracellular	Angiotensin II Norepinephrine Epinephrine Dopamine
Loop of Henle	25	1Na$^+$-1K$^+$-2Cl$^-$ symport	Aldosterone Angiotensin II
Distal tubule	~5	NaCl symport	Aldosterone Angiotensin II
Late distal tubule and collecting duct	~3	Na$^+$ channels	Aldosterone, ANP, BNP, urodilatin, uroguanylin, guanylin, angiotensin II

proteins and are returned to the blood. Normally, this mechanism reabsorbs virtually all of the proteins filtered, and hence the urine is essentially protein free. However, because the mechanism is easily saturated, an increase in filtered proteins causes **proteinuria** (appearance of protein in the urine). Disruption of the glomerular filtration barrier to proteins increases the filtration of proteins and results in proteinuria. Proteinuria is frequently seen with kidney disease.

Urinalysis is an important and routine tool in disease detection. A thorough analysis of the urine includes macroscopic and microscopic assessments. This is performed by visual assessment of the urine, microscopic examination, and chemical evaluation, which is conducted using dipstick reagents strips. The dipstick test is inexpensive and fast (i.e., less than 5 minutes). Dipstick reagent strips test the urine for the presence of many substances including bilirubin, blood, glucose, ketones, pH, and protein. It is normal to find trace amounts of protein in the urine. Trace amounts of protein in the urine can be derived from two sources: (1) filtration and incomplete reabsorption by the proximal tubule and (2) synthesis by the thick ascending limb of the loop of Henle. Cells in the thick ascending limb produce **Tamm-Horsfall glycoprotein** and secrete it into the tubular fluid. Because the mechanism for protein reabsorption is "upstream" of the thick ascending limb (i.e., proximal tubule), the secreted Tamm-Horsfall glycoprotein appears in the urine. However, more than trace amounts of protein in the urine is indicative of renal disease.

Organic Anion and Organic Cation Secretion Cells of the proximal tubule also secrete organic cations and organic anions. Secretion of organic cations and anions by the proximal tubule plays a key role in limiting the body's exposure to toxic compounds derived from endogenous and exogenous sources (i.e., xenobiotics). Many of the organic anions and cations (see Box 4-1 and Box 4-2) secreted by the proximal tubule are end products of metabolism that circulate in the plasma. The proximal tubule also secretes numerous exogenous organic compounds, including numerous drugs and toxic chemicals. Many of these organic compounds can be bound to plasma proteins and are not readily filtered. Therefore, only a small portion of these potentially toxic substances are eliminated from the body by excretion resulting from filtration alone. Such substances are also secreted from the peritubular capillary into the tubular fluid. These secretory mechanisms are very powerful and remove virtually all organic anions and cations from the plasma that enters the kidneys. Hence, these substances are removed from the plasma by both filtration and secretion.

Figure 4-6 illustrates the mechanisms of organic anion (OA$^-$) transport across the proximal tubule. This secretory pathway has a maximum transport rate, a low specificity (i.e., it transports many organic anions), and is responsible for the secretion of all organic anions listed in Box 4-1. OA$^-$s are taken up into the cell, across the basolateral membrane, against their chemical gradient in exchange for α-ketoglutarate (α-KG) by several OA$^-$-α-KG antiport mechanisms (OAT1, OAT2, OAT3). α-KG accumulates inside the cells by metabolism

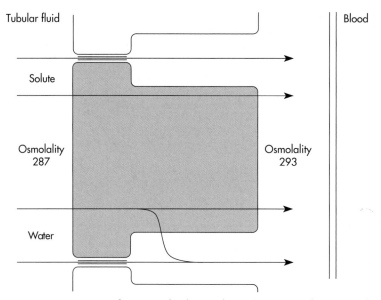

FIGURE 4-5 ■ Routes of water and solute reabsorption across the proximal tubule. The transport of solutes, including Na$^+$, Cl$^-$, and organic solutes, into the lateral intercellular space increases the osmolality of this compartment, which establishes the driving force for osmotic water reabsorption across the proximal tubule. This occurs because some Na$^+$,K$^+$-ATPase and some transporters of organic solutes, HCO$_3^-$, and Cl$^-$ are located on the lateral cell membranes and deposit these solutes between cells. Furthermore, some NaCl also enters the lateral intercellular space by diffusion across the tight junction (i.e., paracellular pathway). An important consequence of osmotic water flow across the transcellular and paracellular pathways in the proximal tubule is that some solutes, especially K$^+$ and Ca^{++}, are entrained in the reabsorbed fluid and are thereby reabsorbed by the process of solvent drag.

BOX 4-1
SOME ORGANIC ANIONS SECRETED BY THE PROXIMAL TUBULE

Endogenous Anions
Cyclic AMP, cyclic GMP
Bile salts
Hippurates
Oxalate
Prostaglandins: PGE$_2$, PGF$_{2\alpha}$
Urate
Vitamins: ascorbate, folate

Drugs
Acetazolamide
Chlorothiazide
Furosemide
Penicillin
Probenecid
Salicylate (aspirin)
Hydrochlorothiazide
Bumetanide
Nonsteroidal anti-inflammatory
    drugs (NSAIDs): indomethacin

Because organic anions compete for the same secretory pathways, elevated plasma levels of one anion often inhibit the secretion of the others. For example, infusing para-amino hippurate (PAH) can reduce penicillin secretion by the proximal tubule. Because the kidneys are responsible for eliminating penicillin, the infusion of PAH into individuals who receive penicillin reduces penicillin excretion and thereby extends the biologic half-life of the drug. In World War II, when penicillin was in short supply, hippurates were given with the penicillin to extend the drug's therapeutic effect.

The histamine H_2 antagonist cimetidine is used to treat gastric ulcers. Organic cation transport mechanisms in the proximal tubule secrete cimetidine. If cimetidine is given to patients also receiving procainamide (a drug used to treat cardiac arrhythmias), cimetidine reduces the urinary excretion of procainamide (also an organic cation) by competing with this antiarrhythmic drug for the secretory pathway. Thus, the coadministration of organic cations can increase the plasma concentrations of both drugs to levels much higher than those seen when the drugs are given alone. This effect can lead to drug toxicity.

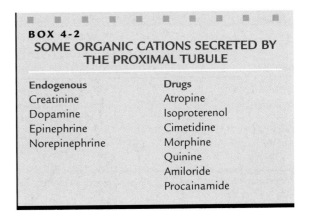

BOX 4-2
SOME ORGANIC CATIONS SECRETED BY THE PROXIMAL TUBULE

Endogenous	Drugs
Creatinine	Atropine
Dopamine	Isoproterenol
Epinephrine	Cimetidine
Norepinephrine	Morphine
	Quinine
	Amiloride
	Procainamide

of glutamate and by an Na^+-α-KG symporter (i.e., an Na^+-dicarboxylate transporter [NaDC]) also present in the basolateral membrane. Thus, OA⁻ uptake into the cell against its electrochemical gradient is coupled to the exit of α-KG out of the cell, down its chemical gradient generated by the Na^+-α-KG antiport mechanism. The resulting high intracellular concentration of OA⁻ provides a driving force for OA⁻ exit across the luminal membrane into the tubular fluid by a poorly

Tubular fluid   Blood

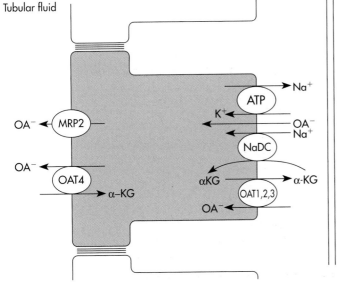

FIGURE 4-6 ■ Organic anion (OA⁻) secretion across the proximal tubule. OA⁻s enter the cell across the basolateral membrane by one of three OA⁻-α-ketoglutarate (α-KG) antiport mechanisms (OAT1, OAT2, OAT3). The uptake of α-KG into the cell, against its chemical concentration gradient, is driven by the movement of Na^+ into the cell by the Na^+-dicarboxylate transporter (NaDC). The [Na^+] inside the cell is low because of the Na^+, K^+-ATPase in the basolateral membrane, which transports Na^+ out the cell in exchange for K^+ (not shown). The α-KG recycles across the basolateral membrane on the OATs in exchange for OA⁻. OA⁻s leave the cell across the apical membrane most likely by MRP2 and OAT4.

TABLE 4-5

Water Transport Along the Nephron

SEGMENT	PERCENTAGE OF FILTERED REABSORBED	MECHANISM OF WATER REABSORPTION	HORMONES THAT REGULATE WATER PERMEABILITY
Proximal tubule	67	Passive	None
Loop of Henle	15	Descending thin limb only; passive	None
Distal tubule	0	No water reabsorption	None
Late distal tubule and collecting duct	~8-17	Passive	ADH, ANP*, BNP*

*Atrial natriuretic peptide (ANP) and brain natriuretic peptide (BNP) inhibit antidiuretic hormone (ADH)-stimulated water permeability.

understood mechanism. However, recent studies suggest that OA⁻s are transported across the apical membrane by OAT4, which is electrogenic, and by MRP2 (multidrug resistance—associated protein 2) (see Figure 4-6).

Figure 4-7 illustrates the mechanism of organic cation (OC⁺) transport across the proximal tubule. Organic cations are taken up into the cell, across the basolateral membrane, by several transporters that have different substrate specificities. One mechanism that has not been completely characterized involves passive diffusion. In addition, organic cations are transported into proximal tubule cells across the basolateral membrane by three related transport proteins (OCT1, OCT2, OCT3). These transporters mediate the diffusive uptake of organic cations into the cell. Uptake by all four mechanisms is driven by the magnitude of the cell-negative potential difference across the basolateral membrane. Organic cation transport across the luminal membrane into the tubular fluid, which is the rate-limiting step in secretion, is mediated by several transporters, including two OC⁺-H⁺ antiporters (OCTN1 and OCTN2), and MDR1 (also known as P-glycoprotein). These transport mechanisms

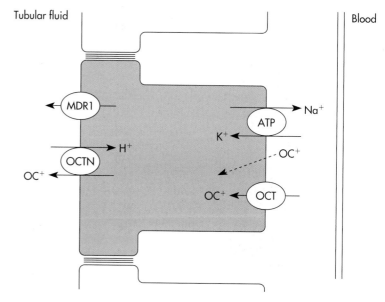

FIGURE 4-7 ■ Organic cation (OC⁺) secretion across the proximal tubule. OC⁺s enter the cell across the basolateral membrane by four transport pathways: passive diffusion and three uniporters (OCT1, OCT2, OCT3, illustrated as one transporter for clarity) that mediate electrogenic uptake. The uptake of OC⁺s into the cell, against their chemical concentration gradient, is driven by the cell-negative potential difference. OC⁺s leave the cell across the apical membrane in exchange with H⁺ by two OC⁺-H⁺ antiporters (OCTN1, OCTN2, illustrated as one transporter for clarity) and MDR1.

mediating organic cation secretion are nonspecific: several organic cations usually compete for each transport pathway. Organic cation secretion is stimulated by protein kinase A and C and by testosterone.

Henle's Loop

Henle's loop reabsorbs approximately 25% of the filtered NaCl and 15% of the filtered water. The reabsorption of NaCl in the loop of Henle occurs in both the thin ascending and thick ascending limbs. The descending thin limb does not reabsorb NaCl. Water reabsorption occurs exclusively in the descending thin limb through AQP-1 water channels. The ascending limb is impermeable to water. In addition, Ca^{++} and

HCO_3^- are reabsorbed in the loop of Henle (see Chapters 8 and 9 for more details).

The thin ascending limb reabsorbs NaCl by a passive mechanism. The reabsorption of water but not NaCl in the descending thin limb increases the [NaCl] in tubule fluid entering the ascending thin limb. As the NaCl-rich fluid moves toward the cortex, NaCl diffuses out of tubule fluid across the ascending thin limb into the medullary interstitial fluid, down a concentration gradient directed from tubule fluid to interstitium.

The key element in solute reabsorption by the thick ascending limb is the Na^+,K^+-ATPase in the basolateral membrane (Figure 4-8). As with reabsorption in the proximal tubule, the reabsorption of every solute by the thick ascending limb is linked to Na^+,K^+-ATPase.

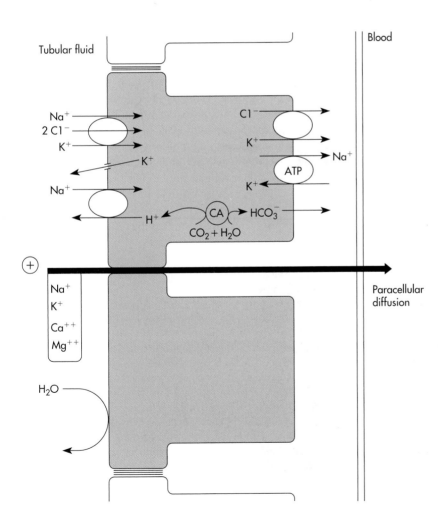

FIGURE 4-8 ■ Transport mechanisms for NaCl reabsorption in the thick ascending limb of the loop of Henle. The positive charge in the lumen plays a major role in driving the passive paracellular reabsorption of cations. Mutations in the apical membrane K^+ channel (ROMK), the apical membrane $1Na^+$-$1K^+$-$2Cl^-$ symporter (NKCC2), or the basolateral Cl^- channel (ClCNKB) cause Bartter's syndrome (see the clinical box on Bartter's syndrome). CA, carbonic anhydrase.

This pump maintains a low intracellular $[Na^+]$, which provides a favorable chemical gradient for the movement of Na^+ from the tubular fluid into the cell. The movement of Na^+ across the apical membrane into the cell is mediated by the $1Na^+$-$1K^+$-$2Cl^-$ symporter (NKCC2), which couples the movement of $1Na^+$ with $1K^+$ and $2Cl^-$. Using the potential energy released by the downhill movement of Na^+ and Cl^-, this symporter drives the uphill movement of K^+ into the cell. The K^+ channel in the apical plasma membrane plays an important role in NaCl reabsorption by the thick ascending limb. This K^+ channel allows the K^+ transported into the cell by the $1Na^+$-$1K^+$-$2Cl^-$ symporter to recycle back into tubule fluid. Because the $[K^+]$ in tubule fluid is relatively low, this K^+ is required for the continued operation of the $1Na^+$-$1K^+$-$2Cl^-$ symporter. A Na^+-H^+ antiporter in the apical cell membrane also mediates Na^+ reabsorption as well as H^+ secretion (HCO_3^- reabsorption) in the thick ascending limb (see also Chapter 8). Na^+ leaves the cell across the basolateral membrane through the Na^+,K^+-ATPase, whereas K^+, Cl^-, and HCO_3^- leave the cell across the basolateral membrane by separate pathways.

The voltage across the thick ascending limb is important for the reabsorption of several cations. The tubular fluid is positively charged relative to blood because of the unique location of transport proteins in the apical and basolateral membranes. Two points are important: (1) increased salt transport by the thick ascending limb increases the magnitude of the positive voltage in the lumen, and (2) this voltage is an important driving force for the reabsorption of several cations, including Na^+, K^+, Mg^{++}, and Ca^{++} across the paracellular pathway (see Figure 4-8). The importance of the paracellular pathway to solute reabsorption is underscored by the observation that inactivating mutations of the tight junction protein claudin-16 reduces Mg^{++} and Ca^{++} reabsorption by the ascending thick limb even when the lumen-positive transepithelial voltage is positive.

As described previously and also in Chapter 2, epithelial cells are joined at their apical surfaces by tight junctions (also knows as **zonula occludens**). A number of proteins have now been identified as components of the tight junction. These include proteins that span the membrane of one cell and link to the extracellular portion of the same molecule in the adjacent cell (e.g., occludins and claudins) as well as cytoplasmic linker proteins (e.g., ZO-1, ZO-2, and ZO-3) that link the membrane-spanning proteins to the cytoskeleton of the cell. Of these junctional proteins, claudins appear to be important in determining the permeability characteristics of the tight junction. As noted, claudin-16 is critical for determining divalent cation permeability of the tight junctions in the thick ascending limb of Henle's loop. Claudin-4 has been shown in cultured kidney cells to control the Na^+ permeability of the tight junction, and claudin-15 determines whether a tight junction is permeable to cations or anions. Thus, the permeability characteristics of the tight junctions in different nephron segments are determined, at least in part, by the specific claudins expressed by the cells in that segment.

In summary, salt reabsorption across the thick ascending limb occurs by the transcellular and paracellular pathways. A total of 50% of NaCl reabsorption is transcellular, and 50% is paracellular. Because the thick ascending limb does not reabsorb water, the reabsorption of NaCl and other solutes reduces the osmolality of tubular fluid to less than 150 mOsm/kg H_2O. Thus, because the thick ascending limb produces a fluid that is dilute relative to plasma, the ascending limb of Henle's loop is called the **diluting segment.**

Bartter's syndrome is a set of autosomal recessive genetic diseases characterized by hypokalemia, metabolic alkalosis, and hyperaldosteronism (see Table 4-3). Inactivating mutations in the gene coding for the $1Na^+$-$1K^+$-$2Cl^-$ (NKCC2 or SLC12A1), the apical K^+ channel (KCNJ1 or ROMK), or the basolateral Cl^- channel (ClCNKB) decrease both NaCl reabsorption and K^+ reabsorption by the ascending thick limb, which in turn causes hypokalemia (i.e., a low plasma $[K^+]$) and a decrease in the extracellular fluid (ECF) volume. The fall in ECF volume stimulates aldosterone secretion, which in turn stimulates NaCl reabsorption and H^+ secretion by the distal tubule and collecting duct (see later).

Distal Tubule and Collecting Duct

The distal tubule and collecting duct reabsorb approximately 8% of the filtered NaCl, secrete variable amounts of K^+ and H^+, and reabsorb a variable amount of water (~8% to 17%). The initial segment of the distal tubule (early distal tubule) reabsorbs Na^+, Cl^-, and Ca^{++} and is impermeable to water (Figure 4-9). NaCl entry into the cell across the apical membrane is mediated by an Na^+-Cl^- symporter (NCC/TSC). Na^+ leaves the cell through the action of Na^+, K^+-ATPase, and Cl^- leaves the cell by diffusion through Cl^- channels. NaCl reabsorption is reduced by thiazide diuretics, which inhibit the Na^+-Cl^- symporter. Thus, dilution of the tubular fluid begins in the thick ascending limb and continues in the early segment of distal tubule.

The last segment of the distal tubule (late distal tubule) and the collecting duct are composed of two cell types: **principal cells** and **intercalated cells.** As illustrated in Figure 4-10, principal cells reabsorb NaCl and water and secrete K^+. Intercalated cells secrete either H^+ or HCO_3^- and are thus important in regulating acid-base balance (see Chapter 8). Intercalated cells also reabsorb K^+ by the operation of an H^+,K^+-ATPase located in the apical plasma membrane. Both Na^+ reabsorption and K^+ secretion by principal cells depend on

the activity of Na^+,K^+-ATPase in the basolateral membrane (see Figure 4-10). By maintaining a low intracellular $[Na^+]$, this pump provides a favorable chemical gradient for the movement of Na^+ from the tubular fluid into the cell. Because Na^+ enters the cell across the apical membrane by diffusion through Na^+-selective channels (ENaC) in the apical membrane, the negative charge inside the cell facilitates Na^+ entry. Na^+ leaves the cell across the basolateral membrane and enters the blood through the action of Na^+,K^+-ATPase. Na^+ reabsorption generates a lumen-negative voltage across the late distal tubule and collecting duct, which provides the driving force for Cl^- reabsorption across the paracellular pathway. A variable amount of water is reabsorbed across principal cells in the late distal tubule and collecting duct. Water reabsorption is mediated by the AQP-2 water channel located in the apical plasma membrane and AQP-3 and AQP-4 located in the basolateral membrane of principal cells. In the presence of antidiuretic hormone (ADH), water is reabsorbed. By contrast, in the absence of ADH, the distal tubule and collecting duct reabsorb little water (see Chapter 5).

K^+ is secreted from the blood into the tubular fluid by principal cells in two steps (see Figure 4-10). First, K^+ uptake across the basolateral membrane is

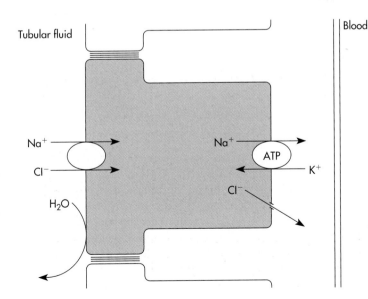

FIGURE 4-9 ■ Transport mechanism for Na^+ and Cl^- reabsorption in the early segment of the distal tubule. This segment is impermeable to water.

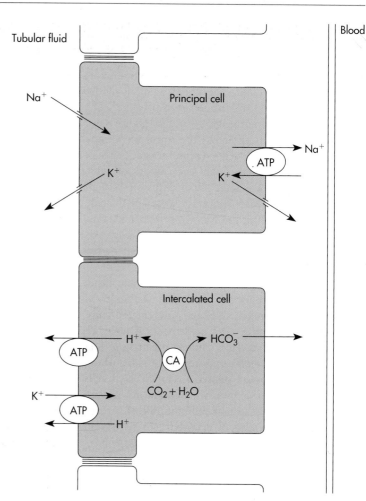

FIGURE 4-10 ■ Transport pathways in principal cells and H⁺-secreting intercalated cells of the distal tubule and collecting duct. CA, carbonic anhydrase.

mediated by the action of the Na⁺,K⁺-ATPase. Second, K⁺ leaves the cell by passive diffusion. Because the K⁺ concentration inside the cells is high (~150 mEq/L) and the K⁺ concentration in tubular fluid is low (~10 mEq/L), K⁺ diffuses down its concentration gradient through apical cell membrane K⁺ channels into the tubular fluid. Although the negative potential inside the cells tends to retain K⁺ within the cell, the electrochemical gradient across the apical membrane favors K⁺ secretion from the cell into the tubular fluid (see Chapter 7). The mechanism of K⁺ reabsorption by intercalated cells is mediated by an H⁺,K⁺-ATPase located in the apical cell membrane.

REGULATION OF NaCl AND WATER REABSORPTION

Quantitatively, angiotensin II, aldosterone, catecholamines, natriuretic peptides, and uroguanylin are the most important hormones that regulate NaCl reabsorption and thereby urinary NaCl excretion (Table 4-6). However, other hormones (including dopamine and adrenomedullin), Starling forces, and the phenomenon of glomerulotubular balance influence NaCl reabsorption. ADH is the only major hormone that directly regulates the amount of water excreted by the kidneys.

TABLE 4-6
Hormones That Regulate NaCl and Water Reabsorption

HORMONE*	MAJOR STIMULUS	NEPHRON SITE OF ACTION	EFFECT ON TRANSPORT
Angiotensin II	↑Renin	PT, TAL, DT/CD	↑NaCl and H_2O reabsorption
Aldosterone	↑Angiotensin II, ↑$[K^+]_p$	TAL, DT/CD	↑NaCl and H_2O reabsorption†
ANP, BNP, urodilatin	↑ECFV	CD	↓H_2O and NaCl reabsorption
Uroguanylin, guanylin	Oral ingestion of NaCl	PT, CD	↓H_2O and NaCl reabsorption
Sympathetic nerves	↓ECFV	PT, TAL, DT/CD	↑NaCl and H_2O reabsorption†
Dopamine	↑ECFV	PT	↓H_2O and NaCl reabsorption
ADH	↑P_{osm}, ↓ECFV	DT/CD	↑H_2O reabsorption†

ANP, atrial natriuretic peptide; BNP, brain natriuretic peptide, BP, blood pressure; CD, collecting duct; DT, distal tubule; ECFV, extracellular fluid volume; $[K^+]_p$, plasma K^+ concentration; P_{osm}, plasma osmolality; PT, proximal tubule; TAL, thick ascending limb.

*All of these hormones act within minutes, except aldosterone, which exerts its action on NaCl reabsorption with a delay of 1 hour. Aldosterone achieves its maximal effect after a few days.

†The effect on H_2O reabsorption does not include the thick ascending limb or the early portion of the distal tubule.

Angiotensin II has a potent stimulatory effect on NaCl and water reabsorption in the proximal tubule. It has also been shown to stimulate Na^+ reabsorption in the thick ascending limb of Henle's loop as well as the distal tubule and collecting duct. Angiotensin II is one of the most potent hormones that stimulates NaCl and water reabsorption in the proximal tubule. A decrease in the ECF volume activates the renin-angiotensin-aldosterone system (see Chapter 6 for more details), thereby increasing the plasma concentration of angiotensin II.

Aldosterone is synthesized by the glomerulosa cells of the adrenal cortex, and it stimulates NaCl reabsorption. It acts on the thick ascending limb of the loop of Henle, distal tubule, and collecting duct. Most of aldosterone's effect on NaCl reabsorption reflects its action on the distal tubule and collecting duct. Aldosterone also stimulates K^+ secretion by the distal tubule and collecting duct (see Chapter 7). Aldosterone enhances NaCl reabsorption across principal cells in the distal tubule and collecting duct by four mechanisms: (1) increasing the amount of Na^+,K^+-ATPase in the basolateral membrane; (2) increasing the expression of the sodium channel (ENaC) in the apical cell membrane; (3) elevating Sgk (**s**erum **g**lucocorticoid–stimulated **k**inase; see Box) levels, which also increases the expression of ENaC in the apical cell membrane; and (4) stimulating CAP1 (**c**hannel-**a**ctivating **p**rotease, also called prostatin), a serine protease, which directly activates ENaC

channels by proteolysis. Taken together these actions increase the uptake of Na^+ across the apical cell membrane and facilitate the exit of Na^+ from the cell interior into the blood. The increase in the reabsorption of Na^+ generates a lumen-negative transepithelial voltage across the distal tubule and collecting duct. This lumen-negative voltage provides the electrochemical driving force for Cl^- reabsorption across the tight junctions (i.e., paracellular pathway) in the distal tubule and collecting duct. Aldosterone secretion is increased by hyperkalemia and by angiotensin II (after activation of the renin-angiotensin system). Aldosterone secretion is decreased by hypokalemia and natriuretic peptides (see later). Through its stimulation of NaCl reabsorption in the collecting duct, aldosterone also indirectly increases water reabsorption by this nephron segment.

Sgk (**s**erum **g**lucocorticoid-stimulated **k**inase), a serine/threonine kinase, plays an important role in maintaining NaCl and K^+ homeostasis by regulating NaCl and K^+ excretion by the kidneys. Studies in Sgk1 knockout mice reveal that this kinase is required for animals to survive severe NaCl restriction and K^+ loading. NaCl restriction and K^+ loading enhance plasma [aldosterone], which rapidly (minutes) increases Sgk1 protein expression and phosphorylation. Phosphorylated Sgk1 enhances ENaC-mediated sodium reabsorption in the collecting duct, primarily by increasing the number of ENaC channels in the apical plasma membrane of principal cells and also by increasing the number of Na+,K+-ATPase pumps in the basolateral membrane. Phosphorylated Sgk1 inhibits Nedd4-2, a ubiquitin ligase, which mono-ubiquitinylates ENaC subunits, targeting them for endocytic removal from the plasma membrane and subsequent destruction in lysosomes. Inhibition of Nedd4-2 by Sgk1 reduces the monoubiquitinylation of ENaC, thereby reducing endocytosis and increasing the number of channels in the membrane. The mechanism whereby Sgk1 stimulates ROMK-mediated K+ excretion has not been elucidated. These effects of Sgk1 precede the aldosterone-stimulated increase in ENaC, ROMK, and Na+,K+-ATPase expression, which leads to a delayed (>4 hours), secondary increase in NaCl and K+ transport by the collecting duct. Activating polymorphisms in Sgk1 cause an increase in blood pressure, presumably by enhanced NaCl reabsorption by the collecting duct, which increases the ECF volume and thereby blood pressure. As noted, CAP1 is a serine protease that directly activates ENaC by proteolysis of the channel proteins.

Liddle's syndrome is a rare genetic disorder characterized by an increase in the extracellular fluid volume that causes an increase in blood pressure (i.e., hypertension). Liddle's syndrome is caused by activating mutations in either the β or γ subunit of the epithelial Na+ channel (ENaC, which is composed of three subunits, α, β, and γ). These mutations increase the number of Na+ channels in the apical cell membrane of principal cells and, thereby, the amount of Na+ reabsorbed by each channel. In Liddle's syndrome the rate of renal Na+ reabsorption is inappropriately high, which leads to an increase in the ECF volume and hypertension.

There are two different forms of **pseudohypoaldosteronism (PHA)** (i.e., the kidneys avidly reabsorb NaCl as they do when aldosterone levels are elevated; however, in PHA aldosterone levels are not elevated). The autosomal recessive form is caused by inactivating mutations in the α, β, or γ subunit of ENaC. The etiology of the autosomal dominant form is an inactivating mutation in the mineralocorticoid receptor. Pseudohypoaldosteronism is characterized by an increase in Na+ excretion, a reduction in the ECF volume, hyperkalemia, and hypotension.

Some individuals with expanded ECF volume and elevated blood pressure are treated with drugs that inhibit **angiotensin-converting enzyme** (ACE inhibitors [e.g., captopril, enalapril, lisinopril]) and thereby lower fluid volume and blood pressure. The inhibition of ACE blocks the degradation of angiotensin I to angiotensin II and thereby lowers plasma angiotensin II levels (see Chapter 6 for details). The decline in plasma angiotensin II concentration has three effects. First, NaCl and water reabsorption by the nephron (especially the proximal tubule) falls. Second, aldosterone secretion decreases, thus reducing NaCl reabsorption in the thick ascending limb, distal tubule, and collecting duct. Third, because angiotensin is a potent vasoconstrictor, a reduction in its concentration permits the systemic arterioles to dilate and thereby lower arterial blood pressure. ACE also degrades the vasodilator hormone bradykinin; ACE inhibitors therefore increase the concentration of bradykinin. Thus, ACE inhibitors decrease the extracellular fluid volume and the arterial blood pressure by promoting renal NaCl and water excretion and by reducing total peripheral resistance.

Atrial natriuretic peptide (ANP), and **brain natriuretic peptide** (BNP) inhibit NaCl and water reabsorption. Secretion of ANP by the cardiac atria and BNP by the cardiac ventricles is stimulated by a rise in blood pressure and an increase in the ECF volume. ANP and BNP reduce the blood pressure by decreasing the total peripheral resistance and by enhancing urinary NaCl and water excretion. These hormones also inhibit NaCl reabsorption by the medullary portion of the collecting duct and inhibit ADH-stimulated water reabsorption across the collecting duct. Moreover, ANP and BNP also reduce the secretion of ADH from the posterior pituitary. These actions of ANP and BNP are mediated by activation of membrane-bound guanylyl cyclase receptors, which increases intracellular levels of the second messenger cyclic guanosine monophosphate (cGMP). ANP induces a more profound natriuresis and diuresis than BNP.

Urodilatin and ANP are encoded by the same gene and have similar amino acid sequences. Urodilatin is a 32-amino-acid hormone that differs from ANP by the addition of four amino acids to the amino terminus.

Urodilatin is secreted by the distal tubule and collecting duct and is not present in the systemic circulation; thus, urodilatin influences only the function of the kidneys. Urodilatin secretion is stimulated by a rise in the blood pressure and an increase in the ECF volume. It inhibits NaCl and water reabsorption across the medullary portion of the collecting duct. Urodilatin is a more potent natriuretic and diuretic hormone than ANP because some of the ANP that enters the kidneys in the blood is degraded by a neutral endopeptidase that has no effect on urodilatin.

Uroguanylin and **guanylin** are produced by neuroendocrine cells in the intestine in response to the oral ingestion of NaCl. These hormones enter the circulation and inhibit NaCl and water reabsorption by the kidneys by activation of membrane-bound guanylyl cyclase receptors, which increases intracellular levels of cGMP. The natriuretic response of the kidneys to a salt load is more pronounced when given orally than when delivered intravenously because oral administration of salt causes the secretion of uroguanylin and guanylin.

Catecholamines stimulate NaCl reabsorption. Catecholamines released from the sympathetic nerves (norepinephrine) and the adrenal medulla (epinephrine) stimulate NaCl and water reabsorption by the proximal tubule, thick ascending limb of the loop of Henle, distal tubule, and collecting duct. Although sympathetic nerves are not active when the ECF volume is normal, when ECF volume declines (e.g., after hemorrhage) sympathetic nerve activity rises and stimulates NaCl and water reabsorption by these four nephron segments.

Dopamine, a catecholamine, is released from dopaminergic nerves in the kidneys and is also synthesized by cells of the proximal tubule. The action of dopamine is opposite to that of norepinephrine and epinephrine. Dopamine secretion is stimulated by an increase in ECF volume, and its secretion directly inhibits NaCl and water reabsorption in the proximal tubule.

Adrenomedullin is a 52-amino-acid peptide hormone that is produced by a variety of organs including the kidneys. Adrenomedullin induces a marked diuresis and natriuresis, and its secretion is stimulated by congestive heart failure and hypertension. The major effect of adrenomedullin on the kidneys is to increase GFR and RBF and, thereby, to stimulate indirectly the excretion of NaCl and water.

ADH regulates water reabsorption. ADH is the most important hormone that regulates water reabsorption in the kidneys (see Chapter 5). This hormone is secreted by the posterior pituitary gland in response to an increase in plasma osmolality (1% or more) or a decrease in the ECF volume (>5% to 10% of normal). ADH increases the permeability of the collecting duct to water. It increases water reabsorption by the collecting duct because of the osmotic gradient that exists across the wall of the collecting duct (see Chapter 5). ADH has little effect on urinary NaCl excretion.

Starling forces regulate NaCl and water reabsorption across the proximal tubule. As previously described, Na$^+$, Cl$^-$, HCO$_3^-$, amino acids, glucose, and water are transported into the intercellular space of the proximal tubule. Starling forces between this space and the peritubular capillaries facilitate the movement of the reabsorbed fluid into the capillaries. Starling forces across the wall of the peritubular capillaries are the hydrostatic pressures in the peritubular capillary (P$_{pc}$) and lateral intercellular space (P$_i$) and the oncotic pressures in the peritubular capillary (π_{pc}) and lateral intercellular space (π_i). Thus, the reabsorption of water, resulting from Na$^+$ transport from tubular fluid into the lateral intercellular space, is modified by the Starling forces. Thus:

$$Q = K_f[(P_i - P_{pc}) + \sigma(\pi_{pc} - \pi_i)] \qquad (4\text{-}2)$$

where Q is flow (positive numbers indicate flow from the intercellular space into blood). Starling forces that favor movement from the interstitium into the peritubular capillaries are π_{pc} and P$_i$ (Figure 4-11). The opposing Starling forces are π_i and P$_{pc}$. Normally, the sum of the Starling forces favors the movement of solute and water from the interstitial space into the capillary. However, some of the solutes and fluid that enter the lateral intercellular space leak back into the proximal tubular fluid. Starling forces do not affect transport by the loop of Henle, distal tubule, and collecting duct because these segments are less permeable to water than the proximal tubule.

A number of factors can alter the Starling forces across the peritubular capillaries surrounding the proximal tubule. For example, dilation of the efferent arteriole increases P$_{pc}$, whereas constriction of the

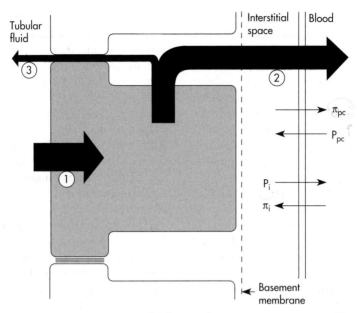

FIGURE 4-11 ■ Routes of solute and water transport across the proximal tubule and the Starling forces that modify reabsorption. 1, Solute and water are reabsorbed across the apical membrane. This solute and water then cross the lateral cell membrane. Some solute and water reenter the tubule fluid (indicated by arrow labeled 3), and the remainder enters the interstitial space and then flows into the capillary (indicated by arrow labeled 2). The width of the arrows is directly proportional to the amount of solute and water moving by the pathways labeled 1 to 3. Starling forces across the capillary wall determine the amount of fluid flowing through pathway 2 versus 3. Transport mechanisms in the apical cell membranes determine the amount of solute and water entering the cell (pathway 1). π_{pc}, peritubular capillary oncotic pressure; P_{pc}, peritubular capillary hydrostatic pressure; π_i, interstitial fluid oncotic pressure; P_i, interstitial hydrostatic pressure. Thin arrows across the capillary wall indicate direction of water movement in response to each force.

efferent arteriole decreases it. An increase in P_{pc} inhibits solute and water reabsorption by increasing the back-leak of NaCl and water across the tight junction, whereas a decrease stimulates reabsorption by decreasing back-leak across the tight junction.

The π_{pc} is partially determined by the rate of formation of the glomerular ultrafiltrate. For example, if one assumes a constant plasma flow in the afferent arteriole, the plasma proteins become less concentrated in the plasma that enters the efferent arteriole and peritubular capillary as less ultrafiltrate is formed

(i.e., as GFR decreases). Hence, the π_{pc} decreases. The π_{pc} is directly related to the **filtration fraction** (FF = GFR/renal plasma flow [RPF]). A fall in the FF resulting from a decrease in GFR, at constant RPF, decreases the π_{pc}. This in turn increases the backflow of NaCl and water from the lateral intercellular space into the tubular fluid and, thereby, decreases net solute and water reabsorption across the proximal tubule. An increase in the FF has the opposite effect.

The importance of Starling forces in regulating solute and water reabsorption by the proximal tubule is underscored by the phenomenon of **glomerulo-tubular (G-T) balance.** Spontaneous changes in GFR markedly alter the filtered load of Na^+ (filtered load = GFR × Na^+ concentration in the filtered fluid). Without rapid adjustments in Na^+ reabsorption to counter the changes in filtration of Na^+, urine Na^+ excretion would fluctuate widely, disturb the Na^+ balance of the body, and thus alter ECF volume and blood pressure (see Chapter 6 for more details). However, spontaneous changes in GFR do not alter the Na^+ excretion in the urine or Na^+ balance because of the phenomenon of G-T balance. When body Na^+ balance is normal (i.e., ECF volume is normal), G-T balance refers to the fact that Na^+ and water reabsorption increases in proportion to the increase in GFR and filtered load of Na^+. Thus, a constant fraction of the filtered Na^+ and water is reabsorbed from the proximal tubule despite variations in GFR. The net result of G-T balance is to reduce the impact of GFR changes on the amount of Na^+ and water excreted in the urine.

Two mechanisms are responsible for G-T balance. One is related to the oncotic and hydrostatic pressure differences between the peritubular capillaries and the lateral intercellular space (i.e., Starling forces). For example, an increase in the GFR (at constant RPF) raises the protein concentration in the glomerular capillary plasma above normal. This protein-rich plasma leaves the glomerular capillaries, flows through the efferent arterioles, and enters th[...] laries. The increased π_{pc} augment[...] solute and fluid from the lateral [...] into the peritubular capillaries. Th[...] net solute and water reabsorptio[...] tubule.

The second mechanism responsible for G-T balance is initiated by an increase in the filtered load of glucose and amino acids. As discussed earlier, the reabsorption of Na^+ in the first half of the proximal tubule is coupled to that of glucose and amino acids. The rate of Na^+ reabsorption therefore partially depends on the filtered load of glucose and amino acids. As the GFR and filtered load of glucose and amino acids increase, Na^+ and water reabsorption also rises.

In addition to G-T balance, another mechanism minimizes changes in the filtered load of Na^+. As discussed in Chapter 3, an increase in the GFR (and, thus, in the amount of Na^+ filtered by the glomerulus) activates the tubuloglomerular feedback mechanism. This action returns the GFR and filtration of Na^+ to normal values. Thus, spontaneous changes in the GFR (e.g., caused by changes in posture and blood pressure) increase the amount of Na^+ filtered for only a few minutes. The mechanisms that underlie G-T balance maintain urinary Na^+ excretion constant and, thereby, maintain Na^+ homeostasis (and ECF volume and blood pressure) until the GFR returns to normal.

SUMMARY

1. The four major segments of the nephron (proximal tubule, Henle's loop, distal tubule, and collecting duct) determine the composition and volume of the urine by the processes of selective reabsorption of solutes and water and secretion of solutes.

2. Tubular reabsorption allows the kidneys to retain the substances that are essential and regulate their levels in the plasma by altering the degree to which they are reabsorbed. The reabsorption of Na^+, Cl^-, other anions, and organic anions and cations together with water constitutes the major function of the nephron. Approximately 25,200 mEq of Na^+ and 179 L of water are reabsorbed each day. The proximal tubule cells reabsorb 67% of the glomerular ultrafiltrate, and cells of Henle's loop reabsorb about 25% of the NaCl that was filtered and about 15% of the water that was filtered. The distal segments of the nephron (distal tubule and collecting duct system) have a more limited reabsorptive capacity. However, the final adjustments in the composition and volume of the urine and most of the regulation by hormones and other factors occur in distal segments.

3. Secretion of substances into tubular fluid is a means for excreting various byproducts of metabolism, and it also serves to eliminate exogenous organic anions and cations (e.g., drugs) and pollutants from the body. Many organic anions and cations

are bound to plasma proteins and are therefore unavailable for ultrafiltration. Thus, secretion is their major route of excretion in the urine.

4. Various hormones (including angiotensin II, aldosterone, ADH, natriuretic peptides [ANP, BNP], and urodilatin), uroguanylin, guanylin, sympathetic nerves, dopamine, and Starling forces regulate NaCl reabsorption by the kidneys. ADH is the major hormone that regulates water reabsorption.

KEY WORDS AND CONCEPTS

- Passive transport (diffusion)
- Solvent drag
- Facilitated diffusion
- Uniport
- Coupled transport
- Symport
- Antiport
- Secondary active transport
- Active transport
- Endocytosis
- Tight junctions
- Transcellular pathway
- Paracellular pathway
- Fanconi syndrome
- Glomerulotubular balance (G-T balance)
- Angiotensin II
- Aldosterone
- Sympathetic nerves
- Catecholamines
- Antidiuretic hormone (ADH)
- Atrial natriuretic peptide (ANP)
- Brain natriuretic peptide (BNP)
- Urodilatin
- Uroguanylin
- Guanylin
- Adrenomedullin
- Peritubular Starling forces

SELF-STUDY PROBLEMS

1. Consider the amount of water and NaCl filtered and reabsorbed by the kidneys each day. What does this tell you about the amount of energy (ATP) expended by the kidneys? Could this explain why the blood flow is so high relative to the size of the kidneys?

2. What are the composition and volume of a normal 24-hour urine?

3. Compare and contrast passive and active transport.

4. If it were possible to inhibit completely the Na^+,K^+-ATPase in the kidney, what would happen to transcellular and paracellular NaCl reabsorption across the proximal tubule? If GFR was unchanged, how much water and NaCl would appear in the urine every day?

5. Describe the mechanisms and pathways of Na^+, glucose, amino acid, Cl^-, and water reabsorption by the proximal tubule. Which pathways occur in the first phase of reabsorption, and which occur in the second phase? How do Starling forces affect solute and water reabsorption in the proximal tubule?

6. Describe how Na^+ and Cl^- are reabsorbed by the thick ascending limb of Henle's loop. If a diuretic that inhibits NaCl reabsorption (e.g., furosemide) in the thick ascending limb was given to an individual, what would happen to water reabsorption by this segment?

7. What is glomerulotubular balance, and what is the physiologic importance of this phenomenon? If the GFR increased without a change in the ECF volume, what would happen to Na^+ balance if glomerulotubular balance did not exist?

8. List the hormones and factors that regulate NaCl and water reabsorption by the kidneys.

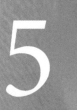

5

REGULATION OF BODY FLUID OSMOLALITY: REGULATION OF WATER BALANCE

OBJECTIVES

Upon completion of this chapter, the student should be able to answer the following questions:

1. Why do changes in water balance result in alterations in the [Na$^+$] of the extracellular fluid (ECF)?

2. How is the secretion of antidiuretic hormone (ADH) controlled by changes in the osmolality of the body fluids and in blood volume and pressure?

3. What are the cellular events associated with the action of ADH on the collecting duct, and how do they lead to an increase in the water permeability of this segment?

4. What is the role of Henle's loop in the production of both dilute and concentrated urine?

5. What is the composition of the medullary interstitial fluid, and how does it participate in the process of producing concentrated urine?

6. What are the roles of the vasa recta in the process of diluting and concentrating the urine?

7. How is the diluting and concentrating ability of the kidneys quantitated?

As described in Chapter 1, water constitutes approximately 60% of the healthy adult human body. The body water is divided into two compartments (i.e., intracellular fluid [ICF] and extracellular fluid [ECF]), which are in osmotic equilibrium. Water intake into the body generally occurs orally. However, in clinical situations, intravenous infusion is an important route of water entry. Regardless of the route of entry (oral versus intravenous), water first enters the ECF and then equilibrates with the ICF. The kidneys are responsible for regulating water balance and under most conditions are the major route for elimination of water from the body (Table 5-1). Other routes of water loss from the body include evaporation from the cells of the skin and respiratory passages. Collectively, water loss by these routes is termed **insensible water loss** because the individual is unaware of its occurrence.

The production of sweat accounts for the loss of additional water. Water loss by this mechanism can increase dramatically in a hot environment, with exercise, or in the presence of fever (Table 5-2). Finally, water can be lost from the gastrointestinal tract. Fecal water loss is normally small (~100 ml/day) but can increase dramatically with diarrhea (e.g., 20 L/day with cholera). Vomiting can also cause gastrointestinal water loss.

Although water loss from sweating, defecation, and evaporation from the lungs and skin can vary depending on the environmental conditions or during pathologic conditions, the loss of water by these routes cannot be regulated. In contrast, the renal excretion of water is tightly regulated to maintain whole-body water balance. The maintenance of water balance requires that water intake and loss from the body are precisely matched.

TABLE 5-1

Normal Routes of Water Gain and Loss in Adults at Room Temperature (23 °C)

ROUTE	ml/DAY
Water Intake	
Fluid*	1200
In food	1000
Metabolically produced from food	300
Total	2500
Water Output	
Insensible	700
Sweat	100
Feces	200
Urine	1500
Total	2500

*Fluid intake varies widely for both social and cultural reasons.

If intake exceeds losses, **positive water balance** exists. Conversely, when intake is less than losses, **negative water balance** exists.

When water intake is low or water losses increase, the kidneys conserve water by producing a small volume of urine that is hyperosmotic with respect to plasma. When water intake is high, a large volume of hypo-osmotic urine is produced. In a normal individual, the urine osmolality (U_{osm}) can vary from approximately 50 to 1200 mOsm/kg H_2O, and the corresponding urine volume can vary from approximately 18 to 0.5 L/day.

It is important to recognize that disorders of water balance are manifested by alterations in the body fluid osmolality, which are usually measured by changes in plasma osmolality (P_{osm}). Because the major determinant of plasma osmolality is Na^+ (with its anions Cl^- and HCO_3^-), these disorders also result in alterations in the plasma [Na^+]. When an abnormal plasma [Na^+] is observed in an individual, it is tempting to suspect a problem in Na^+ balance. However, the problem is most often related to water balance, not Na^+ balance. As described in Chapter 6, changes in Na^+ balance result in alterations in the volume of ECF, not its osmolality.

In the clinical setting, hypo-osmolality (a reduction in plasma osmolality) shifts water into cells, and this process results in cell swelling. Symptoms associated with hypo-osmolality are related primarily to swelling of brain cells. For example, a rapid fall in P_{osm} can alter neurologic function and thereby cause nausea, malaise, headache, confusion, lethargy, seizures, and coma. When P_{osm} is increased (i.e., hyperosmolality), water is lost from cells. The symptoms of an increase in P_{osm} are also primarily neurologic and include lethargy, weakness, seizures, coma, and even death.

The symptoms associated with changes in body fluid osmolality vary depending on how quickly osmolality is changed. Rapid changes in osmolality (i.e., over hours) are less well tolerated than changes that occur more gradually (i.e., over days to weeks). Indeed, individuals who have developed alterations in their body fluid osmolality over an extended period of time may be entirely asymptomatic. This reflects the ability of cells over time either to eliminate intracellular osmoles, as occurs with hypo-osmolality, or to generate new intracellular osmoles in response to

TABLE 5-2

Effect of Environmental Temperature and Exercise on Water Loss and Intake in Adults

WATER LOSS	NORMAL TEMPERATURE	HOT WEATHER*	PROLONGED HEAVY EXERCISE*
Insensible loss			
Skin	350	350	350
Lungs	350	250	650
Sweat	100	1400	5000
Feces	200	200	200
Urine*	1500	1200	500
Total loss	2500	3400	6700

*In hot weather and during prolonged heavy exercise, water balance is maintained by increased water ingestion. Decreased excretion of water by the kidneys alone is insufficient to maintain water balance.

hyperosmolality and thus minimize changes in cell volume of the neurons. This has important clinical implications when treating a patient with an abnormal plasma osmolality. For example, rapid correction of the osmolality of an individual who has had long-standing hypo-osmolality of the body fluids can lead to demyelination, especially of the pons, the results of which are irreversible. Depending on the extent of pontine demyelination, this condition can be fatal.

Under steady-state conditions, the kidneys control water excretion independently of their ability to control the excretion of various other physiologically important substances such as Na+, K+, and urea (Figure 5-1). Indeed, this ability is necessary for survival because it allows water balance to be achieved without upsetting the other homeostatic functions of the kidneys.

This chapter discusses the mechanisms by which the kidneys excrete either hypo-osmotic (dilute) or hyperosmotic (concentrated) urine. The control of vasopressin secretion and its important role in regulating the excretion of water by the kidneys are also explained.

ANTIDIURETIC HORMONE

Antidiuretic hormone (ADH), or **vasopressin,** acts on the kidneys to regulate the volume and osmolality of the urine. When plasma ADH levels are low, a large volume of urine is excreted (diuresis), and the urine is dilute.[1] When plasma levels are high, a small volume of urine is excreted (antidiuresis), and the urine is concentrated. Figure 5-1 illustrates the effect of ADH on the urine flow rate and osmolality. The excretion of total solute (e.g., Na+, K+, urea) by the kidneys is also shown. As already noted, ADH does not appreciably alter the excretion of solute. This underscores the fact that ADH controls water excretion and maintains water balance without altering the excretion and homeostatic control of other substances.

ADH is a small peptide that is nine amino acids in length. It is synthesized in neuroendocrine cells located within the supraoptic and paraventricular nuclei of the hypothalamus.[2] The synthesized hormone is packaged in granules that are transported down the axon of the cell and stored in the nerve terminals located in the neurohypophysis (posterior pituitary). The anatomy of the hypothalamus and pituitary gland is shown in Figure 5-2.

The gene for ADH is found on chromosome 20. It contains approximately 2000 base pairs with three exons and two introns. The gene codes for a prepro-hormone that consists of a signal peptide, the ADH molecule, neurophysin, and a glycopeptide (copeptin). As the cell processes the preprohormone, the signal peptide is cleaved off in the rough endoplasmic reticulum. Once packaged in neurosecretory granules, the preprohormone is further cleaved into ADH, neurophysin, and copeptin molecules.

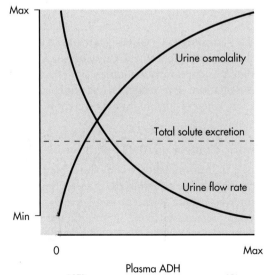

FIGURE 5-1 ■ Relationship between plasma antidiuretic hormone (ADH) levels and urine osmolality, urine flow rate, and total solute excretion.

[1]Diuresis is simply a large urine output. When the urine contains primarily water, it is referred to as a water diuresis. This is in contrast to the diuresis seen with diuretic agents (see Chapter 10). In the latter case, there is a large urine output but the urine contains solute plus water. This is sometimes termed a solute diuresis.

[2]Neurons within the supraoptic and paraventricular nuclei synthesize either ADH or the related peptide oxytocin. ADH-secreting cells predominate in the supraoptic nucleus, and the oxytocin-secreting neurons are found primarily in the paraventricular nucleus.

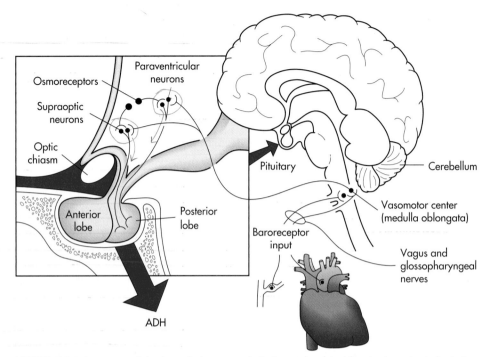

FIGURE 5-2 ■ Anatomy of the hypothalamus and pituitary gland (midsagittal section) depicting the pathways for antidiuretic hormone (ADH) secretion. Also shown are pathways involved in regulating ADH secretion. Afferent fibers from the baroreceptors are carried in the vagus and glossopharyngeal nerves. The closed box illustrates an expanded view of the hypothalamus and pituitary gland.

The neurosecretory granules are then transported down the axon to the posterior pituitary and stored in the nerve endings until released. When the neurons are stimulated to secrete ADH, the action potential opens Ca^{++} channels in the nerve terminal, which raises the intracellular $[Ca^{++}]$ and causes exocytosis of the neurosecretory granules. All three peptides are secreted in this process. Neurophysin and copeptin do not have an identified physiologic function.

The secretion of ADH by the posterior pituitary can be influenced by several factors. The two primary physiologic regulators of ADH secretion are the osmolality of the body fluids (osmotic) and volume and pressure of the vascular system (hemodynamic). Other factors that can alter ADH secretion include nausea (stimulates), atrial natriuretic peptide (inhibits), and angiotensin II (stimulates). A number of drugs, prescription and nonprescription, also affect ADH secretion. For example, nicotine stimulates secretion, whereas ethanol inhibits secretion.

Osmotic Control of ADH Secretion

Changes in the osmolality of body fluids play the most important role in regulating ADH secretion; changes as minor as 1% are sufficient to alter it significantly. Although the neurons in the supraoptic and paraventricular nuclei respond to changes in body fluid osmolality by altering their secretion of ADH, it is clear that there are separate cells in the anterior hypothalamus that are exquisitely sensitive to changes in body fluid osmolality and therefore play an important role in regulating the secretion of ADH.[3] These cells, termed osmoreceptors, appear to behave as osmometers and sense changes in body fluid osmolality by either shrinking or swelling. The osmoreceptors respond only to solutes in plasma that are effective osmoles (see Chapter 1). For example, urea is an ineffective osmole when the function of osmoreceptors is considered. Thus, elevation of the plasma urea concentration alone has little effect on ADH secretion.

When the effective osmolality of the plasma increases, the osmoreceptors send signals to the ADH synthesizing/secreting cells located in the supraoptic and paraventricular nuclei of the hypothalamus, and ADH synthesis and secretion are stimulated. Conversely, when the effective osmolality of the plasma is reduced, secretion is inhibited. Because ADH is rapidly degraded in the plasma, circulating levels can be reduced to zero within minutes after secretion is inhibited. As a result, the ADH system can respond rapidly to fluctuations in body fluid osmolality.

Figure 5-3A illustrates the effect of changes in plasma osmolality on circulating ADH levels. The slope of the relationship is quite steep and accounts for the sensitivity of this system. The set point of the system is the plasma osmolality value at which ADH secretion begins to increase. Below this set point, virtually no ADH is released. The set point varies among individuals and is genetically determined. In healthy adults, it varies from 275 to 290 mOsm/kg H_2O (average ~280 to 285 mOsm/kg H_2O). Several physiologic factors can also change the set point in a given individual. As discussed later, alterations in blood volume and pressure can shift it. In addition, pregnancy is associated with a decrease in the set point.

Hemodynamic Control of ADH Secretion

A decrease in blood volume or pressure also stimulates ADH secretion. The receptors responsible for this response are located in both the low-pressure (left atrium and large pulmonary vessels) and the high-pressure (aortic arch and carotid sinus) sides of the circulatory system. Because the low-pressure receptors are located in the high-compliance side of the circulatory system (i.e., venous) and because the majority of blood is in the venous side of the circulatory system, these low-pressure receptors can be

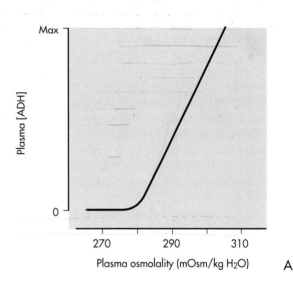

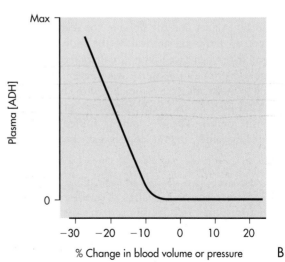

FIGURE 5-3 ■ Osmotic and hemodynamic control of antidiuretic hormone (ADH) secretion. Depicted are the relationships between plasma ADH levels and plasma osmolality (A) and blood volume and pressure (B).

---

[3]Several sites for the location of the osmoreceptors have been identified; one of these sites is the organum vasculosum of the lamina terminalis (OVLT). In addition, the subfornical organ (SFO), which is outside the blood-brain barrier, responds to circulating levels of angiotensin II.

viewed as responding to overall vascular volume. The high-pressure receptors respond to arterial pressure. Both groups of receptors are sensitive to stretch of the wall of the structure in which they are located (e.g., cardiac atrial wall, wall of the aortic arch) and are termed **baroreceptors.** Signals from these receptors are carried in afferent fibers of the vagus and glossopharyngeal nerves to the brainstem (solitary tract nucleus of the medulla oblongata), which is part of the center that regulates heart rate and blood pressure. Signals are then relayed from the brainstem to the ADH secretory cells of the supraoptic and paraventricular hypothalamic nuclei. The sensitivity of the baroreceptor system is less than that of the osmoreceptors, and a 5% to 10% decrease in blood volume or pressure is required before ADH secretion is stimulated. This is illustrated in Figure 5-3B. A number of substances have been shown to alter the secretion of ADH through their effects on blood pressure. These include bradykinin and histamine, which lower pressure and thus stimulate ADH secretion, and norepinephrine, which increases blood pressure and inhibits ADH secretion.

Alterations in blood volume and pressure also affect the response to changes in body fluid osmolality (Figure 5-4). With a decrease in blood volume or pressure, the set point is shifted to lower osmolality values and the slope of the relationship is steeper. In terms of survival of the individual, this means that when faced with circulatory collapse the kidneys continue to conserve water, even though by doing so they reduce the osmolality of the body fluids. With an increase in blood volume or pressure, the opposite occurs. The set point is shifted to higher osmolality values, and the slope is decreased.

Inadequate release of ADH from the posterior pituitary results in excretion of large volumes of dilute urine (polyuria). To compensate for this loss of water, the individual must ingest large volumes of water (polydipsia) to maintain constant body fluid osmolality. If the individual is deprived of water, the body fluids become hyperosmotic. This condition is called central diabetes insipidus or pituitary diabetes insipidus. Central diabetes insipidus can be inherited, although this is rare. It occurs more commonly after head trauma and with brain neoplasms or infections. Individuals with central diabetes insipidus have a urine-concentrating defect that can be corrected by the administration of exogenous ADH.

The inherited (autosomal dominant) form of central diabetes insipidus has been shown to represent multiple mutations in the ADH gene. In patients with this form of central diabetes insipidus, mutations have been identified in all regions of the ADH gene (i.e., ADH, copeptin, and neurophysin). The most common mutation is found in the neurophysin portion of the gene. In each of these situations, there is defective trafficking of the peptide, with abnormal accumulation in the endoplasmic reticulum. It is believed that this abnormal accumulation in the endoplasmic reticulum results in death of the ADH secretory cells of the supraoptic and paraventricular nuclei.

The syndrome of inappropriate ADH secretion **(SIADH)** is a common clinical problem characterized by plasma ADH levels that are elevated above what would be expected on the basis of body fluid osmolality and blood volume and pressure—hence the term inappropriate ADH secretion. In addition, the collecting duct overexpresses water channels (see later), thus augmenting the effect of ADH on the kidney. Individuals with SIADH retain water, and their body fluids become progressively hypo-osmotic. In addition, their urine is more hyperosmotic than expected on the basis of the low body fluid osmolality. SIADH can be caused by infections and neoplasms of the brain, drugs (e.g., antitumor drugs), pulmonary diseases, and carcinoma of the lung. Many of these conditions stimulate ADH secretion by altering neural input to the ADH secretory cells. However, small cell carcinoma of the lung produces and secretes a number of peptides including ADH.

ADH Actions on the Kidneys

The primary action of ADH on the kidneys is to increase the permeability of the collecting duct to water. In addition, and notably, ADH increases the permeability of the medullary portion of the collecting duct to urea.

The actions of ADH on water permeability of the collecting duct have been studied extensively. ADH binds to a receptor on the basolateral membrane of the cell. This receptor is termed the V_2 receptor

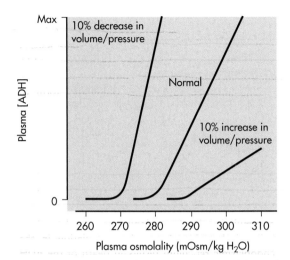

FIGURE 5-4 ■ Interaction between osmotic and hemodynamic stimuli for antidiuretic hormone (ADH) secretion. With decreased blood volume and pressure, the osmotic set point is shifted to lower plasma osmolality values and the slope is increased. An increase in blood volume and pressure has the opposite effects.

(i.e., vasopressin 2 receptor).[4] Binding to this receptor, which is coupled to adenylyl cyclase through a stimulatory G protein (Gs), increases the intracellular levels of cyclic adenosine monophosphate (cAMP). The rise in intracellular cAMP activates protein kinase A (PKA), which ultimately results in the insertion of vesicles containing aquaporin-2 (AQP-2) water channels into the apical membrane of the cell as well as the synthesis of more AQP-2. With the removal of ADH, these water channels are reinternalized into the cell through clathrin-coated pits, and the apical membrane is once again impermeable to water. This shuttling of water channels into and out of the apical membrane provides a rapid mechanism for controlling membrane water permeability. Because the basolateral membrane is freely permeable to water due to the presence of aquaporin-3 (AQP-3) and aquaporin-4 (AQP-4) water channels, any water that enters the cell through apical membrane water

channels exits across the basolateral membrane, resulting in net absorption of water from the tubule lumen.

The gene for the **V₂ receptor** is located on the X chromosome. It codes for a 371-amino-acid protein that is in the family of receptors that have seven membrane-spanning domains and are coupled to heterotrimeric G proteins. As shown in Figure 5-5, binding of ADH to its receptor on the basolateral membrane activates adenylyl cyclase. The increase in intracellular cAMP then activates protein kinase (PKA), which results in phosphorylation of AQP-2 water channels and also results in increased transcription of the AQP-2 gene through activation of a cAMP response element (CRE). Vesicles containing phosphorylated AQP-2 move toward the apical membrane along microtubules driven by the molecular motor dynein. Once near the apical membrane, proteins called SNAREs interact with vesicles containing AQP-2 and facilitate the fusion of these vesicles with the membrane. The addition of AQP-2 to the membrane allows water to enter the cell driven by the osmotic gradient (lumen osmolality < cell osmolality). The water then exits the cell across the basolateral membrane through AQP-3 and AQP-4 water channels, which are constitutively present in the basolateral membrane. When the V₂ receptor is not occupied by ADH, the AQP-2 water channels are removed from the apical membrane by clathrin-mediated endocytosis rendering the apical membrane once again impermeable to water. The endocytosed AQP-2 molecules may be either stored in cytoplasmic vesicles ready for reinsertion into the apical membrane when ADH levels in the plasma increase or degrade.

Recently, individuals have been found who have activating (gain-of-function) mutations in the V₂ receptor gene. Thus, the receptor is constitutively activated even in the absence of ADH. These individuals have laboratory findings similar to those seen in the syndrome of inappropriate ADH secretion (SIADH), including reduced plasma osmolality, hyponatremia (reduced plasma [Na⁺]), and urine more concentrated than would be expected from the reduced body fluid osmolality. However, unlike those with SIADH, in whom circulating levels of ADH are elevated and thus responsible for water retention by the kidneys, these individuals have undetectable levels of ADH in their plasma. This new clinical entity has been termed "nephrogenic syndrome of inappropriate antidiuresis."

---

[4]A different ADH receptor (V1 receptor) is present on vascular smooth muscle. This receptor mediates the vasoconstrictor response to ADH. It is this action that accounts for its alternative name, vasopressin.

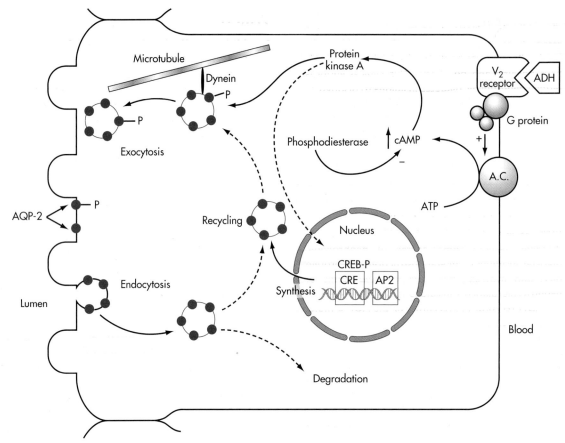

FIGURE 5-5 ■ Action of antidiuretic hormone (ADH) through the V_2 receptor on the principal cell of the late distal tubule and collecting duct. See text for details. AC, adenylyl cyclase; AP2, aquaporin-2 gene; AQP-2, aquaporin-2; cAMP, cyclic adenosine monophosphate; CRE, cAMP response element; CREB-P, phosphorylated cAMP response element binding protein; P, phosphorylated proteins. *(Adopted and modified from Brown D, Nielsen S: The cell biology of vasopressin action. In Brenner BM, editor: The kidney, ed 7. Philadelphia, 2004, WB Saunders.)*

ADH also increases the permeability of the terminal portion of the inner medullary collecting duct to urea. This results in an increase in urea reabsorption and an increase in the osmolality of the medullary interstitial fluid. The apical membrane of medullary collecting duct cells contains two different urea transporters (UT-A1 and UT-A3).[5] ADH, acting through adenylyl cyclase and the cAMP/PKA cascade, increases the permeability of the apical membrane to urea. This increase in permeability is associated with phosphorylation of UT-A1 and perhaps also UT-A3.

Increasing the osmolality of the interstitial fluid of the renal medulla also increases the permeability of the collecting duct to urea. This effect is mediated by the phospholipase C pathway and involves protein kinase C (PKC) phosphorylation. Thus, this effect is separate from and additive to that of ADH.

ADH also stimulates the reabsorption of NaCl by the thick ascending limb of Henle's loop and by the distal tubule and cortical segment of the collecting duct. It is thought that stimulation of thick ascending limb NaCl transport, in particular, may help maintain the hyperosmotic medullary interstitium that is necessary for absorption of water from the medullary portion of the collecting duct (see later).

---

[5]In some species UT-A3 is localized to the basolateral membrane.

The collecting ducts of some individuals do not respond normally to ADH. These individuals cannot maximally concentrate their urine and consequently have polyuria and polydipsia. This clinical entity is termed **nephrogenic diabetes insipidus** to distinguish it from central diabetes insipidus. Nephrogenic diabetes insipidus can result from a number of systemic disorders and, more rarely, occurs as a result of inherited disorders. Many of the acquired forms of nephrogenic diabetes insipidus are the result of decreased expression of AQP-2 in the collecting duct. Decreased expression of AQP-2 has been documented in the urine-concentrating defects associated with hypokalemia, lithium ingestion (35% of individuals who take lithium for bipolar disorder develop some degree of nephrogenic diabetes insipidus), ureteral obstruction, low-protein diet, and hypercalcemia. The inherited forms of nephrogenic diabetes insipidus reflect mutations in the ADH receptor (V_2 receptor) or the AQP-2 molecule. Approximately 90% of hereditary forms of nephrogenic diabetes insipidus are the result of mutations in the V_2 receptor gene, with the other 10% being the result of mutations in the AQP-2 gene. Because the gene for the V_2 receptor is located on the X chromosome, these inherited forms are X linked. To date, more than 150 different mutations in the V_2 receptor gene have been described. Most of the mutations result in trapping of the receptor in the endoplasmic reticulum of the cell; only a few cases result in the surface expression of a V_2 receptor that does not bind ADH. The gene coding for AQP-2 is located on chromosome 12 and is inherited as both an autosomal recessive and an autosomal dominant defect. As noted in Chapters 1 and 4, aquaporins exist as homotetramers. This homotetramer formation explains the difference between the two forms of nephrogenic diabetes insipidus. In the recessive form, heterozygotes produce both normal AQP-2 and defective AQP-2 molecules. The defective AQP-2 monomer cannot bind to other monomers, and thus the homotetramers that do form contain only normal molecules. Thus, mutations in both alleles would be required to produce nephrogenic diabetes insipidus. In the autosomal dominant form, the defective monomers can form tetramers with normal monomers as well as defective monomers. However, these tetramers are nonfunctional.

THIRST

In addition to affecting the secretion of ADH, changes in plasma osmolality and blood volume or pressure lead to alterations in the perception of thirst. When body fluid osmolality is increased or the blood volume or pressure is reduced, the individual perceives thirst. Of these stimuli, hypertonicity is the more potent. An increase in plasma osmolality of only 2% to 3% produces a strong desire to drink, whereas decreases in blood volume and pressure in the range of 10% to 15% are required to produce the same response.

As already discussed, there is a genetically determined threshold for ADH secretion (i.e., a body fluid osmolality above which ADH secretion increases). Similarly, there is a genetically determined threshold for triggering the sensation of thirst. However, the thirst threshold is higher than the threshold for ADH secretion. On average, the threshold for ADH secretion is approximately 285 mOsm/kg H_2O, whereas the thirst threshold is approximately 295 mOsm/kg H_2O. Because of this difference, thirst is stimulated at a body fluid osmolality at which ADH secretion is already maximal.

The neural centers involved in regulating water intake (the thirst center) are located in the same region of the hypothalamus involved with regulating ADH secretion. However, it is not certain if the same cells serve both functions. Indeed, the thirst response, like the regulation of ADH secretion, occurs only in response to effective osmoles (e.g., NaCl). Even less is known about the pathways involved in the thirst response to decreased blood volume or pressure, but it is believed that the pathways are the same as those involved in the volume- and pressure-related regulation of ADH secretion. Angiotensin II, acting on cells of the thirst center (subfornical organ), also evokes the sensation of thirst. Because angiotensin II levels are increased when blood volume and pressure are reduced, this effect of angiotensin II contributes to the homeostatic response that restores and maintains the body fluids at their normal volumes.

The sensation of thirst is satisfied by the act of drinking even before sufficient water is absorbed from the gastrointestinal tract to correct the plasma osmolality. Oropharyngeal and upper gastrointestinal receptors appear to be involved in this response. However, relief of the thirst sensation by these receptors is short lived, and thirst is completely satisfied only when the plasma osmolality or blood volume or pressure is corrected.

It should be apparent that the ADH and thirst systems work in concert to maintain water balance. An increase in the plasma osmolality evokes drinking and, through ADH action on the kidneys, the conservation of water. Conversely, when the plasma osmolality is decreased, thirst is suppressed and, in the absence of ADH, renal water excretion is enhanced. However, most of the time fluid intake is dictated by cultural factors and social situations. This is especially the case when thirst is not stimulated. In this situation, maintaining a normal body fluid osmolality relies solely on the ability of the kidneys to excrete water. How the kidney accomplishes this is discussed in detail in the following sections of this chapter.

With adequate access to water, the thirst mechanism can prevent the development of hyperosmolality. Indeed, it is this mechanism that is responsible for the polydipsia seen in response to the polyuria of both central and nephrogenic diabetes insipidus.

Water intake is also influenced by social and cultural factors. Thus, individuals ingest water even in the absence of the thirst sensation. Normally, the kidneys are able to excrete this excess water because they can excrete up to 18 L/day of urine. However, in some instances, the volume of water ingested exceeds the kidneys' capacity to excrete water, especially over short periods of time. When this occurs, the body fluids become hypo-osmotic. An example of how water intake can exceed the capacity of the kidneys to excrete water is long-distance running. A study of participants in the **Boston Marathon** found that 13% of the runners developed hyponatremia during the course of the race.[6] This reflected the practice of some runners of ingesting water, or other hypotonic drinks, during the race in order to remain "well hydrated." In addition, water is produced from the metabolism of glycogen and triglycerides used as fuels by the exercising muscle. Because over the course of the race they ingested and generated more

water through metabolism than their kidneys were able to excrete, hyponatremia developed. In some racers the hyponatremia was severe enough to elicit the neurologic symptoms described previously.

Throughout the popular media one can find the urging to drink eight 8-oz glasses of water a day (the **8 × 8 recommendation**). Drinking this volume of water is said to provide innumerable health benefits. As a result, it seems that everyone now has a water bottle as his or her constant companion. Although ingesting this volume of water over the course of a day (approximately 2 L) does not harm most individuals, there is no scientific evidence to support the beneficial health claims ascribed to the 8 × 8 recommendation.[7] Indeed, most individuals get adequate amounts of water through the foods they ingest and the fluids taken with those meals.

The maximum amount of water that can be excreted by the kidneys depends on the amount of solute excreted, which in turn depends on food intake. For example, with maximally dilute urine ($U_{osm} = 50$ mOsm/kg H_2O), the maximum urine output of 18 L/day is achieved only if the solute excretion rate is 900 mmol/day.

$$U_{osm} = \text{solute excretion/volume excreted} \qquad (5\text{-}1)$$
$$50 \text{ mOsm/kg } H_2O = 900 \text{ mmol/18 L}$$

If solute excretion is reduced, as commonly occurs in elderly people with reduced food intake, the maximum urine output decreases. For example, if solute excretion is only 400 mmol/day, a maximum urine output (at $U_{osm} = 50$ mOsm/kg H_2O) of only 8 L/day can be achieved. Thus, individuals with reduced food intake have a reduced capacity to excrete water.

RENAL MECHANISMS FOR DILUTION AND CONCENTRATION OF THE URINE

Under normal circumstances, the excretion of water is regulated separately from the excretion of solutes (see Figure 5-1). For this to occur the kidneys must be able to excrete urine that is either hypo-osmotic or hyperosmotic with respect to the body fluids. This ability to

---

[6]Almond CS, Shin AY, Fortescue EB, et al: Hyponatremia among runners in the Boston Marathon. *N Engl J Med* 352:1150-1556, 2005.

[7]Valtin H: "Drink at least eight glasses of water a day." Really? Is there scientific evidence for "8 × 8"? *Am J Physiol Reg Integr Comp Physiol* 283:R993, 2002.

excrete urine of varying osmolality in turn requires that solute be separated from water at some point along the nephron. As discussed in Chapter 4, the reabsorption of solute in the proximal tubule results in the reabsorption of a proportional amount of water. Hence, solute and water are not separated in this portion of the nephron. Moreover, this proportionality between proximal tubule water and solute reabsorption occurs regardless of whether the kidneys excrete dilute or concentrated urine. Thus, the proximal tubule reabsorbs a large portion of the filtered load of solute and water, but it does not produce dilute or concentrated tubular fluid. The loop of Henle, in particular the thick ascending limb, is the major site where solute and water are separated. Thus, the excretion of both dilute and concentrated urine requires normal function of the loop of Henle.

The excretion of hypo-osmotic urine is relatively easy to understand. The nephron must simply reabsorb solute from the tubular fluid and not allow water reabsorption to occur. As just noted, and as described in greater detail in the following, the reabsorption of solute without concomitant water reabsorption occurs in the ascending limb of Henle's loop. Under appropriate conditions (i.e., in the absence of ADH), the distal tubule and collecting duct also dilute the tubular fluid.

The excretion of hyperosmotic urine is more complex and thus more difficult to understand. This process in essence involves removing water from the tubular fluid without solute. Because water movement is passive, driven by an osmotic gradient, the kidney must generate a hyperosmotic compartment that then reabsorbs water osmotically from the tubular fluid. The compartment in the kidney that serves this function is the interstitium of the renal medulla. Henle's loop, in particular the thick ascending limb, is critical for generating the hyperosmotic medullary interstitium. Once established, this hyperosmotic compartment drives water reabsorption from the collecting duct and thereby concentrates the urine.

Figure 5-6 summarizes the essential features of the mechanisms whereby the kidneys excrete either a dilute or a concentrated urine. Table 5-3 also summarizes the transport and passive permeability properties of the nephron segments involved in these processes.

First, how the kidneys excrete dilute urine (**water diuresis**) when ADH levels are low or zero is considered. The following numbers refer to those encircled in Figure 5-6A.

1. Fluid entering the thin descending limb of the loop of Henle from the proximal tubule is isosmotic with respect to plasma. This reflects the essentially isosmotic nature of solute and water reabsorption in the proximal tubule (see Chapter 4).
2. The thin descending limb is highly permeable to water and much less so to solutes such as NaCl and urea. (*Note:* Urea is an ineffective osmole in many tissues, but it is an effective osmole in many portions of the nephron [see Table 5-3].) Consequently, as the fluid in the thin descending limb descends deeper into the hyperosmotic medulla, water is reabsorbed owing to the osmotic gradient set up across the thin descending limb by both NaCl and urea, which are present at high concentrations in the medullary interstitium (see later section). Through this process, tubular fluid at the bend of the loop has an osmolality equal to that of the surrounding interstitial fluid. Although the osmolality of the tubular and interstitial fluids is similar at the bend of the loop, their compositions differ. The tubular fluid NaCl concentration is greater than that of the surrounding interstitial fluid. However, the urea concentration of the tubular fluid is less than that of the interstitial fluid (see later section).
3. The thin ascending limb is impermeable to water but permeable to NaCl and urea. Consequently, as tubular fluid moves up the ascending limb, NaCl is passively reabsorbed (because the tubular fluid NaCl concentration is higher than the interstitial NaCl concentration), whereas urea passively diffuses into the tubular fluid (because the tubular fluid urea concentration is lower than the interstitial urea concentration). The net effect is that the volume of the tubular fluid remains unchanged along the length of the thin ascending limb, but the NaCl concentration decreases and the urea concentration increases. Overall, the movement of NaCl out of the lumen

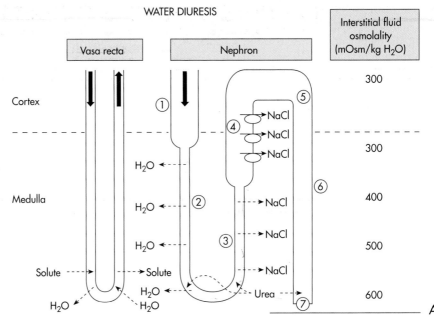

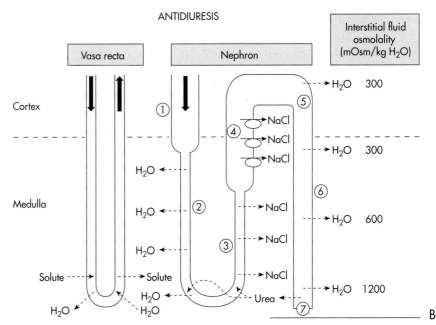

FIGURE 5-6 ■ Schematic of nephron segments involved in dilution and concentration of the urine. Henle's loops of juxtamedullary nephrons are shown. **A,** Mechanism for the excretion of dilute urine (water diuresis). Antidiuretic hormone (ADH) is absent, and the collecting duct is essentially impermeable to water. Note also that during a water diuresis the osmolality of the medullary interstitium is reduced as a result of increased vasa recta blood flow and the entry of some urea into the medullary collecting duct. **B,** Mechanism for the excretion of a concentrated urine (antidiuresis). Plasma ADH levels are maximal, and the collecting duct is highly permeable to water. Under this condition, the medullary interstitial gradient is maximal. See text for details.

TABLE 5-3
Transport and Permeability Properties of Nephron Segments Involved in Urine Concentration and Dilution

Tubule Segment	Active Transport	PASSIVE PERMEABILITY*			Effect of ADH
		NaCl	Urea	H_2O	
Loop of Henle					
Thin descending limb	0	+	+	+++	
Thin ascending limb	0	+++	0	0	
Thick ascending limb	+++	+	0	0	↑NaCl reabsorption
Distal tubule	++	+	0	0	↑H_2O permeability (late portion only)
Collecting duct					
Cortex	+	+	0	0	↑H_2O permeability
Medulla	+	+	++	+	↑H_2O and urea permeability

*Permeability is proportional to the number of plus signs indicated: +, low permeability; +++, high permeability; 0, impermeable.
ADH, antidiuretic hormone.

of the thin ascending limb exceeds the movement of urea into the lumen, and the tubular fluid becomes less concentrated than the surrounding interstitial fluid (i.e., tubular fluid dilution begins).

4. The thick ascending limb of the loop of Henle is impermeable to water and urea. This portion of the nephron actively reabsorbs NaCl from the tubular fluid and thereby dilutes it. Dilution occurs to such a degree that this segment is often referred to as the **diluting segment** of the kidney. Fluid leaving the thick ascending limb is hypo-osmotic with respect to plasma (approximately 150 mOsm/kg H_2O).

5. The distal tubule and cortical portion of the collecting duct actively reabsorb NaCl and are impermeable to urea. In the absence of ADH, these segments are not permeable to water. Thus, when ADH is absent or present at low levels (i.e., decreased plasma osmolality), the osmolality of tubule fluid in these segments is reduced further because NaCl is reabsorbed without water. Under this condition, fluid leaving the cortical portion of the collecting duct is hypo-osmotic with respect to plasma (approximately 50 to 100 mOsm/kg H_2O).

6. The medullary collecting duct actively reabsorbs NaCl. Even in the absence of ADH, this segment is slightly permeable to water and urea. Consequently, some urea enters the collecting duct from the medullary interstitium, and a small volume of water is reabsorbed.

7. The urine has an osmolality as low as approximately 50 mOsm/kg H_2O and contains low concentrations of NaCl and urea. The volume of urine excreted can be as much as 18 L/day or approximately 10% of the glomerular filtration rate.

Next, how the kidneys excrete concentrated urine (**antidiuresis**) when plasma osmolality and plasma ADH levels are high is considered. The following numbers refer to those encircled in Figure 5-6B.

1-4. These steps are similar to those for production of dilute urine. An important point in understanding how a concentrated urine is produced is to recognize that although reabsorption of NaCl by the thin and thick ascending limbs of the loop of Henle dilutes the tubular fluid, the reabsorbed NaCl accumulates in the medullary interstitium and raises the osmolality of this compartment. The accumulation of NaCl in the medullary interstitium is crucial for the production of urine hyperosmotic to plasma because it provides the osmotic driving force for water reabsorption by the medullary collecting duct. The overall process by which the loop of Henle, in particular the thick ascending limb, generates the hyperosmotic medullary interstitial gradient is termed **countercurrent multiplication.**

This term derives from both the form and function of the loop of Henle. The loop of Henle consists of two parallel limbs with tubular fluid flowing in opposite directions (countercurrent flow). Fluid flows into the medulla in the descending limb and out of the medulla in the ascending limb. The ascending limb is impermeable to water and reabsorbs solute from the tubular fluid. Thus, fluid within the ascending limb becomes diluted. This separation of solute and water by the ascending limb is termed the **single effect** of the countercurrent multiplication process. The solute removed from the ascending limb tubular fluid accumulates in the surrounding interstitial fluid and raises its osmolality. Because the descending limb is highly permeable to water, the increased osmolality of the medullary interstitium causes water to be reabsorbed and thereby concentrates the tubular fluid in this segment. The countercurrent flow within the descending and ascending limbs of the loop of Henle magnifies, or "multiplies," the osmotic gradient between the tubule fluid in the descending and ascending limbs of the loop of Henle such that an increasing osmotic gradient is generated throughout the medullary interstitium as illustrated. As already noted, ADH stimulates NaCl reabsorption by the thick ascending limb of Henle's loop. This is thought to maintain the medullary interstitial gradient at a time when water is being added to this compartment from the medullary collecting duct, which would tend to dissipate the gradient.

5. Because of NaCl reabsorption by the ascending limb of the loop of Henle, the fluid reaching the collecting duct is hypo-osmotic with respect to the surrounding interstitial fluid. Thus, an osmotic gradient is established across the collecting duct. In the presence of ADH, which increases the water permeability of the last half of the distal tubule and the collecting duct, water diffuses out of the tubule lumen, and the tubule fluid osmolality increases. This diffusion of water out of the lumen of the collecting duct begins the process of urine concentration. The maximum osmolality that the fluid in the distal tubule and cortical portion of the collecting duct can attain is approximately 290 mOsm/kg H_2O (i.e., the same as that of plasma), which is the osmolality of the interstitial fluid and plasma within the cortex of the kidney. Although the fluid at this point has the same osmolality as that which entered the descending thin limb, its composition has been altered dramatically. Because of NaCl reabsorption by the preceding nephron segments, NaCl accounts for a much smaller portion of the total tubular fluid osmolality. Instead, the tubule fluid osmolality reflects the presence of urea (filtered urea plus urea added to the descending thin limb of the loop of Henle) and other solutes (e.g., K^+, NH_4^+, creatinine).

6. The osmolality of the interstitial fluid in the medulla progressively increases from the junction between the renal cortex and medulla, where it is approximately 300 mOsm/kg H_2O, to the papilla, where it is approximately 1200 mOsm/kg H_2O. Thus, an osmotic gradient exists between tubule fluid and the interstitial fluid along the entire medullary collecting duct. In the presence of ADH, which renders the medullary collecting duct permeable to water, the osmolality of tubule fluid increases as water is reabsorbed. Because the initial portions of the collecting duct (cortical and outer medullary) are impermeable to urea, it remains in the tubular fluid, and its concentration increases. As already noted, in the presence of ADH, the urea permeability of the last portion of the medullary collecting duct (inner medullary) is increased. Because the urea concentration of the tubular fluid has been increased by water reabsorption in the cortex and outer medulla, its concentration in the tubular fluid is greater than its concentration in the interstitial fluid, and some urea diffuses out of the tubule lumen into the medullary interstitium. The maximal osmolality that the fluid in the medullary collecting duct can attain is equal to that of the surrounding interstitial fluid. The major components of the tubular fluid within the medullary collecting ducts are substances that have either escaped reabsorption or been secreted into the tubular fluid. Of these, urea is the most abundant.

7. The urine produced when ADH levels are elevated has an osmolality of 1200 mOsm/kg H_2O and contains high concentrations of urea and other nonreabsorbed solutes. Because urea in the tubular fluid equilibrates with urea in the medullary interstitial fluid, its concentration in the urine is similar to that of the interstitium. The urine volume under this condition can be as low as 0.5 L/day.

As just described, water reabsorption by the proximal tubule (67% of the filtered amount) and the thin descending limb of the loop of Henle (15% of the filtered amount) is essentially the same regardless of whether the urine is dilute or concentrated. As a result, a relatively constant volume of water is delivered to the distal tubule and collecting duct each day. Depending on the plasma ADH concentration, a variable portion of this water is then reabsorbed (8% to 17% of the filtered amount), with water excretion ranging from less than 1% to 10% of the filtered water. During antidiuresis, most of the water is reabsorbed in the distal tubule and cortical and outer medullary portions of the collecting duct. Thus, a relatively small volume of fluid reaches the inner medullary collecting duct, where it is then reabsorbed. This distribution of water reabsorption along the length of the collecting duct (i.e., cortex > outer medulla > inner medulla) allows the maintenance of a hyperosmotic interstitial environment in the inner medulla by minimizing the amount of water entering this compartment.

Water movement across the various segments of the nephron occurs through water channels (aquaporins). The proximal tubule and the thin descending limb of Henle's loop are highly permeable to water, and these segments express high levels of AQP-1 in both the apical and basolateral membranes. The vasa recta are also highly permeable to water and express AQP-1. AQP-7 and AQP-8 are also expressed in the proximal tubule. As already discussed, AQP-2 is responsible for ADH-regulated water movement across the apical membrane of principal cells of the late distal tubule and collecting duct, and AQP-3 and AQP-4 are responsible for water movement across the basolateral membrane.

Mice lacking the AQP-1 gene have been created. These mice have a urine-concentrating defect with increased urine output. Several individuals have been found that also lack the normal AQP-1 gene. Interestingly, these individuals do not have polyuria. However, when challenged by water deprivation, they are able to concentrate their urine to only approximately half of what is seen in a normal individual.

Medullary Interstitium

As noted, the interstitial fluid of the renal medulla is critically important in concentrating the urine. The osmotic pressure of the interstitial fluid provides the driving force for reabsorbing water from both the thin descending limb of the loop of Henle and the collecting duct. The principal solutes of the medullary interstitial fluid are NaCl and urea, but the concentration of these solutes is not uniform throughout the medulla (i.e., a gradient exists from cortex to papilla). Other solutes also accumulate in the medullary interstitium (e.g., NH_4^+ and K^+), but the most abundant solutes are NaCl and urea. For simplicity, this discussion assumes that NaCl and urea are the only solutes.

At the junction of the medulla with the cortex, the interstitial fluid has an osmolality of approximately 300 mOsm/kg H_2O, with virtually all osmoles attributable to NaCl. The concentrations of both NaCl and urea increase progressively with increasing depth into the medulla. When maximally concentrated urine is excreted, the medullary interstitial fluid osmolality is approximately 1200 mOsm/kg H_2O at the papilla (see Figure 5-6B). Of this value, approximately 600 mOsm/kg H_2O are attributed to NaCl and 600 mOsm/kg H_2O to urea. As described later, NaCl is an effective osmole in the inner medulla and thus is responsible for driving water reabsorption from the medullary collecting duct.

The medullary gradient for NaCl results from the accumulation of NaCl reabsorbed by the nephron segments in the medulla during countercurrent multiplication. The most important segment in this regard is the ascending limb (the thick limb more than the thin limb) of the loop of Henle. Urea accumulation within the medullary interstitium is more complex and occurs most effectively when hyperosmotic urine is excreted (i.e., antidiuresis). When dilute urine is produced, especially over extended periods, the osmolality of the medullary interstitium declines (compare Figure 5-6A and B). This reduced osmolality is almost entirely caused by a decrease in the concentration of urea. This decrease reflects washout by the vasa recta (see later section) and diffusion of urea from the interstitium into the tubular fluid within the medullary portion of the collecting duct. Recall that the medullary collecting duct is significantly permeable to urea even in the absence of ADH (see Table 5-3).

Urea is not synthesized in the kidney but is generated by the liver as a product of protein metabolism. It enters the tubular fluid by glomerular filtration. As indicated in Table 5-3, the permeability of most nephron segments involved in urinary concentration and dilution to urea is relatively low. The important exception is the medullary collecting duct, which has a relatively high urea permeability that is further increased by ADH. As fluid moves along the nephron and as water is reabsorbed in the collecting duct, the urea concentration in the tubular fluid increases. When this urea-rich tubular fluid reaches the medullary collecting duct, where the permeability to urea not only is high but also is increased by ADH, urea diffuses down its concentration gradient into the medullary interstitial fluid, where it accumulates. When ADH levels are elevated, the urea within the lumen of the collecting duct and the interstitium equilibrates. The resultant urea concentration of the urine is equal to that of the medullary interstitium at the papilla, or approximately 600 mOsm/kg H_2O.

Some of the urea within the interstitium enters the descending thin limb of the loop of Henle through the UT-A2 urea transporter. This urea is then trapped in the nephron until it again reaches the medullary collecting duct, where it can reenter the medullary interstitium. Thus urea recycles from the interstitium to the nephron and back into the interstitium. This process of recycling facilitates the accumulation of urea in the medullary interstitium.

As described, the hyperosmotic medullary interstitium is essential for concentrating the tubular fluid within the collecting duct. Because water reabsorption from the collecting duct is driven by the osmotic gradient established in the medullary interstitium,

urine can never be more concentrated than the interstitial fluid in the papilla. Thus, any condition that reduces the medullary interstitial osmolality impairs the ability of the kidneys to concentrate the urine maximally. Urea within the medullary interstitium contributes to the total osmolality of the urine. However, because the inner medullary collecting duct is highly permeable to urea, especially in the presence of ADH, urea cannot drive water reabsorption across this nephron segment (i.e., urea is an ineffective osmole).[8] Instead, the urea in the tubular fluid and that in the medullary interstitium equilibrate and a small volume of urine with a high concentration of urea is excreted. It is the medullary interstitial NaCl concentration that is responsible for reabsorbing water from the medullary collecting duct and thereby concentrating the nonurea solutes (e.g., NH_4^+ salts, K^+ salts, creatinine) in the urine.

Vasa Recta Function

The **vasa recta,** the capillary networks that supply blood to the medulla, are highly permeable to solute and water. As with the loop of Henle, the vasa recta form a parallel set of hairpin loops within the medulla (see Chapter 2). Not only do the vasa recta bring nutrients and oxygen to the medullary nephron segments but, more important, they also remove the excess water and solute that is continuously added to the medullary interstitium by these nephron segments. The ability of the vasa recta to maintain the medullary interstitial gradient is flow dependent. A substantial increase in vasa recta blood flow dissipates the medullary gradient (i.e., washout of osmoles from the medullary interstitium). Alternatively, reduced blood flow reduces oxygen delivery to the nephron segments within the medulla. Because transport of salt and other solutes requires oxygen and ATP, reduced medullary blood flow decreases salt and solute transport by nephron segments in the medulla. As a result, the medullary interstitial osmotic gradient cannot be maintained.

---

[8]In contrast to that of the medullary collecting duct, the urea permeability of the thin descending limb of Henle's loop is considerably less, and thus urea, together with the interstitial NaCl, can drive water reabsorption from this segment.

The vasa recta express the UT-B urea transporter. Individuals who lack this transporter have a decreased ability to concentrate their urine. Similarly, UT-B knockout mice cannot maximally concentrate urine. Thus, in the absence of this transporter there is impaired trapping of urea in the medulla by the vasa recta.

ASSESSMENT OF RENAL DILUTING AND CONCENTRATING ABILITY

Assessment of renal water handling includes measurements of urine osmolality and the volume of urine excreted. The range of urine osmolality is from 50 to 1200 mOsm/kg H_2O. The corresponding range in urine volume is 18 to as little as 0.5 L/day. These ranges are not fixed, but they vary from individual to individual and, as noted previously, depend on the amount of solute excreted.

As emphasized in this chapter, the ability of the kidneys to dilute or concentrate the urine requires the separation of solute and water (i.e., the single effect of the countercurrent multiplication process). This separation of solute and water in essence generates a volume of water that is "free of solute." When the urine is dilute, **solute-free water** is excreted from the body. When the urine is concentrated, solute-free water is returned to the body (i.e., conserved). The concept of **free-water clearance** provides a way to calculate the amount of solute-free water generated by the kidneys, either when dilute urine is excreted or when concentrated urine is formed. As its name denotes, free-water clearance is directly derived from the concept of renal clearance discussed in Chapter 3.

To calculate free-water clearance, the clearance of total solute by the kidneys must be calculated. This clearance of total solute (i.e., osmoles, whether effective or ineffective) from plasma by the kidneys is termed the **osmolar clearance (C_{osm})** and can be calculated as follows:

$$C_{osm} = \frac{U_{osm} \times \dot{V}}{P_{osm}} \qquad (5\text{-}2)$$

where U_{osm} is the urine osmolality, $\dot{V}$ is the urine flow rate, and P_{osm} is the osmolality of plasma.

C_{osm} has units of volume/unit time. Free-water clearance (C_{H_2O}) is then calculated as follows:

$$C_{H_2O} = \dot{V} - C_{osm} \qquad (5\text{-}3)$$

By rearranging equation 5-3; it should be apparent that

$$\dot{V} = C_{H_2O} - C_{osm} \qquad (5\text{-}4)$$

In other words, it is possible to partition the total urine output ($\dot{V}$) into two hypothetical components. One component contains all the urine solutes and has an osmolality equal to that of plasma (i.e., $U_{osm} = P_{osm}$). This volume is defined by C_{osm} and represents a volume from which there has been no separation of solute and water. The second component is a volume of solute-free water (i.e., C_{H_2O}).

When dilute urine is produced, the value of C_{H_2O} is positive, indicating that solute-free water is excreted from the body. When concentrated urine is produced, the value of C_{H_2O} is negative, indicating that solute-free water is retained in the body. By convention, negative C_{H_2O} values are expressed as $T^c_{H_2O}$ (**tubular conservation of water**).

Calculating C_{H_2O} and $T^c_{H_2O}$ can provide important information about the function of the portions of the nephron involved in producing dilute and concentrated urine. Whether the kidneys excrete or reabsorb free water depends on the presence of ADH. When ADH is absent or ADH levels are low, solute-free water is excreted. When ADH levels are high, solute-free water is reabsorbed.

The following factors are necessary for the kidneys to excrete a maximal amount of solute-free water (C_{H_2O}):

1. ADH must be absent. Without ADH, the collecting duct does not reabsorb a significant amount of water.
2. The tubular structures that separate solute from water (i.e., dilute the luminal fluid) must function normally. In the absence of ADH, the following nephron segments can dilute the luminal fluid:

- Thin ascending limb of Henle's loop
- Thick ascending limb of Henle's loop
- Distal tubule
- Collecting duct

Because of its high transport rate, the thick ascending limb is quantitatively the most important of these segments involved in the separation of solute and water.

3. An adequate amount of tubular fluid must be delivered to the aforementioned nephron sites for maximal separation of solute and water. Factors that reduce delivery (e.g., decreased GFR or enhanced proximal tubule reabsorption) impair the kidneys' ability to excrete solute-free water.

Similar requirements also apply to the conservation of water by the kidneys ($T^c_{H_2O}$). For the kidneys to conserve water maximally, the following conditions must exist:

1. An adequate amount of tubular fluid must be delivered to the nephron segments in which separation of solute from water occurs. The important segment in the separation of solute and water is the thick ascending limb of Henle's loop. Delivery of tubular fluid to Henle's loop depends on GFR and proximal tubule reabsorption.
2. Reabsorption of NaCl by the nephron segments must be normal; again, the most important segment is the thick ascending limb of Henle's loop.
3. A hyperosmotic medullary interstitium must be present. The interstitial fluid osmolality is maintained by NaCl reabsorption by Henle's loop (conditions 1 and 2) and by effective accumulation of urea. Urea accumulation in turn depends on adequate dietary protein intake.
4. Maximum levels of ADH must be present and the collecting duct must respond normally to ADH.

The concept of free-water clearance as just described does not distinguish between effective and ineffective osmoles, either in the plasma or in the urine. However, urea, which can account for half of total urine osmoles, is not an effective osmole when the movement of water between ICF and ECF is considered (see Chapter 1). Accordingly, when one wants to

understand how the handling of water by the kidneys contributes to the maintenance of whole-body water balance, it is more appropriate to consider only the solutes that are effective osmoles. For plasma (i.e., ECF), the effective osmoles are Na^+ and its attendant anions. For urine, they are the nonurea solutes.

The importance of using effective osmoles in determining the impact of renal water handling on whole-body water balance (i.e., body fluid osmolality) is illustrated by the following example. A patient has an elevated plasma [urea], and his plasma [Na^+] is also increased to 150 mEq/L. His total plasma osmolality (including urea) is 320 mOsm/kg H_2O, but his effective plasma osmolality (calculated as $2 \times$ plasma [Na^+]) is only 300 mOsm/kg H_2O. His urine osmolality is 600 mOsm/kg H_2O, with 300 mOsm/kg H_2O related to urea and 300 mOsm/kg H_2O related to nonurea solutes. His urinary flow rate is 3 L/day.

According to equations 5-2 and 5-3, his total osmolar clearance (C_{osm}) and free-water clearance (C_{H_2O}) are as follows:

$$C_{osm} = \frac{600 \text{ mOsm/kg } H_2O \times 3 \text{ L/day}}{320 \text{ mOsm/kg } H_2O} = 5.6 \text{ L/day} \quad (5\text{-}5)$$

$$C_{H_2O} = 3 \text{ L/day} - 5.6 \text{ L/day} = -2.6 \text{ L/day} \; (T^c_{H_2O}) \quad (5\text{-}6)$$

Thus, it appears that the kidneys are conserving 2.6 L/day of solute-free water, which would be an appropriate response to correct the elevated plasma osmolality. However, when C_{osm} and C_{H_2O} are analyzed from the perspective of effective osmoles, the following results are obtained:

$$C_{osm} = \frac{300 \text{ mOsm/kg } H_2O \times 3 \text{ L/day}}{300 \text{ mOsm/kg } H_2O} = 3 \text{ L/day} \quad (5\text{-}7)$$

$$C_{H_2O} = 3 \text{ L/day} - 3 \text{ L/day} = 0 \text{ L/day} \quad (5\text{-}8)$$

Thus, when viewed from the more appropriate perspective of effective osmoles, it is apparent that the kidneys are not reabsorbing solute-free water and the patient's kidneys are not correcting the hyperosmolality.

S U M M A R Y

1. The osmolality and volume of the body fluids are maintained within a narrow range despite wide variations in water and solute intake. The kidneys play the central role in this regulatory process by virtue of their ability to vary the excretion of water and solutes.

2. Regulation of body fluid osmolality requires that water intake and loss from the body are equal. This involves the integrated interaction of the ADH secretory and thirst centers of the hypothalamus and the ability of the kidneys to excrete urine that is either hypo-osmotic or hyperosmotic with respect to the body fluids.

3. When body fluid osmolality increases, ADH secretion and thirst are stimulated. ADH acts on the kidneys to increase the permeability of the collecting duct to water. Hence, water is reabsorbed from the lumen of the collecting duct, and a small volume of hyperosmotic urine is excreted. This renal conservation of water, together with increased water intake, restores body fluid osmolality to normal.

4. When body fluid osmolality decreases, ADH secretion and thirst are suppressed. In the absence of ADH, the collecting duct is impermeable to water and a large volume of hypo-osmotic urine is excreted. With this increased excretion of water and a decreased intake of water caused by suppression of thirst, the osmolality of the body fluids is restored to normal.

5. Central to the process of concentrating and diluting the urine is Henle's loop. The transport of NaCl by Henle's loop allows the separation of solute and water, which is essential for the elaboration of hypo-osmotic urine. By the same mechanism, the interstitial fluid in the medullary portion of the kidney is rendered hyperosmotic. This hyperosmotic medullary interstitial fluid in turn provides the osmotic driving force for the reabsorption of water from the lumen of the collecting duct when ADH is present.

6. Disorders of water balance result in alterations in body fluid osmolality. Because Na^+ and its attendant anions (Cl^- and HCO_3^-) are the major osmotically active particles in the ECF, changes in body fluid osmolality are manifested by a change in the plasma $[Na^+]$. Positive water balance (intake > excretion) results in a decrease in the body fluid osmolality and thus hyponatremia. Negative water balance (intake < excretion) results in an increase in body fluid osmolality and thus hypernatremia.

7. The handling of water by the kidneys is quantitated by measuring the amount of solute-free water that is either excreted (C_{H_2O}) or reabsorbed ($T^c_{H_2O}$). Maximal excretion of solute-free water requires normal nephron function (especially the thick ascending limb of Henle's loop), adequate delivery of tubular fluid to the nephrons, and the absence of ADH. Maximal reabsorption of solute-free water requires normal nephron function (especially the thick ascending limb of Henle's loop), adequate delivery of tubular fluid to the nephrons, a hyperosmotic medullary interstitium, the presence of ADH, and responsiveness of the collecting duct to ADH.

KEY WORDS AND CONCEPTS

- Insensible water loss
- Antidiuretic hormone (ADH) (vasopressin)
- Diuresis
- Antidiuresis
- Supraoptic nuclei
- Paraventricular nuclei
- Neurohypophysis (posterior pituitary)
- Osmoreceptors
- Effective osmole
- Ineffective osmole
- Set point (for osmotic control of ADH secretion)
- Baroreceptors
- Polyuria
- Polydipsia
- Central diabetes insipidus
- Pituitary diabetes insipidus
- Syndrome of inappropriate secretion of ADH (SIADH)
- Nephrogenic syndrome of inappropriate antidiuresis
- Nephrogenic diabetes insipidus
- Aquaporin (AQP)

- Thirst
- Diluting segment (thick ascending limb of Henle's loop)
- Concurrent multiplication (by Henle's loop)
- Free-water clearance
- Solute-free water excretion (C_{H_2O})
- Tubular conservation of water ($T^c_{H_2O}$)

SELF-STUDY PROBLEMS

1. An individual's blood is drawn, and the following values are obtained (see Appendix B for normal values):

Plasma [Na$^+$]	135 mEq/L
Serum [glucose]	100 mg/dL
Serum [BUN]	100 mg/dL
P_{osm}	310 mOsm/kg H_2O

Would plasma ADH levels in this individual be elevated or suppressed?

2. In the following table, indicate the expected osmolality of tubular fluid in the absence and presence of ADH (assume that the plasma osmolality is 300 mOsm/kg H_2O and osmolality of the medullary interstitium is 1200 mOsm/kg H_2O at the papilla).

Nephron site	0-ADH	Max. ADH
Proximal tubule	_____	_____
Beginning of thin descending limb	_____	_____
Beginning of thin ascending limb	_____	_____
End of thick ascending limb	_____	_____
End of cortical collecting duct	_____	_____
Urine	_____	_____

3. The ability of the kidneys to concentrate the urine maximally is impaired under each of the following conditions:
   a. Decreased renal perfusion (i.e., decreased GFR)
   b. Administration of a diuretic that inhibits active NaCl transport by the thick ascending limb of Henle's loop
   c. Nephrogenic diabetes insipidus
   d. Defect in the urea transporter in the vasa recta

   What are the mechanisms responsible for the observed impairment in the kidneys' concentrating ability during each of these conditions?

4. An individual must excrete 800 mOsm of solute in a 24-hour period. What volume of urine is required if the individual can concentrate the urine to only 400 mOsm/kg H_2O? What volume of urine is required if this individual can concentrate the urine to 1200 mOsm/kg H_2O?

5. An individual excretes 6 L/day of urine having an osmolality of 200 mOsm/kg H_2O. If plasma osmolality is 280 mOsm/kg H_2O, what are the total osmolar clearance and free-water clearance?

6

REGULATION OF EXTRACELLULAR FLUID VOLUME AND NaCl BALANCE

OBJECTIVES

Upon completion of this chapter, the student should be able to answer the following questions:

1. Why do changes in Na$^+$ balance alter the volume of extracellular fluid (ECF)?

2. What is the effective circulating volume, how is it influenced by changes in Na$^+$ balance, and how does it influence renal Na$^+$ excretion?

3. What are the mechanisms by which the body monitors the effective circulating volume?

4. What are the major signals acting on the kidneys to alter their excretion of Na$^+$?

5. How do changes in ECF volume alter Na$^+$ transport in the different segments of the nephron, and how do these changes in transport regulate renal Na$^+$ excretion?

6. What are the mechanisms involved in the formation of edema, and what role do the kidneys play in this process?

The major solutes of the ECF are the salts of Na$^+$. Of these, NaCl is the most abundant. Because NaCl is also the major determinant of ECF osmolality, alterations in Na$^+$ balance are commonly assumed to disturb ECF osmolality. However, under normal circumstances, this is not the case because the ADH and thirst systems maintain body fluid osmolality within a very narrow range. For example, the addition of NaCl to the ECF (without water) increases the Na$^+$ concentration and osmolality of this compartment. (ICF osmolality also increases because of osmotic equilibration with the ECF.) This increase in osmolality in turn stimulates thirst and the release of ADH from the posterior pituitary. The increased ingestion of water in response to thirst, together with the ADH-induced decrease in water excretion by the kidneys, quickly restores ECF osmolality to normal. However, the volume of the ECF increases in proportion to the amount of water

ingested, which in turn depends on the amount of NaCl added to the ECF. Thus, in the new steady state, the addition of NaCl to the ECF is equivalent to adding an isosmotic solution, and the volume of this compartment increases. Conversely, a decrease in the NaCl content of the ECF lowers the volume of this compartment.

The kidneys are the major route for excretion of NaCl from the body. Only about 10% of the Na$^+$ lost from the body each day is lost by nonrenal routes (e.g., in perspiration and feces). Thus, the kidneys are critically important in regulating the volume of the ECF. Under normal conditions, the kidneys keep the volume of the ECF constant by adjusting the excretion of NaCl to match the amount ingested in the diet. If ingestion exceeds excretion, ECF volume increases above normal, whereas the opposite occurs if excretion exceeds ingestion.

Neuroendocrine cells in the intestine produce a peptide hormone called **uroguanylin** in response to NaCl ingestion. This hormone has been shown to cause increased NaCl and water excretion by the kidneys. A related hormone, **guanylin**, is also produced by the intestine. It too increases renal NaCl excretion, but its effect is less than that of uroguanylin. The actions of both uroguanylin and guanylin are mediated by activation of guanylyl cyclase and include inhibition of Na^+ reabsorption by the proximal tubule and the collecting duct. The kidneys also produce uroguanylin and guanylin. The fact that these peptides are produced by the kidneys suggests a role in the intrarenal regulation of NaCl excretion. Interestingly, mice lacking the uroguanylin gene have been found to have a blunted natriuretic response to an oral NaCl load. These mice also have increased blood pressure. Thus, uroguanylin and guanylin may be important hormones involved with others in regulating the renal excretion of NaCl in response to changes in intake.

The typical diet contains approximately 140 mEq/day of Na^+ (8 g of NaCl), and thus daily Na^+ excretion is also about 140 mEq/day. However, the kidneys can vary the excretion of Na^+ over a wide range. Excretion rates as low as 10 mEq/day can be attained when individuals are placed on a low-salt diet. Conversely, the kidneys can increase their excretion rate to more than 1000 mEq/day when challenged by the ingestion of a high-salt diet. These changes in Na^+ excretion can occur with only modest changes in the ECF volume and steady-state Na^+ content of the body.

The response of the kidneys to abrupt changes in NaCl intake typically takes several hours to several days, depending on the magnitude of the change. During this transition period, the intake and excretion of Na^+ are not matched as they are in the steady state. Thus, the individual experiences either **positive Na^+** balance (intake > excretion) or **negative Na^+** balance (intake < excretion). However, by the end of the transition period, a new steady state is established, and intake once again equals excretion. Provided that the ADH and thirst systems are intact and normal, alterations in Na^+ balance change the volume, but not the

Na^+ concentration, of the ECF. Changes in ECF volume can be monitored by measuring body weight because 1 L of ECF equals 1 kg of body weight.

This chapter reviews the physiology of the receptors that monitor ECF volume and explains the various signals that act on the kidneys to regulate NaCl excretion and thereby ECF volume. In addition, the responses of the various portions of the nephron to these signals are considered. Finally, the pathophysiologic mechanisms involved in the formation of edema are presented, with emphasis on the role of NaCl handling by the kidneys.

CONCEPT OF EFFECTIVE CIRCULATING VOLUME

As described in Chapter 1, the ECF is subdivided into two compartments: blood plasma and interstitial fluid. Plasma volume is a determinant of vascular volume and thus blood pressure and cardiac output. The maintenance of Na^+ balance, and thus ECF volume, involves a complex system of sensors and effector signals that act primarily on the kidneys to regulate the excretion of NaCl. As can be appreciated from the dependence of vascular volume, blood pressure, and cardiac output on ECF volume, this complex system is designed to ensure adequate tissue perfusion. Because the primary sensors of this system are located in the large vessels of the vascular system, changes in vascular volume, blood pressure, and cardiac output are the principal factors regulating renal NaCl excretion (see later section).

In a healthy individual, changes in ECF volume result in parallel changes in vascular volume, blood pressure, and cardiac output. Thus, a decrease in ECF volume, a situation termed **volume contraction,** results in reduced vascular volume, blood pressure, and cardiac output. Conversely, an increase in ECF volume, a situation termed **volume expansion,** results in increased vascular volume, blood pressure, and cardiac output. The degree to which these cardiovascular parameters change is dependent upon the degree of volume contraction or expansion and the effectiveness of cardiovascular reflex mechanisms. When a person is in negative Na^+ balance ECF volume is decreased, and renal NaCl excretion is reduced.

Conversely, with positive Na$^+$ balance there is an increase in ECF volume, which results in enhanced renal NaCl excretion (i.e., **natriuresis**).

However, in some pathologic conditions (e.g., congestive heart failure, hepatic cirrhosis), the renal excretion of NaCl does not reflect the ECF volume. In both of these situations the volume of the ECF is increased. However, instead of increased renal NaCl excretion, as would be expected, there is a reduction in the renal excretion of NaCl. In order to explain renal Na$^+$ handling in these situations, it is necessary to understand the concept of **effective circulating volume (ECV)**. Unlike the ECF, the ECV is not a measurable and distinct body fluid compartment. The ECV refers to the portion of the ECF that is contained within the vascular system and is "effectively" perfusing the tissues (effective blood volume is another commonly used term). More specifically, the ECV reflects the activity of volume sensors located in the vascular system (see later section).

Patients with congestive heart failure frequently have an increase in the volume of the ECF, which is manifested as accumulation of fluid in the lungs **(pulmonary edema)** and peripheral tissues **(peripheral edema)**. This excess fluid is the result of NaCl and water retention by the kidneys. The kidneys' response (i.e., retention of NaCl and water) is paradoxical because the ECF volume is increased. However, this fluid is not in the vascular system but is in the interstitial fluid compartment. In addition, blood pressure and cardiac output may be reduced because of poor cardiac performance. Therefore, the sensors located in the vascular system respond as they do in ECF volume contraction and cause NaCl and water retention by the kidneys. In this situation the ECV, as monitored by the volume sensors, is decreased.

Large volumes of fluid accumulate in the peritoneal cavity of patients with advanced hepatic cirrhosis. This fluid, called **ascites,** is a component of the ECF and results from NaCl and water retention by the kidneys. Again, the response of the kidneys in this situation seems paradoxical if only ECF volume is considered. With advanced hepatic cirrhosis, blood pools in the splanchnic circulation (i.e., the damaged liver impedes the drainage of blood from the splanchnic circulation by the portal vein). Thus, volume and pressure are reduced in the portions of the vascular system where the sensors are found, but venous pressure in the portal system increases, which enhances fluid transudation into the peritoneal cavity. Hence, the kidneys respond as they would during ECF volume contraction, which results in NaCl and water retention and the accumulation of ascites fluid. As with congestive heart failure, the ECV in cirrhosis with ascites is decreased.

In healthy individuals, ECV varies directly with the volume of the ECF and in particular the volume of the vascular system (arterial and venous), the arterial blood pressure, and cardiac output. However, as noted, this is not the case in certain pathologic conditions. In the remaining sections of this chapter, the relationship between ECF volume and renal NaCl excretion in normal adults, where changes in ECV and ECF volume occur in parallel, is examined.

VOLUME-SENSING SYSTEMS

The ECF volume (or ECV) is monitored by multiple sensors (Table 6-1). A number of the sensors are located in the vascular system, and they monitor its fullness and pressure. These receptors are typically called volume receptors, or because they respond to pressure-induced stretch of the walls of the receptor (e.g., blood vessels or cardiac atria), they are also referred to as baroreceptors (see also Chapter 5). The sensors

TABLE 6-1
Volume and Na$^+$ Sensors

I. Vascular
  A. Low-pressure
    1. Cardiac atria
    2. Pulmonary vasculature
  B. High-pressure
    1. Carotid sinus
    2. Aortic arch
    3. Juxtaglomerular apparatus of the kidney
II. Central nervous system
III. Hepatic

within the liver and central nervous system (CNS) are less well understood and do not seem to be as important as the vascular sensors in monitoring the ECF volume.

Vascular Low-Pressure Volume Sensors

Volume sensors (i.e., baroreceptors) are located within the walls of the cardiac atria, right ventricle, and large pulmonary vessels and they respond to distention of these structures. Because the low-pressure side of the circulatory system has a high compliance, these sensors respond mainly to the "fullness" of the vascular system. These baroreceptors send signals to the brainstem through afferent fibers in the glossopharyngeal and vagus nerves. The activity of these sensors modulates both sympathetic nerve outflow and ADH secretion. For example, a decrease in filling of the pulmonary vessels and cardiac atria increases sympathetic nerve activity and stimulates ADH secretion. Conversely, distention of these structures decreases sympathetic nerve activity. In general, 5% to 10% changes in blood volume and pressure are necessary to evoke a response.

The cardiac atria possess an additional mechanism related to the control of renal NaCl excretion. The myocytes of the atria synthesize and store a peptide hormone. This hormone, termed **atrial natriuretic peptide (ANP),** is released when the atria are distended, which, by mechanisms outlined later in this chapter, reduces blood pressure and increases the excretion of NaCl and water by the kidneys. The ventricles of the heart also produce a natriuretic peptide termed **brain natriuretic peptide (BNP),** so named because it was first isolated from the brain. Like ANP, BNP is released from the ventricular myocytes by distention of the ventricles. Its actions are similar to those of ANP.

Vascular High-Pressure Volume Sensors

Baroreceptors are also present in the arterial side of the circulatory system, located in the wall of the aortic arch, carotid sinus, and afferent arterioles of the kidneys. The aortic arch and carotid baroreceptors send input to the brainstem through afferent fibers in the glossopharyngeal and vagus nerves. The response to this input alters sympathetic outflow and ADH secretion.

Thus, a decrease in blood pressure increases sympathetic nerve activity and ADH secretion. An increase in pressure tends to reduce sympathetic nerve activity (and activate parasympathetic nerve activity). The sensitivity of the high-pressure baroreceptors is similar to that in the low-pressure side of the vascular system; 5% to 10% changes in pressure are needed to evoke a response.

The **juxtaglomerular apparatus (JG apparatus)** of the kidneys (see Chapter 2), particularly the afferent arteriole, responds directly to changes in pressure. If perfusion pressure in the afferent arteriole is reduced, renin is released from the myocytes. Renin secretion is suppressed when perfusion pressure is increased. As described later in this chapter, renin determines blood levels of angiotensin II and aldosterone, both of which play an important role in regulating renal NaCl excretion.

Constriction of a renal artery by an atherosclerotic plaque, for example, reduces perfusion pressure to that kidney. This reduced perfusion pressure is sensed by the afferent arteriole of the JG apparatus and results in the secretion of renin. The elevated renin levels increase the production of angiotensin II, which in turn increases systemic blood pressure by its vasoconstrictor effect on arterioles throughout the vascular system. The increased systemic blood pressure is sensed by the JG apparatus of the contralateral kidney (i.e., the kidney without stenosis of its renal artery), and renin secretion from that kidney is suppressed. In addition, the high levels of angiotensin II act to inhibit renin secretion by the contralateral kidney (negative feedback). The treatment of patients with constricted renal arteries includes surgical repair of the stenotic artery, administration of angiotensin II receptor blockers, or administration of an inhibitor of angiotensin-converting enzyme (ACE). The ACE inhibitor blocks the conversion of angiotensin I to angiotensin II.

Of the two classes of baroreceptors, those on the high-pressure side of the vascular system appear to be more important in influencing sympathetic tone and ADH secretion. For example, patients with congestive heart failure often have an increased vascular volume with dilation of the atria and ventricles. This would be expected to decrease sympathetic tone and inhibit ADH secretion via the low-pressure baroreceptors. However, sympathetic tone is often increased and ADH secretion stimulated in these patients (the renin-angiotensin-aldosterone system is also activated). This reflects the activity of the high-pressure baroreceptors in response to reduced blood pressure and cardiac output secondary to the failing heart (i.e., the high-pressure baroreceptors detect a reduced ECV).

Hepatic Sensors

Although not as important as the vascular sensors, the liver also contains volume sensors that can modulate renal NaCl excretion. One type of hepatic sensor responds to pressure within the hepatic vasculature and therefore functions in a manner similar to the low- and high-pressure baroreceptors. A second type of sensor also appears to exist in the liver. This sensor responds to the $[Na^+]$ of the portal blood entering the liver. Afferent signals from both types of sensors are sent to the same area of the brainstem where afferent fibers from both the low- and high-pressure baroreceptors converge. Increased pressure within the hepatic vasculature or an increase in portal blood $[Na^+]$ results in a decrease in efferent sympathetic nerve activity.[1] As described later, this decreased sympathetic nerve activity leads to an increase in renal NaCl excretion.

Central Nervous System Na+ Sensors

Like the hepatic sensors, the CNS sensors do not appear to be as important as the vascular sensors in monitoring the ECF volume and controlling renal NaCl excretion. Nevertheless, alterations in the $[Na^+]$ of blood carried to the brain in the carotid arteries or the $[Na^+]$ of the cerebrospinal fluid (CSF) modulate renal NaCl excretion. For example, if the $[Na^+]$ in either the carotid artery blood or the CSF is increased,

there is a decrease in renal sympathetic nerve activity, which in turn leads to an increase in renal NaCl excretion. The hypothalamus appears to be the site where these sensors are located. Angiotensin II and natriuretic peptides are generated in the hypothalamus. These locally generated signals together with systemically generated angiotensin II and natriuretic peptides appear to play a role in modulating the CNS Na^+-sensing system.

Of the volume and Na^+ sensors just described, those located in the vascular system are better understood. Moreover, their function in health and disease explains quite effectively the regulation of renal NaCl excretion. Therefore, the remainder of this chapter focuses on the vascular volume sensors (i.e., baroreceptors) and their role in regulating renal NaCl excretion.

Volume Sensor Signals

When the vascular volume sensors have detected a change in the ECF volume, they send signals to the kidneys, which results in an appropriate adjustment in NaCl and water excretion. Accordingly, when the ECF volume is expanded, renal NaCl and water excretion is increased. Conversely, when the ECF volume is contracted, renal NaCl and water excretion is reduced. The signals involved in coupling the volume sensors to the kidneys are both neural and hormonal. These are summarized in Table 6-2, as are their effects on renal NaCl and water excretion.

Renal Sympathetic Nerves

As described in Chapter 2, sympathetic nerve fibers innervate the afferent and efferent arterioles of the glomerulus as well as the nephron cells. With negative Na^+ balance (i.e., ECF volume contraction), the low- and high-pressure vascular baroreceptors stimulate sympathetic nerve activity including the fibers innervating the kidneys. This has the following effects:

1. The afferent and efferent arterioles are constricted (mediated by α-adrenergic receptors). This vasoconstriction (the effect appears to be greater on the afferent arteriole) decreases the hydrostatic pressure within the glomerular capillary lumen, which results in a decreased GFR.

---

[1]The hepatic sensors also appear to be involved in the regulation of gastrointestinal NaCl absorption. For example, when the $[Na^+]$ of the portal vein blood is increased, there is a reflex reduction in jejunal NaCl absorption.

TABLE 6-2

Signals Involved in the Control of Renal NaCl and Water Excretion

Renal Sympathetic Nerves (↑Activity: ↓NaCl Excretion)
↓GFR
↑Renin secretion
↑Na⁺ reabsorption along the nephron

Renin-Angiotensin-Aldosterone (↑Secretion: ↓NaCl Excretion)
↑Angiotensin II stimulates Na⁺ reabsorption along the nephron
↑Aldosterone stimulates Na⁺ reabsorption in the thick ascending limb of Henle's loop, distal tubule, and collecting duct
↑Angiotensin II stimulates ADH secretion

Natriuretic Peptides: ANP, BNP, and Urodilatin (↑Secretion: ↑NaCl Excretion)
↑GFR
↓Renin secretion
↓Aldosterone secretion (indirect through↓ angiotensin II and direct on adrenal gland)
↓NaCl and water reabsorption by the collecting duct
↓ADH secretion and inhibition of ADH action on the distal tubule and collecting duct

ADH (↑Secretion: ↓H₂O Excretion)
↑H₂O reabsorption by the distal tubule and collecting duct

ADH, antidiuretic hormone; ANP, atrial natriuretic peptide; BNP, brain natriuretic peptide; GFR, glomerular filtration rate.

A new "renal hormone" has been discovered, a flavin adenine dinucleotide–dependent (FAD-dependent) amine oxidase named **renalase**. Renalase is similar in structure to monoamine oxidase and metabolizes cathecholamines (e.g., dopamine, epinephrine, and norepinephrine). Other tissues express renalase (e.g., skeletal muscle, heart, and small intestine), but the kidneys secrete the enzyme into the circulation. Because individuals with chronic renal failure have very low levels of renalase in their plasma, the kidney is probably the primary source of the circulating enzyme. In experimental animals, infusion of renalase decreases blood pressure and heart contractility. Although the precise role of renalase in cardiovascular function and blood pressure regulation is not known, it may be important in modulating the effect of the sympathetic nervous system and especially the effects of the sympathetic nerves on the kidney.

Renin-Angiotensin-Aldosterone System

Cells in the afferent arterioles (**juxtaglomerular cells**) are the site of synthesis, storage, and release of the proteolytic enzyme **renin**. Three factors are important in stimulating renin secretion:

With this decrease in GFR, the filtered load of Na⁺ to the nephrons is reduced.

2. Renin secretion is stimulated by the cells of the afferent arterioles (mediated by β-adrenergic receptors). As described later, renin ultimately increases the circulating levels of angiotensin II and aldosterone.

3. NaCl reabsorption along the nephron is directly stimulated (mediated by α-adrenergic receptors). Quantitatively, the most important segment influenced by sympathetic nerve activity is the proximal tubule.

As a result of these actions, increased renal sympathetic nerve activity decreases NaCl excretion, an adaptive response that works to restore ECF volume to normal, a state termed **euvolemia**. With positive Na⁺ balance (i.e., ECF volume expansion), renal sympathetic nerve activity is reduced. This generally reverses the effects just described.

1. *Perfusion pressure.* The afferent arteriole behaves as a high-pressure baroreceptor. When perfusion pressure to the kidneys is reduced, renin secretion is stimulated. Conversely, an increase in perfusion pressure inhibits renin release.

2. *Sympathetic nerve activity.* Activation of the sympathetic nerve fibers that innervate the afferent arterioles increases renin secretion (mediated by β-adrenergic receptors). Renin secretion is decreased as renal sympathetic nerve activity is decreased.

3. *Delivery of NaCl to the macula densa.* Delivery of NaCl to the macula densa regulates the GFR by a process termed **tubuloglomerular feedback** (see Chapter 3). In addition, the macula densa plays a role in renin secretion. When NaCl delivery to the macula densa is decreased, renin secretion is enhanced. Conversely, an increase in NaCl delivery inhibits renin secretion. It is likely that macula densa–mediated renin secretion

helps to maintain systemic arterial pressure under conditions of a reduced vascular volume. For example, when vascular volume is reduced, perfusion of body tissues (including the kidneys) decreases. This in turn decreases the GFR and the filtered load of NaCl. The reduced delivery of NaCl to the macula densa then stimulates renin secretion, which acts through angiotensin II (a potent vasoconstrictor) to increase the blood pressure and thereby maintain tissue perfusion.

Although many tissues express renin (e.g., brain, heart, and adrenal gland), the primary source of circulating renin is the kidneys. Renin is secreted by juxtaglomerular cells located in the afferent arteriole. At the cellular level, renin secretion is mediated by the fusion of renin-containing granules with the luminal membrane of the cell. This process is stimulated by a decrease in intracellular $[Ca^{++}]$, a response opposite to that of most secretory cells where secretion is stimulated by an increase in intracellular $[Ca^{++}]$. It is also stimulated by an increase in intracellular cAMP levels. Thus, anything that increases intracellular $[Ca^{++}]$ inhibits renin secretion. This includes stretch of the afferent arteriole (myogenic control of renin secretion), angiotensin II (i.e., feedback inhibition), and endothelin. Conversely, anything that increases intracellular cAMP stimulates renin secretion. This includes norepinephrine acting through β-adrenergic receptors and prostaglandin E_2. Increases in intracellular cGMP have been shown to stimulate renin secretion in some situations and to inhibit secretion in others. Notably, two substances that increase intracellular cGMP are ANP and nitric oxide (NO). Both inhibit renin secretion. The control of renin secretion by the macula densa (see also Chapter 3) may involve paracrine factors such as prostaglandin E_2 (stimulates renin secretion when NaCl delivery to the macula densa is decreased) and adenosine (inhibits renin secretion when NaCl delivery to the macular densa is increased).

Figure 6-1 summarizes the essential components of the renin-angiotensin-aldosterone system. Renin alone does not have a physiologic function; it functions solely as a proteolytic enzyme. Its substrate is a circulating protein, **angiotensinogen,** which is produced by the liver. Angiotensinogen is cleaved by renin to yield a 10-amino-acid peptide, **angiotensin I.** Angiotensin I

also has no known physiologic function, and it is further cleaved to an 8-amino-acid peptide, **angiotensin II,** by a converting enzyme (**ACE**) found on the surface of vascular endothelial cells. (Pulmonary and renal endothelial cells are important sites for the conversion of angiotensin I to angiotensin II.) ACE also degrades bradykinin, a potent vasodilator. Angiotensin II has several important physiologic functions, including:

1. Stimulation of aldosterone secretion by the adrenal cortex.
2. Arteriolar vasoconstriction, which increases blood pressure.
3. Stimulation of ADH secretion and thirst.
4. Enhancement of NaCl reabsorption by the proximal tubule, thick ascending limb of Henle's loop, the distal tubule, and even the collecting duct. Of these segments, the effect on the proximal tubule is quantitatively the largest.

Angiotensin II is an important secretagogue for **aldosterone.** An increase in the plasma K^+ concentration is the other important stimulus for aldosterone secretion (see Chapter 7). Aldosterone is a steroid hormone produced by the glomerulosa cells of the adrenal cortex. Aldosterone acts in a number of ways on the kidneys (see also Chapter 4). With regard to the regulation of the ECF volume, aldosterone reduces NaCl excretion by stimulating its reabsorption by the thick ascending limb of the loop of Henle, distal tubule, and collecting duct. The effect of aldosterone on renal NaCl excretion depends mainly on its ability to stimulate Na^+ reabsorption in the distal tubule as well as the collecting duct.

Aldosterone has many cellular actions in responsive cells (see Chapter 4 for details). Notably, it increases the abundance of the apical membrane Na^+-Cl^- symporter in the cells of the early portion of the distal tubule and the abundance of the epithelial Na^+ channel (ENaC) in the apical membrane of principal cells in the late portion of the distal tubule and collecting duct. By this action, Na^+ entry into the cells across the apical membrane is increased. Extrusion of Na^+ from the cell across the basolateral membrane occurs by Na^+, K^+-ATPase, the abundance of which is also increased by aldosterone. Thus, aldosterone increases the reabsorption of Na^+ from the tubular fluid by distal nephron segments, and reduced levels

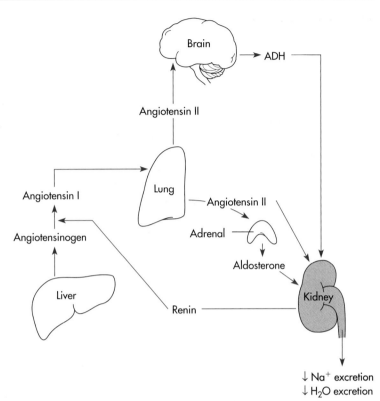

FIGURE 6-1 ■ Schematic representation of the essential components of the renin-angiotensin-aldosterone system. Activation of this system results in a decrease in the excretion of Na^+ and water by the kidneys. *Note*: Angiotensin I is converted to angiotensin II by an angiotensin-converting enzyme, which is present on all vascular endothelial cells. As shown, the endothelial cells within the lungs play a significant role in this conversion process. ADH, antidiuretic hormone. See text for details.

of aldosterone decrease the amount of Na^+ reabsorbed by these segments.

As noted, aldosterone also enhances Na^+ reabsorption by cells of the thick ascending limb of the loop of Henle. This action probably reflects increased entry of Na^+ into the cell across the apical membrane (probably by the apical membrane $1Na^+-1K^+-2Cl^-$ symporter) and increased extrusion from the cell by the basolateral membrane Na^+, K^+-ATPase.

Diseases of the adrenal cortex can alter aldosterone levels and thereby impair the ability of the kidneys to maintain Na^+ balance and euvolemia. With decreased secretion of aldosterone (hypoaldosteronism), the reabsorption of Na^+, mainly by the distal tubule and collecting duct, is reduced, and NaCl is lost in the urine. Because urinary NaCl loss can exceed the amount of NaCl ingested in the diet, negative Na^+

balance ensues, and the ECF volume decreases. In response to the ECF volume contraction, sympathetic tone is increased, and levels of renin, angiotensin II, and ADH are elevated. With increased aldosterone secretion (hyperaldosteronism), the effects are the opposite; Na^+ reabsorption, especially by the distal tubule and collecting duct, is enhanced, and excretion of NaCl is reduced. Consequently, ECF volume is increased, sympathetic tone is decreased, and the levels of renin, angiotensin II, and ADH are decreased. As described later, ANP and BNP levels are also elevated in this setting.

As summarized in Table 6-2, activation of the renin-angiotensin-aldosterone system, as occurs with ECF volume depletion, decreases the excretion of NaCl by the kidneys. This system is suppressed with ECF volume expansion, and renal NaCl excretion is therefore enhanced.

Natriuretic Peptides

The body produces a number of substances that act on the kidneys to increase Na^+ excretion.[2] Of these, natriuretic peptides produced by the heart and kidneys are best understood, and they are the focus of the following discussion.

The heart produces two natriuretic peptides. Atrial myocytes primarily produce and store the peptide hormone **atrial natriuretic peptide (ANP)**, and ventricular myocytes primarily produce and store **brain natriuretic peptide (BNP)**. Both peptides are secreted when the heart dilates (i.e., during volume expansion and with heart failure), and they act to relax vascular smooth muscle and promote NaCl and water excretion by the kidneys. The kidneys also produce a related natriuretic peptide termed urodilatin. Its actions are limited to promoting NaCl excretion by the kidneys. In general, the actions of these natriuretic peptides, as they relate to renal NaCl and water excretion, antagonize those of the renin-angiotensin-aldosterone system. These actions include:

1. Vasodilation of the afferent and vasoconstriction of the efferent arterioles of the glomerulus. This increases the GFR and the filtered load of Na^+.
2. Inhibition of renin secretion by the afferent arterioles.
3. Inhibition of aldosterone secretion by the glomerulosa cells of the adrenal cortex. This occurs by two mechanisms: (a) inhibition of renin secretion by the juxtaglomerular cells, thereby reducing angiotensin II–induced aldosterone secretion, and (b) direct inhibition of aldosterone secretion by the glomerulosa cells of the adrenal cortex.

4. Inhibition of NaCl reabsorption by the collecting duct, which is also caused in part by reduced levels of aldosterone. However, the natriuretic peptides also act directly on the collecting duct cells. Through the second messenger cyclic GMP, natriuretic peptides inhibit Na^+ channels in the apical membrane and thereby decrease Na^+ reabsorption. This effect occurs predominantly in the medullary portion of the collecting duct.
5. Inhibition of ADH secretion by the posterior pituitary and ADH action on the collecting duct. These effects decrease water reabsorption by the collecting duct and thus increase excretion of water in the urine.

These effects of the natriuretic peptides increase the excretion of NaCl and water by the kidneys. Hypothetically, a reduction in the circulating levels of these peptides would be expected to decrease NaCl and water excretion, but convincing evidence for this effect has not been reported.

Antidiuretic Hormone

As discussed in Chapter 5, a decreased ECF volume stimulates ADH secretion by the posterior pituitary. The elevated levels of ADH decrease water excretion by the kidneys, which serves to reestablish euvolemia.

CONTROL OF RENAL NaCl EXCRETION DURING EUVOLEMIA

The maintenance of Na^+ balance and therefore euvolemia requires the precise matching of the amount of NaCl ingested and the amount excreted from the body. As already noted, the kidneys are the major route for NaCl excretion. Accordingly, in a euvolemic individual we can equate daily urine NaCl excretion with daily NaCl intake.

The amount of NaCl excreted by the kidneys can vary widely. Under conditions of salt restriction (i.e., low-NaCl diet), virtually no Na^+ appears in the urine. Conversely, in individuals who ingest large quantities of NaCl, renal Na^+ excretion can exceed 1000 mEq/day. The kidneys require several days to respond maximally

---

[2]Uroguanylin and adrenomedullin are two examples of these substances. As noted earlier, uroguanylin increases renal NaCl excretion and may serve to regulate the renal excretion of ingested NaCl. Adrenomedullin is produced by many tissues including the heart, kidneys, and the adrenal medulla (whence its name is derived). It is secreted in response to a number of factors (e.g., cytokines, angiotensin II, endothelin, and increased shear stress on endothelial cells). Although structurally distinct from ANP and BNP, its actions are similar in that it reduces blood pressure, increases GFR, suppresses angiotensin II–induced secretion of aldosterone, and causes increased NaCl excretion.

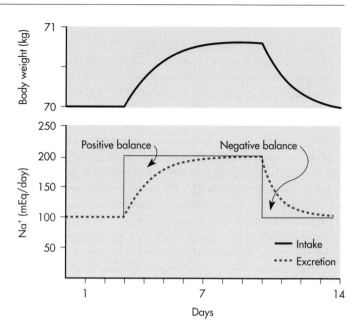

FIGURE 6-2 ■ Response to step increases and decreases in NaCl intake. Na$^+$ excretion by the kidneys (lower panel, dashed line) lags behind abrupt changes in Na$^+$ intake (lower panel, solid line). The change in ECF volume that occurs during the periods of positive and negative Na$^+$ balance is reflected in acute alterations in body weight. See text for details.

to variations in dietary NaCl intake. During the transition period, excretion does not match intake, and the individual is in either positive (intake > excretion) or negative (intake < excretion) Na$^+$ balance. This is illustrated in Figure 6-2. When Na$^+$ balance is altered during these transition periods, the ECF volume changes in parallel. (Water excretion, regulated by the ADH system, is also adjusted to keep plasma osmolality constant, resulting in an isosmotic change in ECF volume.) Thus, with positive Na$^+$ balance, the ECF volume expands (detected as an acute increase in body weight), whereas with negative Na$^+$ balance, the ECF volume contracts (detected as an acute decrease in body weight). Ultimately, renal excretion reaches a new steady state and NaCl excretion once again is matched to intake. The time course for the adjustment of renal NaCl excretion varies (hours to days) and depends on the magnitude of the change in NaCl intake. Adaptation to large changes in NaCl intake requires a longer time than adaptation to small changes in intake.

The general features of Na$^+$ handling along the nephron must be understood to comprehend how renal Na$^+$ excretion is regulated. (See Chapter 4 for the cellular mechanisms of Na$^+$ transport along the nephron.) Most (67%) of the filtered load of Na$^+$ is reabsorbed by the proximal tubule. An additional 25% is reabsorbed by the thick ascending limb of the loop of Henle and

the remainder by the distal tubule and collecting duct (Figure 6-3).

In a normal adult, the filtered load of Na$^+$ is approximately 25,000 mEq/day.

$$\textbf{Filtered load of Na}^+ = (\textbf{GFR})(\textbf{plasma [Na}^+])$$
$$= (\textbf{180 L/day})(\textbf{140 mEq/L}) \quad (6\text{-}1)$$
$$= \textbf{25,200 mEq/day}$$

With a typical diet, less than 1% of this filtered load is excreted in the urine (approximately 140 mEq/day).[3] Because of the large filtered load of Na$^+$, small changes in Na$^+$ reabsorption by the nephron can profoundly affect Na$^+$ balance and, thus, the volume of the ECF. For example, an increase in Na$^+$ excretion from 1% to 3% of the filtered load represents an additional loss of approximately 500 mEq/day of Na$^+$. Because the ECF Na$^+$ concentration is 140 mEq/L, such a Na$^+$ loss would decrease the ECF volume by more than 3 L (i.e., water excretion would parallel the loss of Na$^+$ to maintain body fluid osmolality constant: (500 mEq/day)/(140 mEq/L) = 3.6 L/day of fluid loss). Such fluid loss in a 70-kg individual would represent a 26% decrease in the ECF volume (see Chapter 1).

---

[3]The percentage of the filtered load excreted in the urine is termed fractional excretion. In this example, the fractional excretion of Na$^+$ is **140 mEq/day ÷ 25,200 mEq/day = 0.005 or 0.5%**.

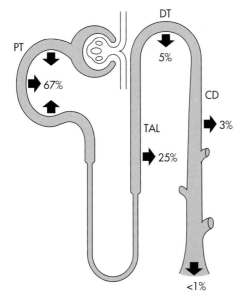

FIGURE 6-3 ■ Segmental Na$^+$ reabsorption. The percentage of the filtered load of Na$^+$ reabsorbed by each nephron segment is indicated. CD, collecting duct; DT, distal tubule; PT, proximal tubule; TAL, thick ascending limb.

In euvolemic subjects, the nephron segments distal to the loop of Henle (distal tubule and collecting duct) are the main nephron segments where Na$^+$ reabsorption is adjusted to maintain excretion at a level appropriate for dietary intake. However, this does not mean that the other portions of the nephron are not involved in this process. Because the reabsorptive capacity of the distal tubule and collecting duct is limited, these other portions of the nephron (i.e., proximal tubule and loop of Henle) must reabsorb the bulk of the filtered load of Na$^+$. Thus, during euvolemia, Na$^+$ handling by the nephron can be explained by two general processes:

1. Na$^+$ reabsorption by the proximal tubule and loop of Henle is regulated so that a relatively constant portion of the filtered load of Na$^+$ is delivered to the distal tubule. The combined action of the proximal tubule and loop of Henle reabsorbs approximately 92% of the filtered load of Na$^+$, and thus 8% of the filtered load is delivered to the distal tubule.
2. Reabsorption of this remaining portion of the filtered load of Na$^+$ by the distal tubule and collecting duct is regulated so that the

amount of Na$^+$ excreted in the urine matches the amount ingested in the diet. Thus, these later nephron segments make final adjustments in Na$^+$ excretion to maintain the euvolemic state.

Mechanisms for Maintaining the Delivery of Na$^+$ to the Distal Tubule Constant

A number of mechanisms maintain delivery of a constant fraction of the filtered load of Na$^+$ to the beginning of the distal tubule. These processes are autoregulation of the GFR (and thus the filtered load of Na$^+$), glomerulotubular balance, and load dependence of Na$^+$ reabsorption by the loop of Henle.

Autoregulation of the GFR (see Chapter 3) allows maintenance of a relatively constant filtration rate over a wide range of perfusion pressures. Because the filtration rate is constant, the filtered load of Na$^+$ to the nephrons is also kept constant.

Despite the autoregulatory control of the GFR, small variations occur. If these changes were not compensated for by an appropriate adjustment in Na$^+$ reabsorption by the nephron, Na$^+$ excretion would change markedly. Fortunately, Na$^+$ reabsorption in the euvolemic state, especially by the proximal tubule, changes in parallel with changes in the GFR. This phenomenon is termed **glomerulotubular (G-T) balance** (see Chapter 4). Thus, if the GFR increases, the amount of Na$^+$ reabsorbed by the proximal tubule also increases. The opposite occurs if the GFR decreases.

The final mechanism that helps maintain the constant delivery of Na$^+$ to the beginning of the collecting duct involves the ability of the loop of Henle to increase its reabsorptive rate in response to increased delivery of Na$^+$.

Regulation of Distal Tubule and Collecting Duct Na$^+$ Reabsorption

When delivery of Na$^+$ is constant, small adjustments in distal tubule and, to a lesser degree, collecting duct Na$^+$ reabsorption are sufficient to balance excretion with intake. (As already noted, as little as a 2% change in fractional Na$^+$ excretion produces more than a 3 L change in the volume of the ECF.) Aldosterone is the primary regulator of Na$^+$ reabsorption by the distal tubule and collecting duct and, thus, of Na^+ excretion under this condition. When aldosterone levels are elevated, Na^+ reabsorption by these segments is increased (excretion decreased). When aldosterone levels are decreased, Na^+ reabsorption is decreased (excretion increased).

In addition to aldosterone, a number of other factors, including natriuretic peptides, prostaglandins, uroguanylin, adrenomedullin, and sympathetic nerves, alter Na^+ reabsorption by the distal tubule and collecting duct. However, the relative effects of these other factors on the regulation of Na^+ reabsorption by these segments during euvolemia are unclear.

As long as variations in the dietary intake of NaCl are minor, the mechanisms previously described can regulate renal Na^+ excretion appropriately and thereby maintain euvolemia. However, these mechanisms cannot effectively handle significant changes in NaCl intake. When NaCl intake changes significantly, ECF volume expansion or ECF volume contraction occurs. In such cases, additional factors are invoked to act on the kidneys to adjust Na^+ excretion and thereby reestablish the euvolemic state.

CONTROL OF Na^+ EXCRETION WITH VOLUME EXPANSION

During ECF volume expansion, the high-pressure and low-pressure vascular volume sensors send signals to the kidneys. These signals result in increased excretion of NaCl and water. The signals acting on the kidneys include:

1. Decreased activity of the renal sympathetic nerves
2. Release of ANP and BNP from the heart and urodilatin in the kidneys
3. Inhibition of ADH secretion from the posterior pituitary and decreased ADH action on the collecting duct
4. Decreased renin secretion and thus decreased production of angiotensin II
5. Decreased aldosterone secretion, which is caused by reduced angiotensin II levels, and elevated natriuretic peptide levels

The integrated response of the nephron to these signals is illustrated in Figure 6-4. Three general

responses to ECF volume expansion occur (the numbers correlate with those encircled in Figure 6-4):

1. *The GFR increases.* The GFR increases mainly as a result of the decrease in sympathetic nerve activity. Sympathetic fibers innervate the afferent and efferent arterioles of the glomerulus and control their diameter. Decreased sympathetic nerve activity leads to arteriolar dilation. Because the effect appears to be greater on the afferent arterioles, the hydrostatic pressure within the glomerular capillary is increased, thereby increasing the GFR (because the renal plasma flow increases to a greater degree than the GFR, the filtration fraction decreases). Natriuretic peptides also increase the GFR by dilating the afferent and constricting the efferent arterioles. Thus, the increased natriuretic peptide levels that occur during ECF volume expansion contribute to this response. With the increase in the GFR, the filtered load of Na^+ increases.

2. *The reabsorption of Na^+ decreases in the proximal tubule and loop of Henle.* Several mechanisms may act to reduce Na^+ reabsorption by the proximal tubule, but the precise role of each of these mechanisms remains controversial. Because activation of the sympathetic nerve fibers that innervate this nephron segment stimulates Na^+ reabsorption, the decreased sympathetic nerve activity that results from ECF volume expansion decreases Na^+ reabsorption. In addition, angiotensin II directly stimulates Na^+ reabsorption by the proximal tubule. Because angiotensin II levels are also reduced under this condition, proximal tubule Na^+ reabsorption decreases as a result. The increased hydrostatic pressure within the glomerular capillaries also tends to increase the hydrostatic pressure within the peritubular capillaries. In addition, the decrease in filtration fraction reduces the peritubular oncotic pressure. These alterations in the capillary Starling forces reduce the absorption of solute (e.g., NaCl) and water from the lateral intercellular space and, thus, reduce tubular reabsorption. (See Chapter 4 for a complete description of this mechanism.) Both the increase in the filtered load and the

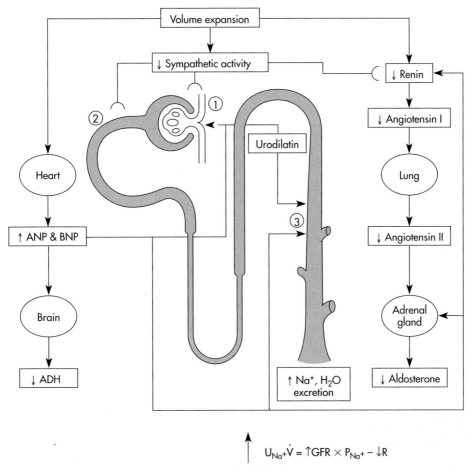

$$U_{Na^+}\dot{V} = \uparrow GFR \times P_{Na^+} - \downarrow R$$

FIGURE 6-4 ■ Integrated response to extracellular fluid volume expansion. Numbers refer to the description of the response in the text. ANP, atrial natriuretic peptide; BNP, brain natriuretic peptide; GFR, glomerular filtration rate; P_{Na^+}, plasma [Na^+]; R, tubular reabsorption of Na^+; $U_{Na^+}\dot{V}$, Na^+ excretion rate.

decrease in NaCl reabsorption by the proximal tubule result in the delivery of more NaCl to the loop of Henle. Because activation of the sympathetic nerves and aldosterone stimulates NaCl reabsorption by the loop of Henle, the reduced nerve activity and low aldosterone levels that occur with ECF volume expansion serve to reduce NaCl reabsorption by this nephron segment. Thus, the fraction of the filtered load delivered to the distal tubule is increased.

3. *Na⁺ reabsorption decreases in the distal tubule and collecting duct.* As noted, the amount of Na⁺ delivered to the distal tubule exceeds that observed in the euvolemic state (the amount of Na⁺ delivered to the distal tubule varies in proportion to the degree of ECF volume expansion). This increased load of Na⁺ overwhelms the reabsorptive capacity of the distal tubule and the collecting duct, and this capacity is even further impaired by the actions of natriuretic peptides and by the decrease in the circulating levels of aldosterone.

The final component in the response to ECF volume expansion is the excretion of water. As Na⁺ excretion increases, plasma osmolality begins to fall. This decreases the secretion of ADH. ADH secretion is also decreased in response to the elevated levels of natriuretic peptides. In addition, these natriuretic peptides inhibit the action of ADH on the collecting duct. Together, these effects decrease water reabsorption by the collecting duct and thereby increase water excretion by the kidneys. Thus, the excretion of Na^+ and water occurs in concert; euvolemia is restored, and body fluid osmolality remains constant. The time course of this response (hours to days) depends on the magnitude of the ECF volume expansion. Thus, if the degree of ECF volume expansion is small, the mechanisms just described generally restore euvolemia within 24 hours. However, with large degrees of ECF volume expansion, the response can take several days.

In brief, the renal response to ECF volume expansion involves the integrated action of all parts of the nephron: (1) the filtered load of Na^+ is increased, (2) the proximal tubule and loop of Henle reabsorption is reduced (the glomerular filtration rate is increased, whereas proximal reabsorption is decreased; thus G-T balance does not occur under this condition), and (3) the delivery of Na^+ to the distal tubule is increased. This increased delivery, along with the inhibition of distal tubule and collecting duct reabsorption, results in the excretion of a larger fraction of the filtered load of Na^+ and thus restores euvolemia.

CONTROL OF Na^+ EXCRETION WITH VOLUME CONTRACTION

During ECF volume contraction, the high-pressure and low-pressure vascular volume sensors send signals to the kidneys that reduce NaCl and water excretion. The signals that act on the kidneys include:

1. Increased renal sympathetic nerve activity
2. Increased secretion of renin, which results in elevated angiotensin II levels and, thus, increased secretion of aldosterone by the adrenal cortex
3. Inhibition of ANP and BNP secretion by the heart and urodilatin production by the kidneys
4. Stimulation of ADH secretion by the posterior pituitary

The integrated response of the nephron to these signals is illustrated in Figure 6-5. The general response

is as follows (the numbers correlate with those encircled in Figure 6-5):

1. *The GFR decreases.* Afferent and efferent arteriolar constriction occurs as a result of increased renal sympathetic nerve activity. The effect appears to be greater on the afferent than on the efferent arteriole. This causes the hydrostatic pressure in the glomerular capillary to fall and thereby decreases the GFR (because the renal plasma flow decreases more than the GFR, filtration fraction increases). The decrease in the GFR reduces the filtered load of Na^+.

2. *Na^+ reabsorption by the proximal tubule and loop of Henle is increased.* Several mechanisms augment Na^+ reabsorption in the proximal tubule. For example, increased sympathetic nerve activity and angiotensin II levels directly stimulate Na^+ reabsorption. The decreased hydrostatic pressure within the glomerular capillaries also leads to a decrease in the hydrostatic pressure within the peritubular capillaries. In addition, the increased filtration fraction results in an increase in the peritubular oncotic pressure. These alterations in the capillary Starling forces facilitate the movement of fluid from the lateral intercellular space into the capillary and thereby stimulate the reabsorption of solute (e.g., NaCl) and water by the proximal tubule. (See Chapter 4 for a complete description of this mechanism.) The reduced filtered load and enhanced proximal tubule reabsorption decrease the delivery of Na^+ to the loop of Henle. Increased sympathetic nerve activity, as well as elevated levels of angiotensin II and aldosterone, stimulates Na^+ reabsorption by the thick ascending limb. Because sympathetic nerve activity is increased and angiotensin II and aldosterone levels are elevated during ECF volume contraction, increased Na^+ reabsorption by this segment is expected. Thus, less Na^+ is delivered to the distal tubule.

3. *Na^+ reabsorption by the distal tubule and collecting duct is enhanced.* The small amount of Na^+ that is delivered to the distal tubule is almost completely reabsorbed because transport in this segment and the collecting duct is

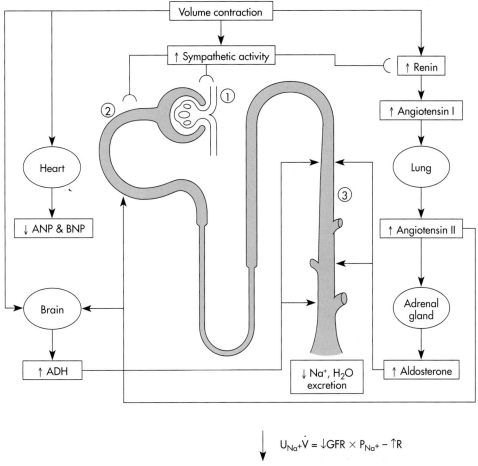

$$\downarrow \quad U_{Na^+}\dot{V} = \downarrow GFR \times P_{Na^+} - \uparrow R$$

FIGURE 6-5 ■ Extracellular fluid volume contraction. Numbers refer to the description of the response in the text. ANP, atrial natriuretic peptide; BNP, brain natriuretic peptide; GFR, glomerular filtration rate; P_{Na^+}, plasma [Na^+]; R, tubular reabsorption of Na^+. $U_{Na^+}\dot{V}$, Na^+ excretion rate.

enhanced. This stimulation of Na^+ reabsorption by the distal tubule and collecting duct is induced mainly by increased aldosterone levels. In addition, plasma levels of natriuretic peptides, which inhibit collecting duct reabsorption, are reduced.

Finally, water reabsorption by the late portion of the distal tubule and the collecting duct is enhanced by ADH, the levels of which are elevated through activation of the low- and high-pressure vascular volume sensors as well as by the elevated levels of angiotensin II. As a result, water excretion is reduced. Because both water and Na^+ are retained by the kidneys in equal

proportions, euvolemia is reestablished, and body fluid osmolality remains constant. The time course of this expansion of the ECF (hours to days) and the degree to which euvolemia is attained depend on the magnitude of the ECF volume contraction as well as the dietary intake of Na^+. Thus, the kidneys reduce Na^+ excretion, and euvolemia can be restored more quickly if additional NaCl is ingested in the diet.

In brief, the nephron's response to ECF volume contraction involves the integrated action of all its segments: (1) the filtered load of Na^+ is decreased, (2) proximal tubule and loop of Henle reabsorption is enhanced (the GFR is decreased, whereas proximal reabsorption is increased; thus G-T balance does not occur under this condition), (3) and the delivery of Na$^+$ to the distal tubule is reduced. This decreased delivery, together with enhanced Na$^+$ reabsorption by the distal tubule and collecting duct, virtually eliminates Na$^+$ from the urine.

EDEMA

Edema is the accumulation of excess fluid within the interstitial space. As described in Chapter 1, Starling forces across the capillary wall determine the movement of fluid into and out of the vascular compartment as well as the interstitial compartment. Alterations of these forces under pathologic conditions can lead to increased movement of fluid from the vascular space into the interstitium, resulting in edema formation.

The role of the kidneys in the formation of edema can be appreciated by recognizing that the interstitial compartment must contain 2 to 3 L of excess fluid before edema is detectable clinically (e.g., swelling of the ankles). The source of this fluid is the vascular compartment (i.e., plasma), which has a volume of 3 to 4 L in the healthy individual. Thus, the movement of 2 to 3 L of fluid out of the vascular compartment into the interstitial compartment would result in a marked decrease in blood pressure. This fall in blood pressure would in turn alter the Starling forces and prevent further movement of fluid from the vascular compartment into the interstitial compartment. However, retention of NaCl and water by the kidneys maintains volume of the vascular compartment and thereby maintains the blood pressure. As a result, accumulation of fluid in the interstitial compartment can continue, and edema can then develop.

Alterations in Starling Forces

In Chapter 1, the Starling forces and their determination of fluid movement across the capillary wall were explained. Edema results from a change in the Starling forces that alter these fluid dynamics. Recall that fluid movement across the capillary wall is driven by hydrostatic and oncotic pressure gradients:

$$\text{Filtration rate} = K_f \left[(P_c - P_i) - \sigma(\pi_c - \pi_i) \right] \quad \text{(6-2)}$$

where K_f = The filtration coefficient of the capillary wall (a measure of the intrinsic permeability and the surface area available for fluid flow)

P_c and P_i = the hydrostatic pressures within the lumen of the capillary and the interstitium, respectively

σ = the reflection coefficient for protein across the capillary wall (approximately 0.9 for skeletal muscle)

π_c and π_i = the oncotic pressures generated by protein within the capillary lumen and the interstitium, respectively

Capillary Hydrostatic Pressure (P$_c$) Increasing the P_c favors the movement of fluid out of the capillary or retards its movement into the capillary, thereby promoting edema formation. Normally, the resistance of the precapillary arteriole is well regulated such that changes in systemic blood pressure do not result in marked alterations in P_c. However, postcapillary resistance is not regulated to the same degree. Therefore, alterations in the pressure within the venous side of the circulation do have significant effects on P_c. Consequently, an increase in the venous pressure elevates P_c. This increases the movement of fluid into the interstitium, resulting in the accumulation of edema fluid. Common causes for increased venous pressure include venous thrombosis and congestive heart failure.

Plasma Oncotic Pressure (π$_c$) A decrease in π_c would be expected to favor movement of fluid out of the capillary lumen and inhibit its reabsorption from the interstitium. Because albumin is the most abundant plasma protein, alterations in π_c result primarily from changes in the plasma [albumin]. However, it is important to remember that changes in plasma protein concentration result in parallel changes in the protein concentration of the interstitial fluid. This reflects the fact that the reflection coefficient for protein is 0.9 and thus, proteins can cross the capillary wall. Because of the parallel changes in capillary and interstitial fluid protein concentration, the oncotic pressure gradient across the capillary wall $(\pi_c - \pi_i)$ may not change appreciably.

Lymphatic Obstruction As noted in Chapter 1, the lymphatic system serves to return interstitial fluid formed by capillary filtration to the vascular system. Obstruction of a lymphatic duct interferes with this process, and as a result interstitial fluid accumulates in the portion of the body drained by the obstructed duct (i.e., edema forms). As this interstitial fluid accumulates, the interstitial hydrostatic pressure (P_i) increases, and eventually a new steady state is reached where the Starling forces are once again balanced and no additional fluid accumulates. However, unless the obstruction is corrected, the area drained by the obstructed lymphatic duct remains edematous even in this new steady state.

Capillary Permeability An increase in capillary permeability favors increased movement of fluid across the capillary wall and, thus, accumulation of excess fluid in the interstitial compartment. The increased permeability can also alter the capillary reflection coefficient for protein(s), allowing more protein across the capillary and thus altering the protein oncotic pressure gradient ($\pi_c - \pi_i$).

Edema can be classified as localized or generalized. Localized edema, as the name denotes, represents the abnormal accumulation of interstitial fluid in a specific area or region of the body. Common causes of localized edema include insect stings and lymphatic obstruction. The venom of many stinging or biting insects contains substances that either directly increase capillary permeability or cause the release of mediators of inflammation that have a similar effect. In addition, the venom or the mediators of inflammation may cause vasodilation. Increasing the permeability of the capillary, or in some cases the postcapillary venule, increases the filtration coefficient (K_f) and can also decrease the protein reflection coefficient. Both effects can increase fluid movement out of the capillary, with the latter effect also altering the Starling forces by changing the protein oncotic pressure gradient. Starling forces are further altered in response to the vasodilation (i.e., P_c is increased). The net effect of these changes is that more fluid moves out of the capillary into the interstitium, and localized swelling occurs. Lymphatic obstruction often accompanies surgical treatment of tumors. For example, in some women with breast cancer, regional lymph nodes that drain the affected breast are surgically

removed. When those located in the axilla are removed, the draining of lymph from that arm may be impaired. As a result, the arm may develop edema.

Generalized edema results when Starling forces across all capillary beds are altered. Edema may be present in the lungs (i.e., **pulmonary edema**) or throughout the systemic circulation (i.e., **peripheral edema**). Peripheral edema is most commonly observed in the feet, ankles, and legs, where the force of gravity magnifies the changes in Starling forces (i.e., further increases P_c) and thereby causes more fluid to leave the capillary and enter the interstitium. One of the most common causes of generalized edema is congestive heart failure. In this condition, blood accumulates in the venous side of the circulation, raising P_c, which in turn causes fluid to move out of the capillary into the interstitium.

Generalized edema is also seen with renal diseases that produce the **nephrotic syndrome.** In the nephrotic syndrome the permeability of the glomerular capillary is abnormally high, causing large quantities of albumin to be filtered and lost in the urine (i.e., **proteinuria**). If the rate of loss exceeds the rate at which albumin is synthesized by the liver, the plasma [albumin] falls. The reduction in plasma protein concentration, and thus π_c, was thought to be the primary cause of edema formation in patients with the nephrotic syndrome. Because the oncotic pressure gradient across the capillary wall may not change appreciably (i.e., interstitial protein oncotic pressure also falls), it is likely that other factors are responsible for, or at least contribute to, the abnormal accumulation of fluid in the interstitial compartment. Recent evidence suggests that there is primary NaCl and water retention by the kidneys in patients with the nephrotic syndrome. This NaCl and water retention increases vascular volume and thereby leads to an increase in P_c, increased movement of fluid into the interstitial compartment, and, thus, edema formation. The distal tubule appears to be one nephron site where Na^+ reabsorption is increased; however, the factor or factors causing this increased reabsorption have not been identified.

The Role of the Kidneys

The role of the kidneys in edema-forming states is best illustrated by considering the situation that exists with heart failure (Figure 6-6). Because of decreased cardiac performance, venous pressure is elevated and perfusion

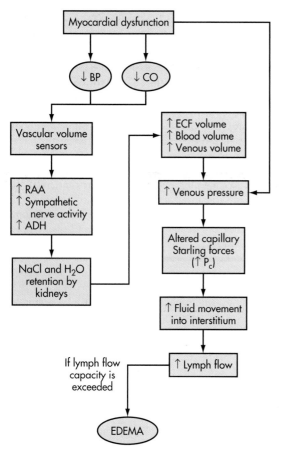

FIGURE 6-6 ■ Mechanisms involved in the formation of generalized edema with congestive heart failure. As indicated, edema forms when the capacity of the lymphatic system to return interstitial fluid to the systemic circulation is exceeded. ADH, antidiuretic hormone; BP, blood pressure; CO, cardiac output; ECF, extracellular fluid; P_c, capillary hydrostatic pressure; RAA, renin-angiotensin-aldosterone.

of the kidneys impaired. The increase in venous pressure alters the Starling forces (i.e., increased P_c) and causes fluid to accumulate in the interstitium. At the same time, decreased cardiac performance (decreased cardiac output and blood pressure) is detected by the body's vascular volume sensors as a decrease in ECV. This in turn activates the renal sympathetic nerves and the renin-angiotensin-aldosterone system and causes ADH secretion. In response to these signals the kidneys retain NaCl and water, as already described. This retention of isotonic fluid expands the ECF volume and thus blood volume. This volume expansion contributes to the increase in P_c and the accumulation of fluid in the interstitium.

As fluid begins to accumulate in the interstitium, it is taken up by the lymphatics and returned to the systemic circulation. As noted in Chapter 1, thoracic duct and right lymphatic duct flow is approximately 1 to 4 L/day. The lymphatic system can increase this flow up to 20 L/day. Because a significant amount of lymph returns to the circulation at the level of regional lymph nodes, the actual amount of interstitial fluid returned to the systemic circulation by the lymphatic system exceeds 20 L/day. Nevertheless, there is a limit to the capacity of the lymphatic system. When this limit is reached, edema fluid begins to accumulate.

The importance of NaCl retention by the kidneys in edema formation provides two approaches for treatment. The first involves dietary manipulation. The ultimate source of NaCl is the diet. Thus, if dietary intake of NaCl is restricted, the amount that can be retained by the kidneys is reduced and edema formation is limited. The second approach is to inhibit the kidneys' ability to retain NaCl. This is accomplished by the use of diuretics, which, as described in Chapter 10, inhibit Na^+ transport mechanisms in the nephron. Thus, NaCl excretion is increased and NaCl retention blunted.

SUMMARY

1. The volume of the ECF is determined by Na^+ balance. When intake of Na^+ exceeds excretion, the ECF volume increases (positive Na^+ balance). Conversely, when excretion of Na^+ exceeds intake, the ECF volume decreases (negative Na^+ balance).

The kidneys are the primary route for Na^+ excretion.

2. The kidneys adjust NaCl excretion in response to changes in ECV. The ECV reflects adequate tissue perfusion and is dependent on the ECF volume,

vascular volume, arterial blood pressure, and cardiac output. It is sensed primarily by the vascular volume sensors. In the absence of disease, ECV, ECF volume, vascular volume, arterial blood pressure, and cardiac output change in parallel (increase with positive Na$^+$ balance and decrease with negative Na$^+$ balance). In some pathologic conditions (e.g., congestive heart failure), changes in ECV, ECF volume, vascular volume, arterial blood pressure, and cardiac output do not occur in parallel. The kidneys always adjust Na$^+$ excretion to changes in the ECV (decreased Na$^+$ excretion with decreased ECV and increased Na$^+$ excretion with increased ECV) as detected by the vascular volume sensors.

3. The coordination of Na$^+$ intake and excretion, and thus the maintenance of a normal ECF volume, involves neural (renal sympathetic nerves) as well as hormonal (renin-angiotensin-aldosterone, uroguanylin, natriuretic peptides, and ADH) regulatory factors and mechanisms.

4. Under normal conditions (euvolemia), Na$^+$ excretion by the kidneys is matched to the amount of Na$^+$ ingested in the diet. The kidneys accomplish this by reabsorbing virtually all of the filtered load of Na$^+$ (typically less than 1% of the filtered load is excreted). During euvolemia, the distal tubule and collecting duct are responsible for making small adjustments in urinary Na$^+$ excretion to effect Na$^+$ balance. The major factor regulating distal tubule and collecting duct Na$^+$ reabsorption is aldosterone, which acts to stimulate Na$^+$ reabsorption.

5. With ECF volume expansion, low- and high-pressure volume sensors initiate a response that ultimately leads to increased excretion of Na$^+$ by the kidneys and a return to the euvolemic state. The components of this response include a decrease in sympathetic outflow to the kidney, a suppression of the renin-angiotensin-aldosterone system, and release of natriuretic peptides from the heart (ANP and BNP) and kidneys (urodilatin). By the actions of these effectors, GFR is enhanced, which increases the filtered load of Na$^+$, and Na$^+$ reabsorption by the nephron is reduced. Together, these changes in renal Na$^+$ handling enhance NaCl excretion.

6. With ECF volume contraction, the aforementioned sequence of events is reversed (increased sympathetic outflow to the kidney, activation of the renin-angiotensin-aldosterone system, and suppression of natriuretic peptide secretion). This decreases the GFR, enhances reabsorption of Na$^+$ by the nephron, and thus reduces NaCl excretion.

7. The development of generalized edema requires alterations in the Starling forces across capillary walls favoring the accumulation of fluid in the interstitium and retention of NaCl and water by the kidneys.

KEY WORDS AND CONCEPTS

- Extracellular fluid (ECF)
- Effective circulating volume (ECV)
- Natriuresis
- Fractional Na$^+$ excretion
- Positive Na$^+$ balance
- Negative Na$^+$ balance
- Congestive heart failure
- Euvolemia
- ECF volume expansion
- ECF volume contraction
- Atrial natriuretic peptide (ANP)
- Brain natriuretic peptide (BNP)
- Urodilatin
- Uroguanylin
- Adrenomedullin
- Renalase
- Juxtaglomerular apparatus
- Sympathetic nerve fibers
- Renin-angiotensin-aldosterone system
- Angiotensinogen
- Angiotensin-converting enzyme (ACE)
- Aldosterone
- Hypoaldosteronism
- Hyperaldosteronism
- Pulmonary edema
- Generalized edema
- Localized edema
- Nephrotic syndrome

SELF-STUDY PROBLEMS

1. An individual experiences an acute episode of vomiting and diarrhea and loses 3 kg in body weight over a 24-hour period. A blood sample

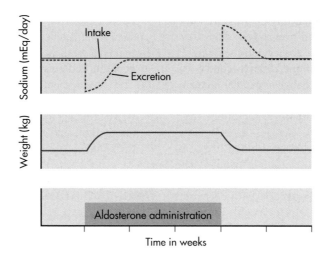

shows that the plasma [Na$^+$] is normal at 142 mEq/L. Indicate whether the following parameters would be increased, decreased, or unchanged (i.e., normal values) from what they were before this illness.

Plasma osmolality _____
ECF volume _____
ECV _____
Plasma ADH levels _____
Urine osmolality _____
Sensation of thirst _____

2. An individual is euvolemic and ingests a diet containing 100 mEq/day of Na$^+$ on average. What would be the estimated Na$^+$ excretion rate for this individual over a 24-hour period?

3. Indicate whether the regulatory signals listed are increased or decreased in response to changes in ECF volume.

	Volume expansion	Volume contraction
Renal sympathetic nerve activity	_____	_____
ANP and BNP levels	_____	_____
Angiotensin II levels	_____	_____
Aldosterone levels	_____	_____
Vasopressin levels	_____	_____

4. A 65-year-old man with congestive heart failure has developed pulmonary and peripheral edema. Over the past 2 weeks, his weight has increased by 4 kg and his serum [Na$^+$] has remained unchanged at 145 mEq/L. Assuming that the entire weight gain is the result of accumulation of edema fluid, calculate the following:

Volume of accumulated edema
  fluid _____ L
Amount of Na$^+$ retained by the
  kidneys _____ mEq

5. As shown in the illustration above, administration of high dosages of aldosterone to a normal individual leads to a transient retention of Na$^+$ by the kidneys (i.e., positive Na$^+$ balance). However, after several days, Na$^+$ excretion increases to the level at which it was before hormone administration. When the hormone is stopped, Na$^+$ excretion transiently increases (i.e., negative Na$^+$ balance) but returns to its initial level over several days. Delineate the mechanisms involved in these transient changes in Na$^+$ excretion.

6. A 55-year-old woman has congestive heart failure. On physical examination she is found to have peripheral and pulmonary edema. Her serum $[Na^+]$ is normal at 142 mEq/L. For each of the following, predict whether the values would be increased, decreased, or unchanged from what would be predicted for a healthy individual.

ECF volume	_____
ECV	_____
Plasma osmolality	_____
Fractional Na^+ excretion	_____
Renal sympathetic nerve activity	_____
ANP and BNP levels	_____
Angiotensin II levels	_____
Aldosterone levels	_____
Vasopressin levels	_____

7 REGULATION OF POTASSIUM BALANCE

OBJECTIVES

Upon completion of this chapter, the student should be able to answer the following questions:

1. How does the body maintain K$^+$ homeostasis?

2. What is the distribution of K$^+$ within the body compartments? Why is this distribution important?

3. What are the hormones and factors that regulate plasma K$^+$ levels? Why is this regulation important?

4. How do the various segments of the nephron transport K$^+$, and how does the mechanism of K$^+$ transport by these segments determine how much K$^+$ is excreted in the urine?

5. Why are the distal tubule and collecting duct so important in regulating K$^+$ excretion?

6. How do plasma K$^+$ levels, aldosterone, ADH, tubular fluid flow rate, and acid-base balance influence K$^+$ excretion?

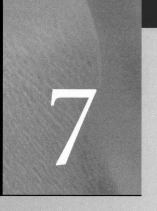K$^+$ is one of the most abundant cations in the body, and it is critical for many cell functions including cell volume regulation, intracellular pH regulation, DNA and protein synthesis, growth, enzyme function, resting membrane potential, and cardiac and neuromuscular activity. Despite wide fluctuations in dietary K$^+$ intake, its concentration ([K$^+$]) in cells and extracellular fluid (ECF) remains remarkably constant. Two sets of regulatory mechanisms safeguard K$^+$ homeostasis. First, several mechanisms regulate the [K$^+$] in the ECF. Second, other mechanisms maintain the amount of K$^+$ in the body constant by adjusting renal K$^+$ excretion to match dietary K$^+$ intake. It is the kidneys that regulate K$^+$ excretion.

OVERVIEW OF K$^+$ HOMEOSTASIS

Total body K$^+$ is 50 mEq/kg of body weight, or 3500 mEq for a 70-kg individual. A total of 98% of the K$^+$ in the body is located within cells, where its average [K$^+$] is 150 mEq/L. A high intracellular [K$^+$] is required for many cell functions, including cell growth and division and volume regulation. Only 2% of total body K$^+$ is located in the ECF, where its normal concentration is approximately 4 mEq/L. A [K$^+$] in the ECF that exceeds 5.0 mEq/L constitutes **hyperkalemia.** Conversely, a [K$^+$] in the ECF of less than 3.5 mEq/L constitutes **hypokalemia.**

Hypokalemia is one of the most common electrolyte disorders in clinical practice and can be observed in

113

as many as 20% of hospitalized patients. The most common causes of hypokalemia include administration of diuretic drugs (see Chapter 10), surreptitious vomiting (i.e., bulimia), and severe diarrhea. Gitelman's syndrome (a genetic defect in the Na^+-Cl^- symporter in the apical membrane of distal tubule cells) also causes hypokalemia (see Chapter 4, Table 4-3). Hyperkalemia is also a common electrolyte disorder and is seen in 1% to 10% of hospitalized patients. Hyperkalemia is often seen in patients with renal failure, in patients taking drugs including ACE inhibitors and K^+-sparing diuretics, in patients with hyperglycemia (i.e., high blood sugar), and in elderly patients. **Pseudohyperkalemia,** a falsely high plasma $[K^+]$, is caused by traumatic lysis of red blood cells during a blood drawing. Red blood cells, like all cells, contain K^+, and lysis of red blood cells releases K^+ into the plasma, artificially elevating plasma $[K^+]$.

The large concentration difference of K^+ across cell membranes (approximately 146 mEq/L) is maintained by the operation of Na^+, K^+-ATPase. This K^+ gradient is important in maintaining the potential difference across cell membranes. Thus, K^+ is critical for the excitability of nerve and muscle cells as well as for the contractility of cardiac, skeletal, and smooth muscle cells (Figure 7-1).

Cardiac arrhythmias are produced by both hypokalemia and hyperkalemia. The electrocardiogram (ECG; Figure 7-2) monitors the electrical activity of the heart and is a fast and easy way to determine whether changes in the plasma $[K^+]$ influence the heart and other excitable cells. In contrast, measurements of the plasma $[K^+]$ by the clinical laboratory require a blood sample, and values are often not immediately available. The first sign of hyperkalemia is the appearance of tall, thin T waves in the ECG. Further increases in the plasma $[K^+]$ prolong the PR interval, depress the ST segment, and lengthen the QRS interval of the ECG. Finally, as the plasma $[K^+]$ approaches 10 mEq/L, the P wave disappears, the QRS interval broadens, the ECG appears as a sine wave, and the ventricles fibrillate (i.e., manifest rapid, uncoordinated contractions of muscle fibers). Hypokalemia prolongs the QT interval, inverts the T wave, and lowers the ST segment of the ECG.

After a meal, the K^+ absorbed by the gastrointestinal tract enters the ECF within minutes (Figure 7-3). If the K^+ ingested during a normal meal ($\approx$33 mEq) were to remain in the ECF compartment (14 L),

FIGURE 7-1 ■ The effects of variations in plasma $[K^+]$ on the resting membrane potential of skeletal muscle. Hyperkalemia causes the membrane potential to become less negative and decreases the excitability by inactivating fast Na^+ channels, which are responsible for the depolarizing phase of the action potential. Hypokalemia hyperpolarizes the membrane potential and thereby reduces excitability.

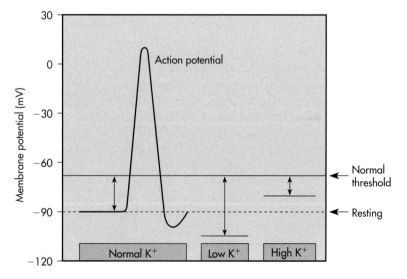

the plasma [K$^+$] would increase by a potentially lethal 2.4 mEq/L (33 mEq added to 14 L of ECF):

$$33 \text{ mEq}/14 \text{ L} = 2.4 \text{ mEq/L} \qquad (7\text{-}1)$$

This rise in the plasma [K$^+$] is prevented by the rapid (minutes) uptake of K$^+$ into cells. Because the excretion of K$^+$ by the kidneys after a meal is relatively slow (hours), the uptake of K$^+$ by cells is essential to prevent life-threatening hyperkalemia. Maintaining total body K$^+$ constant requires that all the K$^+$ absorbed by the gastrointestinal tract is eventually excreted by the kidneys. This process requires about 6 hours.

REGULATION OF PLASMA [K$^+$]

As illustrated in Figure 7-3 and Table 7-1, several hormones, including epinephrine, insulin, and aldosterone, increase K$^+$ uptake into skeletal muscle, liver, bone, and red blood cells by stimulating Na$^+$,K$^+$-ATPase, the Na$^+$-K$^+$-2Cl$^-$ symporter, and the Na$^+$-Cl$^-$ symporter in these cells. Acute stimulation of K$^+$ uptake (i.e., within minutes) is mediated by an increased turnover rate of existing Na$^+$,K$^+$-ATPase, Na$^+$-K$^+$-2Cl$^-$, and Na$^+$-Cl$^-$ transporters, whereas the chronic increase in K$^+$ uptake (i.e., within hours to days) is mediated by an increase in the quantity of Na$^+$,K$^+$-ATPase. A rise in the plasma [K$^+$] that follows K$^+$ absorption by the gastrointestinal tract stimulates insulin secretion from the pancreas, aldosterone release from the adrenal cortex, and epinephrine secretion from the adrenal medulla. In contrast, a decrease in the plasma [K$^+$] inhibits the release of these hormones. Whereas insulin and epinephrine act within a few minutes, aldosterone requires about an hour to stimulate K$^+$ uptake into cells.

FIGURE 7-2 ■ Electrocardiograms from individuals with varying plasma [K$^+$]. Hyperkalemia increases the height of the T wave, and hypokalemia inverts the T wave. See the text for details. (Modified from Barker L, Burton J, Zieve P: Principles of ambulatory medicine, ed 5, Baltimore, 1999, Williams & Wilkins.)

	Serum potassium mEq/L	ECG	
Hyperkalemia	10		Ventricular fibrillation
	9		Auricular standstil, intraventricular block
	8		Prolonged PR interval, depressed ST segment, high T wave
	7		High T wave
Normal	4–5		Normal
Hypokalemia	3.5		Low T wave
	3		Low T wave, high U wave
	2.5		Low T wave, high U wave, low ST segment

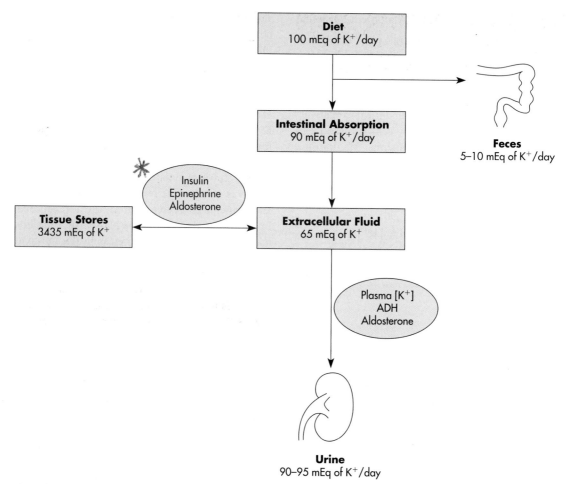

FIGURE 7-3 ■ Overview of potassium homeostasis. An increase in plasma insulin, epinephrine, or aldosterone stimulates K+ movement into cells and decreases plasma [K+], whereas a fall in the plasma concentration of these hormones increases plasma [K+]. The amount of K+ in the body is determined by the kidneys. An individual is in K+ balance when dietary intake and urinary output (plus output by the gastrointestinal tract) are equal. The excretion of K+ by the kidneys is regulated by plasma [K+], aldosterone, and antidiuretic hormone (ADH).

Epinephrine

Catecholamines affect the distribution of K+ across cell membranes by activating α- and β_2-adrenergic receptors. The stimulation of α-adrenoceptors releases K+ from cells, especially in the liver, whereas the stimulation of β_2-adrenceptors promotes K+ uptake by cells.

For example, the activation of β_2-adrenoceptors after exercise is important in preventing hyperkalemia. The rise in plasma [K+] after a K+-rich meal is greater if the patient has been pretreated with propranolol, a β_2-adrenoceptor antagonist. Furthermore, the release of epinephrine during stress (e.g., myocardial ischemia) can rapidly lower the plasma [K+].

Insulin

Insulin also stimulates K+ uptake into cells. The importance of insulin is illustrated by two observations.

TABLE 7-1
Major Factors, Hormones, and Drugs Influencing the Distribution of K$^+$ between the Intracellular and Extracellular Fluid Compartments

Physiologic: Keep Plasma [K$^+$] Constant
Epinephrine
Insulin
Aldosterone

Pathophysiologic: Displace Plasma [K$^+$] from Normal
Acid-base balance
Plasma osmolality
Cell lysis
Exercise

Drugs That Induce Hyperkalemia
Dietary potassium supplements
Angiotensin-converting enzyme (ACE) inhibitors
K$^+$-sparing diuretics
Heparin

First, the rise in plasma [K$^+$] after a K$^+$-rich meal is greater in patients with diabetes mellitus (i.e., insulin deficiency) than in healthy people. Second, insulin (and glucose to prevent insulin-induced hypoglycemia) can be infused to correct hyperkalemia. Insulin is the most important hormone that shifts K$^+$ into cells after the ingestion of K$^+$ in a meal.

Aldosterone

Aldosterone, like catecholamines and insulin, also promotes K$^+$ uptake into cells. A rise in aldosterone levels (e.g., primary aldosteronism) causes hypokalemia, whereas a fall in aldosterone levels (e.g., Addison's disease) causes hyperkalemia. As discussed later, aldosterone also stimulates urinary K$^+$ excretion. Thus, aldosterone alters the plasma [K$^+$] by acting on K$^+$ uptake into cells and by altering urinary K$^+$ excretion.

ALTERATIONS OF PLASMA [K$^+$]

Several factors can alter the plasma [K$^+$] (see Table 7-1). These factors are not involved in the regulation of the plasma [K$^+$] but rather alter the movement of K$^+$ between the ICF and ECF and thus cause the development of hypo- or hyperkalemia.

Acid-Base Balance

In general, metabolic acidosis increases the plasma [K$^+$], whereas metabolic alkalosis decreases it. In contrast, respiratory acid-base disorders have little or no effect on the plasma [K$^+$]. Metabolic acidosis produced by the addition of inorganic acids (e.g., HCl, H$_2$SO$_4$) increases the plasma [K$^+$] much more than an equivalent acidosis produced by the accumulation of organic acids (e.g., lactic acid, acetic acid, keto acids). The reduced pH (i.e., increased [H$^+$]) promotes the movement of H$^+$ into cells and the reciprocal movement of K$^+$ out of cells to maintain electroneutrality. This effect of acidosis occurs in part because acidosis inhibits the transporters that accumulate K$^+$ inside cells, including the Na$^+$,K$^+$-ATPase and the Na$^+$-K$^+$-2Cl$^-$ symporter. In addition, the movement of H$^+$ into cells occurs as the cells buffer changes in the [H$^+$] of the ECF (see Chapter 8). As H$^+$ moves across the cell membranes, K$^+$ moves in the opposite direction, and, thus, cations are neither gained nor lost across cell membranes. Metabolic alkalosis has the opposite effect; the plasma [K$^+$] decreases as K$^+$ moves into cells and H$^+$ exits.

Although organic acids produce a metabolic acidosis, they do not cause significant hyperkalemia. Two explanations have been suggested for the reduced ability of organic acids to cause hyperkalemia. First, the organic anion may enter the cell with H$^+$ and thereby eliminate the need for K$^+$/H$^+$ exchange across the membrane. Second, organic anions may stimulate insulin secretion, which moves K$^+$ into cells. This movement may counteract the direct effect of the acidosis, which moves K$^+$ out of cells.

Plasma Osmolality

The osmolality of the plasma also influences the distribution of K$^+$ across cell membranes. An increase in the osmolality of the ECF enhances K$^+$ release by cells and, thus, increases extracellular [K$^+$]. The plasma [K$^+$] may increase by 0.4 to 0.8 mEq/L for an elevation of 10 mOsm/kg H$_2$O in plasma osmolality. In patients with diabetes mellitus who do not take insulin, plasma K$^+$ is often elevated in part because of the lack of insulin and in part because of the increase in plasma [glucose] (i.e., from a normal value of ~100 mg/dL to as high as ~1200 mg/dL), which increases plasma osmolality. Hypo-osmolality has the opposite action.

The alterations in plasma [K$^+$] associated with changes in osmolality are related to changes in cell volume. For example, as plasma osmolality increases, water leaves cells because of the osmotic gradient across the plasma membrane (see Chapter 1). Water leaves cells until the intracellular osmolality equals that of the ECF. This loss of water shrinks cells and causes the cell [K$^+$] to rise. The rise in intracellular [K$^+$] provides a driving force for the exit of K$^+$ from cells. This sequence increases plasma [K$^+$]. A fall in plasma osmolality has the opposite effect.

Cell Lysis

Cell lysis causes hyperkalemia, which results from the addition of intracellular K$^+$ to the ECF. Severe trauma (e.g., burns) and some conditions such as **tumor lysis syndrome** (i.e., chemotherapy-induced destruction of tumor cells) and **rhabdomyolysis** (i.e., destruction of skeletal muscle) destroy cells and release K$^+$ and other cell solutes into the ECF. In addition, gastric ulcers may cause the seepage of red blood cells into the gastrointestinal tract. The blood cells are digested, and the K$^+$ released from the cells is absorbed and can cause hyperkalemia.

Exercise

During exercise, more K$^+$ is released from skeletal muscle cells than during rest. The ensuing hyperkalemia depends on the degree of exercise. In people walking slowly, the plasma [K$^+$] increases by 0.3 mEq/L. The plasma [K$^+$] may increase by 2.0 mEq/L with vigorous exercise.

Exercise-induced changes in the plasma [K$^+$] usually do not produce symptoms and are reversed after several minutes of rest. However, exercise can lead to life-threatening hyperkalemia in individuals (1) who have endocrine disorders that affect the release of insulin, epinephrine, or aldosterone; (2) whose ability to excrete K$^+$ is impaired (e.g., renal failure); or (3) who take certain medications, such as β_2-adrenergic blockers. For example, during exercise, the plasma [K$^+$] may increase by at least 2 to 4 mEq/L in individuals who take β_2-adrenergic receptor antagonists for hypertension.

Because acid-base balance, plasma osmolality, cell lysis, and exercise do not maintain the plasma [K$^+$] at a normal value, they do not contribute to K$^+$ homeostasis (see Table 7-1). The extent to which these pathophysiologic states alter the plasma [K$^+$] depends on the integrity of the homeostatic mechanisms that regulate plasma [K$^+$] (e.g., the secretion of epinephrine, insulin, and aldosterone).

K$^+$ EXCRETION BY THE KIDNEYS

The kidneys play a major role in maintaining K$^+$ balance. As illustrated in Figure 7-3, the kidneys excrete 90% to 95% of the K$^+$ ingested in the diet. Excretion equals intake even when intake increases by as much as 10-fold. This balance of urinary excretion and dietary intake underscores the importance of the kidneys in maintaining K$^+$ homeostasis. Although small amounts of K$^+$ are lost each day in feces and sweat (approximately 5% to 10% of the K$^+$ ingested in the diet), this amount is essentially constant, is not regulated, and therefore is relatively less important than the K$^+$ excreted by the kidneys. K$^+$ secretion from the blood into the tubular fluid by the cells of the distal tubule and collecting duct system is the key factor in determining urinary K$^+$ excretion (Figure 7-4).

Because K$^+$ is not bound to plasma proteins, it is freely filtered by the glomerulus. When individuals ingest 100 mEq of K$^+$ per day, urinary K$^+$ excretion is about 15% of the amount filtered. Accordingly, K$^+$ must be reabsorbed along the nephron. When dietary K$^+$ intake increases, however, K$^+$ excretion can exceed the amount filtered. Thus, K$^+$ can also be secreted.

The proximal tubule reabsorbs about 67% of the filtered K$^+$ under most conditions. Approximately 20% of the filtered K$^+$ is reabsorbed by the loop of Henle, and, as with the proximal tubule, the amount reabsorbed is a constant fraction of the amount filtered. In contrast to these segments, which can only reabsorb K$^+$, the distal tubule and collecting duct are able to reabsorb or secrete K$^+$. The rate of K$^+$ reabsorption or secretion by the distal tubule and collecting

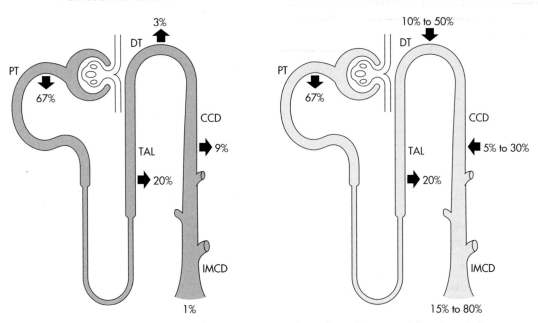

FIGURE 7-4 ■ K⁺ transport along the nephron. K⁺ excretion depends on the rate and direction of K⁺ transport by the distal tubule and collecting duct. Percentages refer to the amount of filtered K⁺ reabsorbed or secreted by each nephron segment. **Left,** Dietary K⁺ depletion. An amount of K⁺ equal to 1% of the filtered load of K⁺ is excreted. **Right,** Normal and increased dietary K⁺ intake. An amount of K⁺ equal to 15% to 80% of the filtered load is excreted. CCD, cortical collecting duct; DT, distal tubule; IMCD, inner medullary collecting duct; PT, proximal tubule; TAL, thick ascending limb.

duct depends on a variety of hormones and factors. When ingesting 100 mEq/day of K⁺, K⁺ is secreted by these nephron segments. A rise in dietary K⁺ intake increases K⁺ secretion. K⁺ secretion can increase the amount of K⁺ that appears in the urine so that it approaches 80% of the amount filtered (see Figure 7-4). In contrast, a low-K⁺ diet activates K⁺ reabsorption along the distal tubule and collecting duct so that urinary excretion falls to about 1% of the K⁺ filtered by the glomerulus (see Figure 7-4). The kidneys cannot reduce K⁺ excretion to the same low levels as they can for Na⁺ (i.e., 0.2%). Therefore, hypokalemia can develop in individuals placed on a K⁺-deficient diet. Because the magnitude and direction of K⁺ transport by the distal tubule and collecting duct are variable, the overall rate of urinary K⁺ excretion is determined by these tubular segments.

In individuals with advanced **renal disease,** the kidneys are unable to eliminate K⁺ from the body. Therefore, the plasma [K⁺] rises. The resulting hyperkalemia reduces the resting membrane potential (i.e., the voltage becomes less negative), which decreases the excitability of neurons, cardiac cells, and muscle cells by inactivating fast Na⁺ channels, which are critical for the depolarization phase of the action potential (see Figure 7-1). Severe, rapid increases in the plasma [K⁺] can lead to cardiac arrest and death. In contrast, in patients taking diuretic drugs for hypertension, urinary K⁺ excretion often exceeds dietary K⁺ intake. Accordingly, the K⁺ balance is negative, and hypokalemia develops. This decline in the extracellular [K⁺] hyperpolarizes the resting cell membrane (i.e., the voltage becomes more negative) and reduces the excitability of neurons, cardiac cells, and muscle cells.

Severe hypokalemia can lead to paralysis, cardiac arrhythmias, and death. Hypokalemia can also impair the ability of the kidneys to concentrate the urine and can stimulate the renal production of NH_4^+, which affects acid-base balance (see Chapter 8). Therefore, the maintenance of a high intracellular $[K^+]$, a low extracellular $[K^+]$, and a high K^+ concentration gradient across cell membranes is essential for a number of cellular functions.

CELLULAR MECHANISMS OF K⁺ SECRETION BY PRINCIPAL CELLS IN THE DISTAL TUBULE AND COLLECTING DUCT

Figure 7-5 illustrates the cellular mechanism of K^+ secretion by principal cells in the distal tubule and collecting duct. Secretion from the blood into the tubule lumen is a two-step process: (1) K^+ uptake from the blood across the basolateral membrane by Na^+, K^+-ATPase and (2) diffusion of K^+ from the cell into the tubular fluid through K^+ channels. The Na^+, K^+-ATPase creates a high intracellular $[K^+]$, which provides the chemical driving force for K^+ exit across the apical membrane through K^+ channels. Although K^+ channels are also present in the basolateral membrane, K^+ preferentially leaves the cell across the apical membrane and enters the tubular fluid. K^+ transport follows this route for two reasons. First, the electrochemical gradient of K^+ across the apical membrane favors its downhill movement into the tubular fluid. Second, the permeability of the apical membrane to K^+ is greater than that of the basolateral membrane. Therefore, K^+ preferentially diffuses across the apical membrane into the tubular fluid. The three major factors that control the rate of K^+ secretion by the distal tubule and the collecting duct are:

1. The activity of Na^+, K^+-ATPase
2. The driving force (electrochemical gradient) for K^+ movement across the apical membrane
3. The permeability of the apical membrane to K^+

Every change in K^+ secretion results from an alteration in one or more of these factors.

Intercalated cells reabsorb K^+ by a H^+, K^+-ATPase transport mechanism located in the apical membrane (see Chapter 4). This transporter mediates K^+ uptake in exchange for H^+. The pathway of K^+ exit from intercalated cells into the blood is unknown. The reabsorption of K^+ is activated by a low-K^+ diet.

REGULATION OF K⁺ SECRETION BY THE DISTAL TUBULE AND COLLECTING DUCT

The regulation of K^+ excretion is achieved mainly by alterations in K^+ secretion by principal cells of the distal tubule and collecting duct. Plasma $[K^+]$ and aldosterone are the major physiologic regulators of K^+ secretion. Antidiuretic hormone (ADH) also stimulates K^+ secretion; however, it is less important than the plasma $[K^+]$ and aldosterone. Other factors, including the flow rate of tubular fluid and acid-base balance, influence K^+ secretion by the distal tubule and collecting duct. However, they are not homeostatic mechanisms because they disturb K^+ balance (Table 7-2).

Plasma [K⁺]

Plasma $[K^+]$ is an important determinant of K^+ secretion by the distal tubule and collecting duct (Figure 7-6). Hyperkalemia (e.g., resulting from a high-K^+ diet or from rhabdomyolysis) stimulates K^+ secretion within minutes. Several mechanisms are involved. First, hyperkalemia stimulates Na^+, K^+-ATPase and thereby increases K^+ uptake across the basolateral membrane. This uptake raises the intracellular $[K^+]$ and increases the electrochemical driving force for K^+ exit across the apical membrane. Second, hyperkalemia also increases the permeability of the apical membrane to K^+. Third, hyperkalemia stimulates aldosterone secretion by the adrenal cortex, which, as discussed later, acts synergistically with the plasma $[K^+]$ to stimulate K^+ secretion. Fourth, hyperkalemia also increases the flow rate of tubular fluid, which, as discussed subsequently, stimulates K^+ secretion by the distal tubule and collecting duct.

Hypokalemia (e.g., caused by a low-K^+ diet or K^+ loss in diarrhea fluid) decreases K^+ secretion by actions opposite to those described for hyperkalemia.

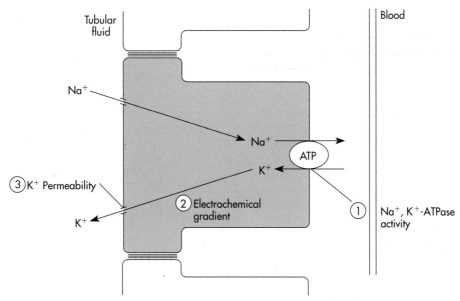

FIGURE 7-5 ■ Cellular mechanism of K$^+$ secretion by a principal cell in the distal tubule and collecting duct. The numbers indicate the sites where K$^+$ secretion is regulated. 1, Na$^+$, K$^+$-ATPase; 2, electrochemical gradient of K$^+$ across the apical membrane; 3, K$^+$ permeability of the apical membrane.

Hence, hypokalemia inhibits Na$^+$, K$^+$-ATPase, decreases the electrochemical driving force for K$^+$ efflux across the apical membrane, reduces the permeability of the apical membrane to K$^+$, and reduces plasma aldosterone levels.

Chronic hypokalemia (plasma [K$^+$] < 3.5 mEq/L) occurs most often in patients who receive diuretics for hypertension. Hypokalemia also occurs in patients who vomit, have nasogastric suction, have diarrhea, abuse laxatives, or have hyperaldosteronism. Hypokalemia occurs because the excretion of K$^+$ by the kidneys exceeds the dietary intake of K$^+$. Vomiting, nasogastric suction, diuretics, and diarrhea all can decrease the ECF volume, which in turn stimulates aldosterone secretion (see Chapter 6). Because aldosterone stimulates K$^+$ excretion by the kidneys, its action contributes to the development of hypokalemia.

   Chronic hyperkalemia (plasma [K$^+$] > 5.0 mEq/L) occurs most frequently in individuals with reduced urine flow, low plasma aldosterone levels, and renal disease in which the glomerular filtration rate falls below 20% of normal. In these individuals, hyperkalemia occurs because the excretion of K$^+$ by the kidneys is less than the dietary intake of K$^+$. Less common causes for hyperkalemia occur in people with deficiencies of insulin, epinephrine, and aldosterone secretion or in people with metabolic acidosis caused by inorganic acids.

TABLE 7-2
Major Factors and Hormones Influencing K$^+$ Excretion

Physiologic: Keep K$^+$ Balance Constant
Plasma [K$^+$]
Aldosterone
Antidiuretic hormone (ADH)

Pathophysiologic: Displace K$^+$ Balance
Flow rate of tubule fluid
Acid-base balance
Glucocorticoids

Aldosterone

A chronic (i.e., 24 hours or more) elevation in the plasma aldosterone concentration enhances K^+ secretion across principal cells in the distal tubule and collecting duct (Figure 7-7) by five mechanisms: (1) increasing the amount of Na^+,K^+-ATPase in the basolateral membrane; (2) increasing the expression of the sodium channel (ENaC) in the apical cell membrane; (3) elevating SGK1 (*s*erum *g*lucocorticoid stimulated *k*inase) levels, which also increases the expression of ENaC in the apical membrane and activates K^+ channels; (4) stimulating CAP1 (*c*hannel *a*ctivating *p*rotease, also called **prostatin**), which directly activates ENaC; and (5) stimulating the permeability of the apical membrane to K^+.

The cellular mechanisms by which aldosterone affects the expression and activity of Na^+,K^+-ATPase and ENaC (preceding actions 1 to 4) have been described (see Chapter 4). Aldosterone increases the apical membrane K^+ permeability by increasing the number of K^+ channels in the membrane. However, the cellular mechanisms involved in this response

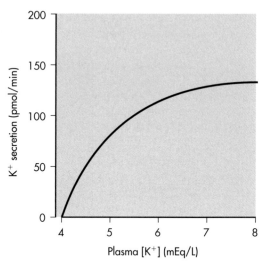

FIGURE 7-6 ■ The relationship between plasma $[K^+]$ and K^+ secretion by the distal tubule and the cortical collecting duct.

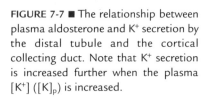

FIGURE 7-7 ■ The relationship between plasma aldosterone and K^+ secretion by the distal tubule and the cortical collecting duct. Note that K^+ secretion is increased further when the plasma $[K^+]$ ($[K]_p$) is increased.

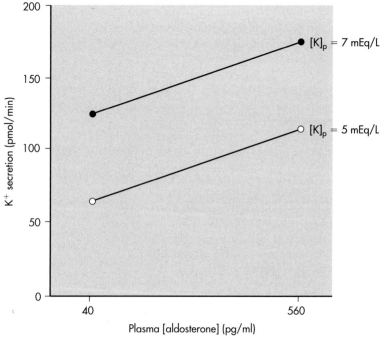

are not completely known. Increased expression of the Na^+, K^+-ATPase facilitates K^+ uptake across the basolateral membrane into cells and thereby elevates intracellular $[K^+]$. The increase in the number and activity of Na^+ channels enhances Na^+ entry into the cell from tubule fluid, an effect that depolarizes the apical membrane voltage. The depolarization of the apical membrane and increased intracellular $[K^+]$ enhance the electrochemical driving force for K^+ secretion from the cell into the tubule fluid. Taken together, these actions increase the cell $[K^+]$ and enhance the driving force for K^+ exit across the apical membrane. Aldosterone secretion is increased by hyperkalemia and by angiotensin II (after activation of the renin-angiotensin system). Aldosterone secretion is decreased by hypokalemia and natriuretic peptides released from the heart.

Although an acute (i.e., within hours) increase in aldosterone levels enhances the activity of Na^+, K^+-ATPase, K^+ excretion does not increase. The reason for this is related to the effect of aldosterone on Na^+ reabsorption and tubular flow. Aldosterone stimulates Na^+ reabsorption and water reabsorption and, thus, decreases tubular flow. The decrease in flow in turn decreases K^+ secretion (as discussed in more detail later). However, chronic stimulation of Na^+ reabsorption expands the ECF and thereby returns tubular flow to normal. These actions allow the direct stimulatory effect of aldosterone on the distal tubule and collecting duct to enhance K^+ excretion.

Antidiuretic Hormone

Although ADH does not affect urinary K^+ excretion, this hormone does stimulate K^+ secretion by the distal tubule and collecting duct (Figure 7-8). ADH increases the electrochemical driving force for K^+ exit across the apical membrane of principal cells by stimulating Na^+ uptake across the apical membrane of principal cells. The increased Na^+ uptake reduces the electrical potential difference across the apical membrane (i.e., the interior of the cell becomes less negatively charged). Despite this effect, ADH does not change K^+ secretion by these nephron segments. The reason for this is

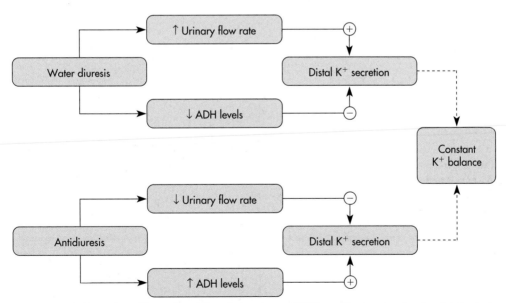

FIGURE 7-8 ■ Opposing effects of antidiuretic hormone (ADH) on K^+ secretion by the distal tubule and cortical collecting duct. Secretion is stimulated by an increase in the electrochemical gradient for K^+ across the apical membrane and by an increase in the K^+ permeability of the apical membrane. In contrast, secretion is reduced by a fall in the flow rate of tubular fluid. Because these effects oppose each other, net K^+ secretion is not affected by ADH.

related to the effect of ADH on tubular fluid flow. ADH decreases tubular fluid flow by stimulating water reabsorption. The decrease in tubular flow in turn reduces K^+ secretion (explained later). The inhibitory effect of decreased flow of tubular fluid offsets the stimulatory effect of ADH on the electrochemical driving force for K^+ exit across the apical membrane (see Figure 7-8). If ADH did not increase the electrochemical gradient favoring K^+ secretion, urinary K^+ excretion would fall as ADH levels increase and urinary flow rates decrease. Hence, K^+ balance would change in response to alterations in water balance. Thus, the effects of ADH on the electrochemical driving force for K^+ exit across the apical membrane and tubule flow enable urinary K^+ excretion to be maintained constant despite wide fluctuations in water excretion.

FACTORS THAT PERTURB K^+ EXCRETION

Whereas plasma [K^+], aldosterone, and ADH play important roles in regulating K^+ balance, the factors and hormones discussed next perturb K^+ balance (see Table 7-2).

Flow of Tubular Fluid

A rise in the flow of tubular fluid (e.g., with diuretic treatment, ECF volume expansion) stimulates K^+ secretion within minutes, whereas a fall (e.g., ECF volume contraction caused by hemorrhage, severe vomiting, or diarrhea) reduces K^+ secretion by the distal tubule and collecting duct (Figure 7-9). Increments in tubular fluid flow are more effective in stimulating K^+ secretion as dietary K^+ intake is increased. Studies of the primary cilium in principal cells have elucidated some of the mechanisms whereby increased flow stimulates K^+ secretion. As described in Chapter 2, increased flow bends the primary cilium in principal cells, which activates the PKD1/PKD2 Ca^{++} conducting channel complex. This allows more Ca^{++} to enter principal cells and increases intracellular [Ca^{++}]. The increase in [Ca^{++}] activates K^+ channels in the apical plasma membrane, which enhances K^+ secretion from the cell into the tubule fluid. Increased flow may also stimulate K^+ secretion by other mechanisms. As flow increases, for example, following the administration of diuretics or as the result of an increase in the ECF volume, so does the Na^+ concentration of tubule fluid. This increase in [Na^+] facilitates Na^+ entry across

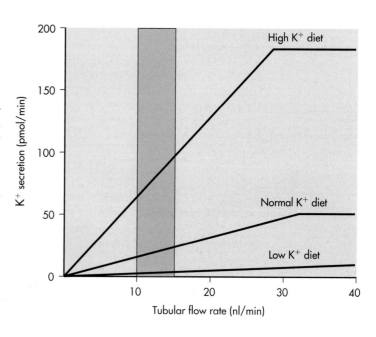

FIGURE 7-9 ■ Relationship between tubular flow rate and K^+ secretion by the distal tubule and cortical collecting duct. A diet high in K^+ increases the slope of the relationship between flow rate and secretion and increases the maximum rate of secretion. A diet low in K^+ has the opposite effects. The shaded bar indicates the flow rate under most physiologic conditions.

the apical membrane of distal tubule and collecting duct cells, thereby decreasing the cell interior negative membrane potential. This depolarization of the cell membrane potential increases the electrochemical driving force that promotes K$^+$ secretion across the apical cell membrane into tubule fluid. In addition, increased Na$^+$ uptake into cells activates the Na$^+$,K$^+$-ATPase in the basolateral membrane, thereby increasing K$^+$ uptake across the basolateral membrane and elevating [K$^+$]. However, it is important to note that an increase in flow rate during a water diuresis does not have a significant effect on K$^+$ excretion (see Figure 7-9), most likely because during a water diuresis the [Na$^+$] of tubule fluid does not increase as flow rises.

ROMK (*KCNJ1*) is the primary channel in the apical membrane responsible for K$^+$ secretion. Four ROMK subunits make up a single channel. In addition, a maxi-K$^+$ channel (*rbsol1*), which is activated by elevations in intracellular [Ca^{++}], is expressed in the apical membrane. The maxi-K$^+$ channel mediates the flow-dependent increase in K$^+$ secretion, as discussed previously. Interestingly, knockout of the *KCNJ1* gene (ROMK) causes increased NaCl and K$^+$ excretion by the kidneys, leading to reduced ECF volume and hypokalemia. Although this effect is somewhat perplexing, it should be noted that ROMK is also expressed in the apical membrane of the thick ascending limb of Henle's loop, where is plays a very important role in K$^+$ recycling across the apical membrane, an effect that is critical for the operation of the Na$^+$-K$^+$-2Cl$^-$ symporter (see Chapter 4). In the absence of ROMK, NaCl reabsorption by the thick ascending limb is reduced, which leads to NaCl loss in the urine. Reduction of NaCl reabsorption by the thick ascending limb also reduces the lumen-positive transepithelial voltage, which is the driving force for K$^+$ reabsorption by this nephron segment. Thus, the reduction in paracellular K$^+$ reabsorption by the thick ascending limb increases urinary K$^+$ excretion, even when the cortical collecting duct is unable to secrete the normal amount of K$^+$ because of a lack of ROMK channels. The cortical collecting duct, however, does secrete K$^+$ even in ROMK knockout mice through the flow and Ca^{++}-dependent maxi-K$^+$ channels and possibly by the operation of a K$^+$-Cl$^-$ symporter expressed in the apical membrane of principal cells.

Acid-Base Balance

Another factor that modulates K$^+$ secretion is the [H$^+$] of the ECF (Figure 7-10). Acute alterations (within minutes to hours) in the pH of the plasma influence K$^+$ secretion by the distal tubule and collecting duct. Alkalosis (i.e., a plasma pH above normal) increases K$^+$ secretion, whereas acidosis (i.e., a plasma pH below normal) decreases it. An acute acidosis reduces K$^+$ secretion by two mechanisms: (1) it inhibits Na$^+$, K$^+$-ATPase and thereby reduces the cell [K$^+$] and the electrochemical driving force for K$^+$ exit across the apical membrane, and (2) it reduces the permeability of the apical membrane to K$^+$. Alkalosis has the opposite effects.

The effect of a metabolic acidosis on K$^+$ excretion is time dependent. When metabolic acidosis lasts for several days, urinary K$^+$ excretion is stimulated (see Figure 7-11). This occurs because chronic metabolic acidosis decreases the reabsorption of water and solutes (e.g., NaCl) by the proximal tubule by inhibiting Na$^+$,K$^+$-ATPase. Hence, the flow of tubular fluid is augmented along the distal tubule and collecting duct. The inhibition of proximal tubular water and NaCl reabsorption also decreases the ECF volume and, thereby, stimulates aldosterone secretion. In addition, chronic acidosis, caused by inorganic acids, increases the plasma [K$^+$], which stimulates aldosterone secretion. The rise in tubular fluid flow, plasma [K$^+$], and

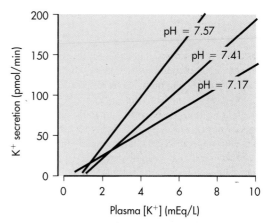

FIGURE 7-10 ■ Effect of plasma pH on the relationship between plasma [K$^+$] and K$^+$ secretion by the distal tubule and collecting duct.

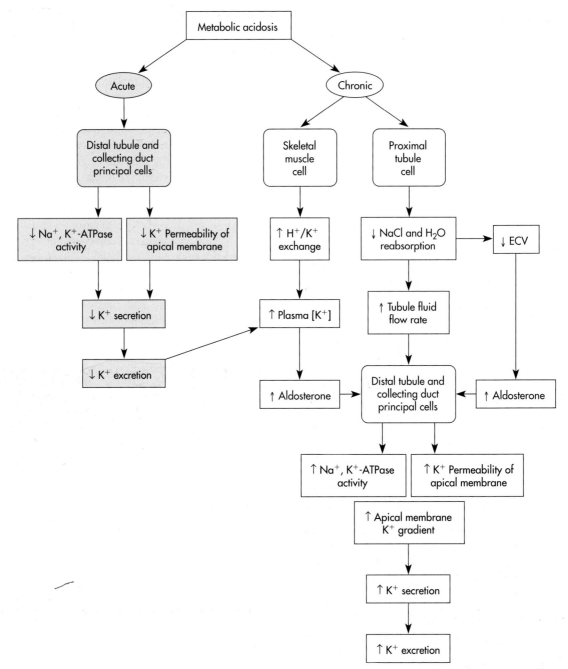

FIGURE 7-11 ■ Acute versus chronic effect of metabolic acidosis on K+ excretion. See text for details. ECV, effective circulating volume.

aldosterone levels offsets the effects of acidosis on the cell [K$^+$] and apical membrane permeability, and K$^+$ secretion rises. Thus, metabolic acidosis may either inhibit or stimulate K$^+$ excretion, depending on the duration of the disturbance. Renal K$^+$ excretion remains elevated during chronic metabolic acidosis and may even increase further depending on the cause of the acidosis.

As noted, acute metabolic alkalosis stimulates K$^+$ excretion. Chronic metabolic alkalosis, especially in association with ECF volume contraction, increases significantly renal K$^+$ excretion because of the associated increased levels of aldosterone.

The cellular mechanisms whereby changes in the K$^+$ content of the diet and acid-base balance regulate K$^+$ secretion by the distal tubule and collecting duct have been elucidated. Elevated K$^+$ intake increases K$^+$ secretion by several mechanisms, all related to increased serum [K$^+$]. Hyperkalemia increases the activity of the ROMK channel in the apical plasma membrane of principal cells. Moreover, hyperkalemia inhibits proximal tubule NaCl and water reabsorption, thereby increasing distal tubule and collecting duct flow rate, a potent stimulus to K$^+$ secretion. Hyperkalemia also enhances [aldosterone], which increases K$^+$ secretion by three mechanisms. First, aldosterone increases the number of K$^+$ channels in the apical plasma membrane. Second, aldosterone stimulates K$^+$ uptake across the basolateral membrane by enhancing the number of Na$^+$, K$^+$-ATPase pumps, thereby enhancing the electrochemical gradient driving K$^+$ secretion across the apical membrane. Third, aldosterone increases Na$^+$ entry across the apical membrane, which depolarizes the apical plasma membrane voltage, thereby increasing the electrochemical gradient promoting K$^+$ secretion.

A low-K$^+$ diet dramatically reduces K$^+$ secretion by the distal tubule and collecting duct by increasing the activity of protein tyrosine kinase, which causes ROMK channels to be endocytosed from the apical plasma membrane, thereby reducing K$^+$ secretion.

Acidosis decreases K$^+$ secretion by stimulating the activity of ROMK channels, whereas alkalosis stimulates K$^+$ secretion by enhancing ROMK channel activity.

Glucocorticoids (cortisol, aldo.)

Glucocorticoids increase urinary K$^+$ excretion. This effect is in part mediated by an increase in GFR, which enhances urinary flow rate, a potent stimulus of K$^+$ excretion, and by stimulating Sgk1 activity (see earlier).

As discussed earlier, the rate of urinary K$^+$ excretion is frequently determined by simultaneous changes in hormone levels, acid-base balance, or the flow rate of tubule fluid (Table 7-3). The powerful effect of flow often enhances or opposes the response of the distal tubule and collecting duct to hormones and changes in acid-base balance. This interaction can be beneficial in the case of hyperkalemia, in which the change in flow enhances K$^+$ excretion and thereby restores K$^+$ homeostasis. However, this interaction can also be detrimental, as in the case of alkalosis, in which changes in flow and acid-base status alter K$^+$ homeostasis.

TABLE 7-3

Net Effects of Hormones and Other Factors on K$^+$ Secretion by the Distal Tubule and Collecting Duct

CONDITION	DIRECT OR INDIRECT	FLOW	URINARY EXCRETION
Hyperkalemia	Increase	Increase	Increase
Aldosterone			
Acute	Increase	Decrease	No change
Chronic	Increase	No change	Increase
Glucocorticoids	No change	Increase	Increase
ADH	Increase	Decrease	No change
Acidosis			
Acute	Decrease	No change	Decrease
Chronic	Decrease	Large increase	Increase
Alkalosis	Increase	Increase	Large increase

Modified from Field MJ, Berliner RW, Giebisch GH: Regulation of renal potassium metabolism. In Narins R, editor: *Textbook of nephrology: clinical disorders of fluid and electrolyte metabolism,* ed 5. New York, 1994, McGraw-Hill.

SUMMARY

1. K⁺ homeostasis is maintained by the kidneys, which adjust K⁺ excretion to match dietary K⁺ intake, and by the hormones insulin, epinephrine, and aldosterone, which regulate the distribution of K⁺ between the ICF and ECF.

2. Other events, such as cell lysis, exercise, and changes in acid-base balance and plasma osmolality, disturb K⁺ homeostasis and the plasma [K⁺].

3. K⁺ excretion by the kidneys is determined by the rate and direction of K⁺ transport by the distal tubule and collecting duct. K⁺ secretion by these tubular segments is regulated by the plasma [K⁺], aldosterone, and ADH. In contrast, changes in tubular fluid flow and acid-base disturbances perturb K⁺ excretion by the kidneys. In K⁺-depleted states, K⁺ secretion is inhibited and the distal tubule and collecting duct reabsorb K⁺.

KEY WORDS AND CONCEPTS

- Hyperkalemia
- Hypokalemia
- Aldosterone
- Epinephrine
- Insulin
- Bartter's syndrome

SELF-STUDY PROBLEMS

1. What would happen to the rise in plasma [K⁺] following an intravenous K⁺ load if the subject had a combination of sympathetic blockade and insulin deficiency?

2. What effect would aldosterone deficiency have on urinary K⁺ excretion? What would happen to plasma [K⁺], and what effect would this have on K⁺ excretion?

3. Describe the homeostatic mechanisms involved in maintaining the plasma [K⁺] following ingestion of a meal rich in K⁺.

4. If the GFR declined by 50% (e.g., because of a loss of one kidney) and the filtered load of K⁺ also declined by 50%, would the remaining kidney be able to maintain K⁺ balance? If so, how would this occur? If not, would the subject become hyperkalemic?

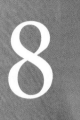

8 REGULATION OF ACID-BASE BALANCE

OBJECTIVES

Upon completion of this chapter, the student should be able to answer the following questions:

1. How does the HCO_3^- system operate as a buffer, and why is it an important buffer of the extracellular fluid (ECF)?

2. How does metabolism of food produce acid and alkali, and what effect does the composition of the diet have on systemic acid-base balance?

3. What is the difference between volatile and nonvolatile acids?

4. How do the kidneys, lungs, and liver contribute to systemic acid-base balance?

5. Why are urinary buffers necessary for the excretion of acid by the kidneys?

6. What are the mechanisms for H^+ transport in the various segments of the nephron, and how are these mechanisms regulated?

7. How do the various segments of the nephron contribute to the process of reabsorbing the filtered HCO_3^-?

8. How do the kidneys produce new HCO_3^-?

9. How is ammonium produced by the kidneys, and how does its excretion contribute to renal acid excretion?

10. What are the major mechanisms by which the body defends itself against changes in acid-base balance?

11. What are the differences between simple metabolic and respiratory acid-base disorders, and how are they differentiated by blood gas measurements?

The concentration of H^+ in the body fluids is low compared with that of other ions. For example, Na^+ is present at a concentration some 3 million times greater than that of H^+ ($[Na^+] = 140$ mEq/L; $[H^+] = 40$ nEq/L). Because of the low $[H^+]$ of the body fluids, it is commonly expressed as the negative logarithm, or pH.

Virtually all cellular, tissue, and organ processes are sensitive to pH. Indeed, life cannot exist outside a range of body fluid pH from 6.8 to 7.8 (160 to 16 nEq/L of H^+). Each day, acid and alkali are ingested in the diet. Also, cellular metabolism produces a number of substances that have an impact on the pH of body fluids. Without appropriate mechanisms to deal with

this daily acid and alkali load and thereby maintain acid-base balance, many processes necessary for life could not occur. This chapter reviews the maintenance of whole-body acid-base balance. Although the emphasis is on the role of the kidneys in this process, the roles of the lungs and liver are also considered. In addition, the impact of diet and cellular metabolism on acid-base balance is presented. Finally, disorders of acid-base balance are considered, primarily to illustrate the physiologic processes involved. Throughout this chapter, **acid** is defined as any substance that adds H^+ to the body fluids, whereas **alkali** is defined as a substance that removes H^+ from the body fluids.

TBW = 42

THE HCO_3^- BUFFER SYSTEM

Bicarbonate (HCO_3^-) is an important buffer of the extracellular fluid (ECF). With a normal plasma [HCO_3^-] of 23 to 25 mEq/L and a volume of 14 L (for a 70-kg individual), the ECF can potentially buffer 350 mEq of H^+. The HCO_3^- buffer system differs from the other buffer systems of the body (e.g., phosphate) because it is regulated by both the lungs and the kidneys. This is best appreciated by considering the following reaction.

$$CO_2 + H_2O \overset{Slow}{\leftrightarrow} H_2CO_3 \overset{Fast}{\leftrightarrow} H^+ + HCO_3^- \quad (8\text{-}1)$$

As indicated, the first reaction (hydration/dehydration of CO_2) is the rate-limiting step. This normally slow reaction is greatly accelerated in the presence of carbonic anhydrase.[1] The second reaction, the ionization of H_2CO_3 to H^+ and HCO_3^-, is virtually instantaneous.

The Henderson-Hasselbalch equation (8-2) is used to quantitate how changes in CO_2 and HCO_3^- affect pH.

$$pH = pK' + \log \frac{HCO_3^-}{\alpha P_{CO_2}} \quad (8\text{-}2)$$

or

$$pH = 6.1 + \log \frac{HCO_3^-}{0.03 P_{CO_2}} \quad (8\text{-}3)$$

In these equations, the amount of CO_2 is determined from the partial pressure of CO_2 (P_{CO_2}) and its solubility (α). For plasma at 37° C, α has a value of 0.03. Also, pK' is the negative logarithm of the overall dissociation constant for the reaction in equation 8-1 and has a value for plasma at 37° C of 6.1. Alternatively, the relationship between HCO_3^-, CO_2, and [H^+] can be determined as follows.

$$[H^+] = \frac{24 \times P_{CO_2}}{[HCO_3^-]} \quad (8\text{-}4)$$

Inspection of equations 8-3 and 8-4 shows that the pH and the [H^+] vary when either the [HCO_3^-] or the P_{CO_2} is altered. Disturbances of acid-base balance that result from a change in the [HCO_3^-] are termed metabolic acid-base disorders, whereas those that result

from a change in the P_{CO_2} are termed respiratory acid-base disorders. These disorders are considered in more detail in a subsequent section. The kidneys are primarily responsible for regulating the [HCO_3^-] of the ECF, whereas the lungs control the P_{CO_2}.

OVERVIEW OF ACID-BASE BALANCE

The diet of humans contains many constituents that are either acid or alkali. In addition, cellular metabolism produces acid and alkali. Finally, alkali is normally lost each day in the feces. As described later, the net effect of these processes is the addition of acid to the body fluids. For acid-base balance to be maintained, acid must be excreted from the body at a rate equivalent to its addition. If acid addition exceeds excretion, **acidosis** results. Conversely, if acid excretion exceeds addition, **alkalosis** results.

The major constituents of the diet are carbohydrates and fats. When tissue perfusion is adequate, O_2 is available to tissues, and insulin is present at normal levels, carbohydrates and fats are metabolized to CO_2 and H_2O. On a daily basis, 15 to 20 moles of CO_2 are generated through this process. Normally, this large quantity of CO_2 is effectively eliminated from the body by the lungs. Therefore, this metabolically derived CO_2 has no impact on acid-base balance. CO_2 is usually termed **volatile acid,** reflecting the fact that it has the potential to generate H^+ after hydration with H_2O (see equation 8-1). Acid not derived directly from the hydration of CO_2 is termed **nonvolatile acid** (e.g., lactic acid).

The cellular metabolism of other dietary constituents also has an impact on acid-base balance. For example, cysteine and methionine, sulfur-containing amino acids, yield sulfuric acid when metabolized, whereas hydrochloric acid results from the metabolism of lysine, arginine, and histidine. A portion of this nonvolatile acid load is offset by the production of HCO_3^- through the metabolism of the amino acids aspartate and glutamate. On average, the metabolism of dietary amino acids yields net nonvolatile acid production. The metabolism of certain organic anions (e.g., citrate) results in the production of HCO_3^-, which offsets nonvolatile acid production to some degree. Overall, in individuals ingesting a meat-containing diet, acid

---

[1]Carbonic anhydrase (CA) actually catalyzes the following reaction:
$$H_2O \rightarrow H^+ + OH^- + CO_2 \rightarrow HCO_3^- + H^+ \rightarrow H_2CO_3$$

production exceeds HCO_3^- production. In addition to the metabolically derived acids and alkalis, the foods ingested contain acid and alkali. For example, the presence of phosphate ($H_2PO_4^-$) in ingested food increases the dietary acid load. Finally, during digestion, some HCO_3^- is normally lost in the feces. This loss is equivalent to the addition of nonvolatile acid to the body. Together, dietary intake, cellular metabolism, and fecal HCO_3^- loss result in the addition of approximately 1 mEq/kg body weight of nonvolatile acid to the body each day (50 to 100 mEq/day for most adults).

When insulin levels are normal, carbohydrates and fats are completely metabolized to $CO_2 + H_2O$. However, if insulin levels are abnormally low (e.g., **diabetes mellitus**), the metabolism of carbohydrates leads to the production of several organic keto acids (e.g., β-hydroxybutyric acid).

In the absence of adequate levels of O_2 **(hypoxia),** anaerobic metabolism by cells can also lead to the production of organic acids (e.g., lactic acid) rather than $CO_2 + H_2O$. This frequently occurs in healthy individuals during vigorous exercise. Poor tissue perfusion, such as that which occurs with reduced cardiac output, can also lead to anaerobic metabolism by cells and thus to acidosis. In these conditions, the organic acids accumulate and the pH of the body fluids decreases (acidosis). Treatment (e.g., administration of insulin in the case of diabetes) or improved delivery of adequate levels of O_2 to the tissues (e.g., in the case of poor tissue perfusion) results in the metabolism of these organic acids to $CO_2 + H_2O$, which consumes H^+ and thereby helps correct the acid-base disorder.

Nonvolatile acids do not circulate throughout the body but are immediately neutralized by the HCO_3^- in the ECF.

$$H_2SO_4 + 2NaHCO_3 \leftrightarrow Na_2SO_4 + 2CO_2 + 2H_2O \qquad (8\text{-}5)$$

$$HCl + NaHCO_3 \leftrightarrow NaCl + CO_2 + H_2O \qquad (8\text{-}6)$$

This neutralization process yields the Na^+ salts of the strong acids and removes HCO_3^- from the ECF. Thus, HCO_3^- minimizes the effect of these strong acids on the pH of the ECF. As noted previously, the ECF contains approximately 350 mEq of HCO_3^-. If this

HCO_3^- was not replenished, the daily production of nonvolatile acids ($\approx$70 mEq/day) would deplete the ECF of HCO_3^- within 5 days. To maintain acid-base balance, the kidneys must replenish the HCO_3^- that is lost by neutralization of the nonvolatile acids.

NET ACID EXCRETION BY THE KIDNEYS

Under normal conditions, the kidneys excrete an amount of acid equal to the nonvolatile acid production and in so doing replenish the HCO_3^- that is lost by neutralization of the nonvolatile acids. In addition, the kidneys must prevent the loss of HCO_3^- in the urine. The latter task is quantitatively more important because the filtered load of HCO_3^- is approximately 4320 mEq/day (24 mEq/L × 180 L/day = 4320 mEq/day), compared with only 50 to 100 mEq/day needed to balance nonvolatile acid production.

Both the reabsorption of filtered HCO_3^- and the excretion of acid are accomplished by H^+ secretion by the nephrons. Thus, in a single day the nephrons must secrete approximately 4390 mEq of H^+ into the tubular fluid. Most of the secreted H^+ serves to reabsorb the filtered load of HCO_3^-. Only 50 to 100 mEq of H^+, an amount equivalent to nonvolatile acid production, is excreted in the urine. As a result of this acid excretion, the urine is normally acidic.

The kidneys cannot excrete urine more acidic than pH 4.0 to 4.5. Even at a pH of 4.0, only 0.1 mEq/L of H^+ can be excreted. Therefore, in order to excrete sufficient acid, the kidneys excrete H^+ with urinary buffers such as phosphate (Pi).[2] Other constituents of the urine can also serve as buffers (e.g., creatinine), although their role is less important than that of Pi. Collectively, the various urinary buffers are termed **titratable acid.** This term is derived from the method by which these buffers are quantitated in the laboratory. Typically, alkali (OH^-) is added to a urine sample to titrate its pH to that of plasma (i.e., 7.4). The amount of alkali added is equal to the H^+ titrated by these urine buffers and is termed titratable acid.

The excretion of H^+ as a titratable acid is insufficient to balance the daily nonvolatile acid load. An additional

---

[2]The titration reaction is $HPO_4^{-2} + H^+ \leftrightarrow H_2PO_4^-$. This reaction has a pK of approximately 6.8.

and important mechanism by which the kidneys contribute to the maintenance of acid-base balance is through the synthesis and excretion of **ammonium (NH$_4^+$).** The mechanisms involved in this process are discussed in more detail later in this chapter. With regard to the renal regulation of acid-base balance, each NH$_4^+$ excreted in the urine results in the return of one HCO$_3^-$ to the systemic circulation, which replenishes the HCO$_3^-$ lost during neutralization of the nonvolatile acids. Thus, the production and excretion of NH$_4^+$, like the excretion of titratable acid, are equivalent to the excretion of acid by the kidneys.

In brief, the kidneys contribute to acid-base homeostasis by reabsorbing the filtered load of HCO$_3^-$ and excreting an amount of acid equivalent to the amount of nonvolatile acid produced each day. This overall process is termed **net acid excretion (NAE),** and it can be quantitated as follows:

$$\text{NAE} = [(U_{NH_4^+} \times \dot{V}) + (U_{TA} \times \dot{V})] - (U_{HCO_3^-} \times \dot{V}) \quad \text{(8-7)}$$

where $(U_{NH_4^+} \times \dot{V})$ and $(U_{TA} \times \dot{V})$ are the rates of excretion (mEq/day) of NH$_4^+$ and titratable acid (TA) and $(U_{HCO_3^-} \times \dot{V})$ is the amount of HCO$_3^-$ lost in the urine (equivalent to adding H$^+$ to the body).[3] Again, maintenance of acid-base balance means that the net acid excretion must equal nonvolatile acid production. Under most conditions, very little HCO$_3^-$ is excreted in the urine. Thus, net acid excretion essentially reflects titratable acid and NH$_4^+$ excretion. Quantitatively, titratable acid accounts for approximately one third and NH$_4^+$ for two thirds of net acid excretion.

HCO$_3^-$ REABSORPTION ALONG THE NEPHRON

As indicated by equation 8-7, net acid excretion is maximized when little or no HCO$_3^-$ is excreted in the urine. Indeed, under most circumstances, very little HCO$_3^-$ appears in the urine. Because HCO$_3^-$ is freely filtered at the glomerulus, approximately 4320 mEq/day are delivered to the nephrons and are then reabsorbed.

[3]This equation ignores the small amount of free H$^+$ excreted in the urine. As already noted, urine with pH = 4.0 contains only 0.1 mEq/L of H$^+$.

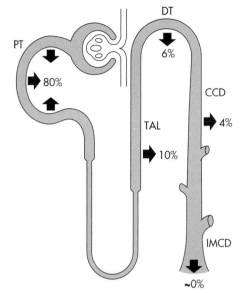

FIGURE 8-1 ■ Segmental reabsorption of HCO$_3^-$. The fraction of the filtered load of HCO$_3^-$ reabsorbed by the various segments of the nephron is shown. Normally, the entire filtered load of HCO$_3^-$ is reabsorbed and little or no HCO$_3^-$ appears in the urine. CCD, cortical collecting duct; DT, distal tubule; IMCD, inner medullary collecting duct; PT, proximal tubule; TAL, thick ascending limb.

Figure 8-1 summarizes the contribution of each nephron segment to the reabsorption of the filtered HCO$_3^-$.

The proximal tubule reabsorbs the largest portion of the filtered load of HCO$_3^-$. Figure 8-2 summarizes the primary transport processes involved. H$^+$ secretion across the apical membrane of the cell occurs by both a Na$^+$-H$^+$ antiporter and a H$^+$-ATPase. The Na$^+$-H$^+$ antiporter (NHE3) is the predominant pathway for H$^+$ secretion and uses the lumen-to-cell [Na$^+$] gradient to drive this process (i.e., secondary active secretion of H$^+$). Within the cell, H$^+$ and HCO$_3^-$ are produced in a reaction catalyzed by carbonic anhydrase. The H$^+$ is secreted into the tubular fluid, whereas the HCO$_3^-$ exits the cell across the basolateral membrane and returns to the peritubular blood. HCO$_3^-$ movement out of the cell across the basolateral membrane is coupled to other ions. The majority of HCO$_3^-$ exits through a symporter that couples the efflux of 1Na$^+$ with 3HCO$_3^-$ (sodium bicarbonate cotransporter, NBC1).

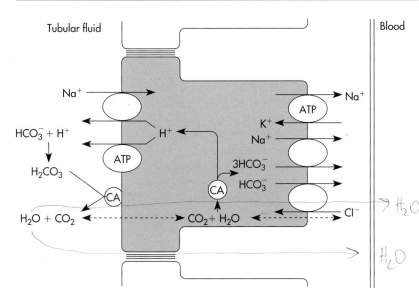

Tubular fluid

Blood

Na^+

Na^+

ATP

K^+

$HCO_3^- + H^+$

H^+

Na^+

H_2CO_3

$3HCO_3^-$

HCO_3^-

ATP

CA

CA

$H_2O + CO_2$

$CO_2 + H_2O$

Cl^-

H_2O

H_2O

FIGURE 8-2 ■ Cellular mechanism for the reabsorption of filtered HCO_3^- by cells of the proximal tubule. ATP, adenosine triphosphate; CA, carbonic anhydrase.

In addition, some of the HCO_3^- may exit in exchange for Cl^- (via a Cl^--HCO_3^- antiporter). As noted in Figure 8-2, carbonic anhydrase is also present in the brush border of the proximal tubule cells. This enzyme catalyzes the dehydration of H_2CO_3 in the luminal fluid and thereby facilitates the reabsorption of HCO_3^-.

Carbonic anhydrases are zinc-containing enzymes that catalyze the hydration of CO_2 (see equation 8-1). The isoform CA-I is found in red blood cells and is critical for the cells' ability to carry CO_2. Two isoforms, CA-II and CA-IV, play important roles in urine acidification. The CA-II isoform is localized to the cytoplasm of many cells along the nephron, including the proximal tubule, thick ascending limb of Henle's loop, and intercalated cells of the distal tubule and collecting duct. The CA-IV isoform is membrane bound and exposed to the contents of the tubular fluid. It is found in the apical membrane of both the proximal tubule and thick ascending limb of Henle's loop, where it facilitates the reabsorption of the large amount of HCO_3^- reabsorbed by these segments. CA-IV has also been demonstrated in the basolateral membrane of the proximal tubule and thick ascending limb of Henle's loop. Its function at this site is thought to facilitate in some way the exit of HCO_3^- from the cell.

The cellular mechanism for HCO_3^- reabsorption by the thick ascending limb of the loop of Henle is very similar to that in the proximal tubule. H^+ is secreted by a Na^+-H^+ antiporter and a H^+-ATPase. As in the proximal tubule, the Na^+-H^+ antiporter is the predominant pathway for H^+ secretion. HCO_3^- exit from the cell involves both a Na^+ HCO_3^- symporter (although the isoform is different from that of the proximal tubule) and a Cl^--HCO_3^- antiporter (anion exchanger, AE-2). Recently, evidence has been obtained for the presence of a K^+- HCO_3^- symporter in the basolateral membrane, which may also contribute to HCO_3^- exit from the cell.

The distal tubule[4] and collecting duct reabsorb the small amount of HCO_3^- that escapes reabsorption by the proximal tubule and loop of Henle. Figure 8-3 shows the cellular mechanism of HCO_3^- reabsorption by the collecting duct, where H^+ secretion occurs through the intercalated cell (see Chapter 2). Within the cell, H^+ and HCO_3^- are produced by the hydration of CO_2; this reaction is catalyzed by carbonic anhydrase.

---

[4]Here and in the remainder of the chapter we focus on the function of intercalated cells. The early portion of the distal tubule, which does not contain intercalated cells, also reabsorbs HCO_3^-. The cellular mechanism is similar to that already described for the thick ascending limb of Henle's loop, although transporter isoforms may be different.

H⁺-secreting cell

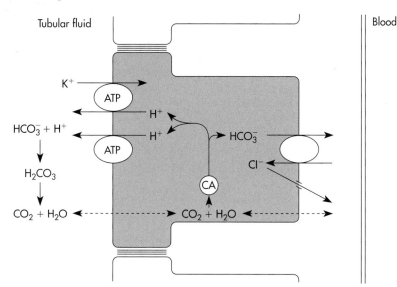

FIGURE 8-3 ■ Cellular mechanisms for the reabsorption and secretion of HCO_3^- by intercalated cells of the collecting duct. ATP, adenosine triphosphate; CA, carbonic anhydrase.

HCO_3^--secreting cell

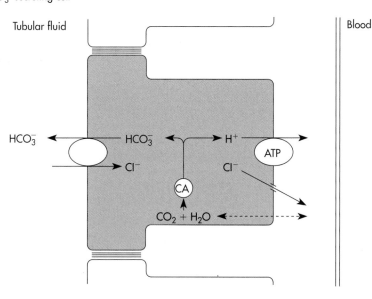

H^+ is secreted into the tubular fluid by two mechanisms. The first involves an apical membrane H^+-ATPase. The second couples the secretion of H^+ with the reabsorption of K^+ through an H^+,K^+-ATPase similar to that found in the stomach. The HCO_3^- exits the cell across the basolateral membrane in exchange for Cl^- (through a Cl^-- HCO_3^- antiporter, AE-1) and enters the peritubular capillary blood.

A second population of intercalated cells within the collecting duct secretes HCO_3^- rather than H^+ into the tubular fluid. In these intercalated cells, in contrast to the intercalated cells previously described, the H^+-ATPase is located in the basolateral membrane, and a Cl^-- HCO_3^- antiporter is located in the apical membrane (see Figure 8-3). The apical membrane Cl^-- HCO_3^- antiporter is different from the one found in the basolateral membrane of H^+-secreting intercalated cell and has been identified as pendrin. The activity of the HCO_3^--secreting intercalated cell is increased during metabolic alkalosis, when the kidneys must excrete excess HCO_3^-. However, under normal conditions H^+ secretion predominates in the collecting duct.

The apical membrane of collecting duct cells is not very permeable to H^+ and thus, the pH of the tubular fluid can become quite acidic. Indeed, the most acidic tubular fluid along the nephron (pH = 4.0 to 4.5) is produced there. In comparison, the permeability of the proximal tubule to H^+ and HCO_3^- is much higher, and the tubular fluid pH falls to only 6.5 in this segment. As explained later, the ability of the collecting duct to lower the pH of the tubular fluid is critically important for the excretion of urinary titratable acids and NH_4^+.

REGULATION OF H$^+$ SECRETION

A number of factors regulate the secretion of H^+, and thus the reabsorption of HCO_3^-, by the cells of the nephron (Table 8-1). From a physiologic perspective, the primary factor that regulates H^+ secretion by the nephron is a change in systemic acid-base balance. Thus, acidosis stimulates H^+ secretion, whereas H^+ secretion is reduced during alkalosis. The response of the kidneys to changes in acid-base balance includes both immediate changes in the activity or number of transporters in the membrane, or both, and longer term changes in the synthesis of transporters. For example, with metabolic acidosis, whether produced by a decrease in the $[HCO_3^-]$ of the ECF or by an increase in the partial pressure of carbon dioxide (P_{CO_2}), the pH of the cells of the nephron decreases. This stimulates H^+ secretion by multiple mechanisms, depending on the particular nephron segment. First, the decrease in intracellular pH creates a more favorable cell-to-tubular fluid H^+ gradient and thereby makes the secretion of H^+ across the apical membrane more energetically favorable. Second, the decrease in

TABLE 8-1	
Factors Regulating H$^+$ Secretion (HCO$_3^-$ Reabsorption) by the Nephron	
FACTOR	**PRIMARY SITE OF ACTION**
Increased H$^+$ Secretion	
Primary	
Decrease in ECF [HCO$_3^-$] ($\downarrow$pH)	Entire nephron
Increase in arterial P$_{CO_2}$	Entire nephron
Cortisol	Proximal tubule*
Endothelin	Proximal tubule*
Secondary	
Increase in filtered load of HCO$_3^-$	Proximal tubule
ECF volume contraction	Proximal tubule
Angiotensin II	Proximal and distal tubules
Aldosterone	Distal tubule and collecting duct
Hypokalemia	Proximal tubule
PTH (chronic)	Thick ascending limb; distal tubule
Decreased H$^+$ Secretion	
Primary	
Increase in ECF [HCO$_3^-$] ($\uparrow$pH)	Entire nephron
Decrease in arterial P$_{CO_2}$	Entire nephron
Secondary	
Decrease in filtered load of HCO$_3^-$	Proximal tubule
ECF volume expansion	Proximal tubule
Hypoaldosteronism	Distal tubule and collecting duct
Hyperkalemia	Proximal tubule
PTH (acute)	Proximal tubule

*Effect on the proximal tubule is established. It may also regulate H^+ secretion in other nephron segments.
ECF, extracellular fluid; P_{CO_2}, partial pressure of CO_2; PTH, parathyroid hormone.

pH may lead to allosteric changes in transport proteins, thereby altering their kinetics. This has been reported for the Na^+-H^+ antiporter (NHE3) in the proximal tubule. Lastly, transporters may be shuttled to the membrane from intracellular vesicles. This mechanism occurs in both the intercalated cells of the collecting duct, where acidosis stimulates the exocytotic insertion of H^+-ATPase into the apical membrane, and the proximal tubule, where apical membrane insertion of the Na^+-H^+ antiporter and the H^+-ATPase has been reported. With long-term acidosis, the abundance of transporters is increased, either by increased transcription of appropriate transporter genes or by increased translation of transporter mRNA. Examples of this include the Na^+-H^+ antiporter and Na^+-3HCO_3^-

symporter in the proximal tubule and the H^+-ATPase in the intercalated cell.

Although some of the effects just described may be attributable directly to the decrease in intracellular pH, most of these changes in cellular H^+ transport are mediated by hormones or other factors. Two important mediators of the renal response to acidosis are endothelin and cortisol. **Endothelin (ET-1)** is produced by endothelial and proximal tubule cells, and, thus, it exerts its effects by autocrine and paracrine mechanisms. With acidosis, ET-1 secretion is enhanced. In the proximal tubule ET-1 stimulates the phosphorylation and subsequent insertion into the apical membrane of the Na^+-H^+ antiporter and insertion of the Na^+-$3HCO_3^-$ symporter into the basolateral membrane. ET-1 may mediate the response to acidosis in other nephron segments as well. Acidosis also stimulates the secretion of the glucocorticoid hormone **cortisol** by the adrenal cortex. It, in turn, acts on the kidneys to increase the transcription of the Na^+-H^+ antiporter and Na^+-$3HCO_3^-$ symporter genes in the proximal tubule and also to increase translation of mRNA of these transporters.

Alkalosis, caused by an increase in the $[HCO_3^-]$ of the ECF, or a decrease in the P_{CO_2}, inhibits H^+ secretion secondary to an increase in the intracellular pH of the nephron cells. Thus, the responses just described for the renal adaptation to acidosis are reversed.

Table 8-1 also lists other factors that influence the secretion of H^+ by the cells of the nephron. However, these factors are not directly related to the maintenance of acid-base balance. Because H^+ secretion in the proximal tubule and thick ascending limb of the loop of Henle is linked to the reabsorption of Na^+ (through the Na^+-H^+ antiporter), factors that alter Na^+ reabsorption secondarily affect H^+ secretion. For example, the process of GT balance ensures that the reabsorption rate of the proximal tubule is matched to the GFR (see Chapter 4). Thus, when the GFR is increased, the filtered load to the proximal tubule is increased, and more fluid (including HCO_3^-) is reabsorbed. Conversely, a decrease in the filtered load results in decreased reabsorption of fluid and thus HCO_3^-.

Alterations in Na^+ balance, through changes in the ECF volume, also have an impact on H^+ secretion. With volume contraction (negative Na^+ balance), H^+ secretion is enhanced. This occurs by several mechanisms. One mechanism involves the renin-angiotensin-aldosterone

system, which is activated by volume contraction, and leads to enhanced Na^+ reabsorption by the nephron (see Chapter 6). Angiotensin II acts on the proximal tubule to stimulate the apical membrane Na^+-H^+ antiporter as well as the basolateral Na^+-$3HCO_3^-$ symporter. This stimulatory effect includes increased activity of the transporters and exocytotic insertion of transporters into the membrane. To a lesser degree, angiotensin II stimulates H^+ secretion in the early portion of the distal tubule, a process also mediated by the Na^+-H^+ antiporter. Aldosterone's primary action on the distal tubule and collecting duct is to stimulate Na^+ reabsorption by principal cells (see Chapter 6). However, it also stimulates intercalated cells in these segments to secrete H^+. The effect is both indirect and direct. By stimulating Na^+ reabsorption by principal cells, aldosterone hyperpolarizes the transepithelial voltage (i.e., the lumen becomes more electrically negative). This change in transepithelial voltage then facilitates the secretion of H^+ by the intercalated cells. In addition to this indirect effect, aldosterone acts directly on intercalated cells to stimulate H^+ secretion. The precise mechanisms for this stimulatory effect are not fully understood. Another mechanism by which ECF volume contraction enhances H^+ secretion (HCO_3^- reabsorption) is through changes in peritubular capillary Starling forces. As described in Chapters 4 and 6, ECF volume contraction alters the peritubular capillary Starling forces such that overall proximal tubule reabsorption is enhanced. With this enhanced reabsorption, more of the filtered load of HCO_3^- is reabsorbed. With volume expansion (positive Na^+ balance), H^+ secretion is reduced because of low levels of angiotensin II and aldosterone as well as because of alterations in the peritubular Starling forces that reduce overall proximal tubule reabsorption.

Parathyroid hormone (PTH) has both inhibitory and stimulatory effects on renal H^+ secretion. Acutely, PTH inhibits H^+ secretion by the proximal tubule by inhibiting the activity of the Na^+-H^+ antiporter and also by causing the antiporter to be endocytosed from the apical membrane. In the long term, PTH stimulates renal acid excretion by acting on the thick ascending limb of Henle's loop and the distal tubule. Because PTH secretion is increased during acidosis, this long-term stimulatory effect on renal acid excretion is a component of the renal response to acidosis.

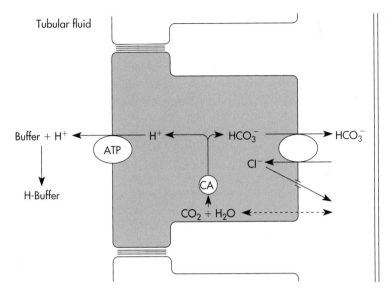

Tubular fluid

Blood

FIGURE 8-4 ■ General scheme for the excretion of H^+ with non-HCO_3^- urinary buffers (titratable acid). The primary urinary buffer is phosphate (HPO_4^{-2}). An H^+-secreting intercalated cell is shown. For simplicity, only the H^+-ATPase is depicted. H^+ secretion by the H^+, K^+-ATPase also titrates luminal buffers. ATP, adenosine triphosphate; CA, carbonic anhydrase.

The stimulatory effect of PTH on acid excretion is due in part to the delivery of increased amounts of Pi to more distal nephron sites, where it is then titrated and excreted as titratable acid.[5]

Finally, K^+ balance influences the secretion of H^+ by the proximal tubule. Hypokalemia stimulates and hyperkalemia inhibits H^+ secretion. It is thought that K^+-induced changes in intracellular pH are responsible, at least in part, for this effect, with hypokalemia acidifying and hyperkalemia alkalinizing the cells. Hypokalemia also stimulates H^+ secretion by the collecting duct. This occurs as a result of increased expression of the H^+,K^+-ATPase in intercalated cells.

FORMATION OF NEW HCO_3^-

As discussed previously, reabsorption of the filtered load of HCO_3^- is important for maximizing net acid excretion. However, HCO_3^- reabsorption alone does not replenish the HCO_3^- lost during the buffering of the nonvolatile acids produced during metabolism. To maintain acid-base balance, the kidneys must replace this lost HCO_3^- with new HCO_3^-. A portion of the new

HCO_3^- is produced when urinary buffers (primarily Pi) are being excreted as titratable acid. This process is illustrated in Figure 8-4. In the distal tubule and collecting duct, where the tubular fluid contains little or no HCO_3^- because of "upstream" reabsorption, H^+ secreted into the tubular fluid combines with a urinary buffer. Thus, H^+ secretion results in the excretion of H^+ with a buffer, and the HCO_3^- produced in the cell from the hydration of CO_2 is added to the blood. The amount of Pi excreted each day and, therefore, available to serve as a urinary buffer is not sufficient to allow adequate generation of new HCO_3^-. However, as noted, increased excretion of Pi does occur with acidosis and therefore contributes to the kidneys' response to the acidosis. Nevertheless, this amount of Pi is insufficient to allow the kidneys to excrete sufficient net acid. In comparison, NH_4^+ is produced by the kidneys and its synthesis, and subsequent excretion, adds HCO_3^- to the ECF. In addition, the synthesis of NH_4^+ and the subsequent production of HCO_3^- are regulated in response to the acid-base requirements of the body. Because of this, NH_4^+ excretion is critically involved in the formation of new HCO_3^-.

NH_4^+ is produced in the kidneys through the metabolism of **glutamine**. Essentially, the kidneys metabolize glutamine, excrete NH_4^+, and add HCO_3^- to the body. However, the formation of new HCO_3^- by this process depends on the kidneys' ability to excrete

[5]As described in Chapter 9, one of the important actions of PTH to inhibit the reabsorption of Pi by the proximal tubule. In so doing, more Pi is delivered to downstream nephron segments, where it is available for titration and excretion as titratable acid.

NH_4^+ in the urine. If NH_4^+ is not excreted in the urine but enters the systemic circulation instead, it is converted into urea by the liver. This conversion process generates H^+, which is then buffered by HCO_3^-. Thus, the production of urea from renally generated NH_4^+ consumes HCO_3^- and negates the formation of HCO_3^- through the synthesis and excretion of NH_4^+ by the kidneys.

The process by which the kidneys excrete NH_4^+ is complex. Figure 8-5 illustrates the essential features of this process. NH_4^+ is produced from glutamine in the cells of the proximal tubule, a process termed **ammoniagenesis.** Each glutamine molecule produces two molecules of NH_4^+ and the divalent anion 2-oxoglutarate^{-2}. The metabolism of this anion ultimately provides two molecules of HCO_3^-. The HCO_3^- exits the cell across the basolateral membrane and enters the peritubular blood as new HCO_3^-. NH_4^+ exits the cell across the apical membrane and enters the tubular fluid. The primary mechanism for the secretion of NH_4^+ into the tubular fluid involves the Na^+-H^+ antiporter, with NH_4^+ substituting for H^+. In addition, NH_3 can diffuse out of the cell across the plasma membrane into the tubular fluid, where it is protonated to NH_4^+.

A significant portion of the NH_4^+ secreted by the proximal tubule is reabsorbed by the loop of Henle. The thick ascending limb is the primary site of this NH_4^+ reabsorption, with NH_4^+ substituting for K^+ on the $1Na^+$-$1K^+$-$2Cl^-$ symporter. In addition, the lumen-positive transepithelial voltage in this segment drives the paracellular reabsorption of NH_4^+ (see Chapter 4).

The NH_4^+ reabsorbed by the thick ascending limb of the loop of Henle accumulates in the medullary interstitium, where it exists in chemical equilibrium with NH_3 (pK = 9.0). NH_4^+ is then secreted into the tubular fluid of the collecting duct. The mechanisms by which NH_4^+ is secreted by the collecting duct include (1) transport into intercalated cells by the Na^+, K^+-ATPase (NH_4^+ substituting for K^+) and exit from the cell across the apical membrane of intercalated cells by the H^+,K^+-ATPase (NH_4^+ substituting for H^+) and (2) the process of **nonionic diffusion** and **diffusion trapping.** Of these mechanisms for NH_4^+ secretion, quantitatively the most important is nonionic diffusion and diffusion trapping. By this mechanism, NH_3 diffuses from the medullary interstitium into the lumen of the collecting duct. As previously described,

H^+ secretion by the intercalated cells of the collecting duct acidifies the luminal fluid (a luminal fluid pH as low as 4.0 to 4.5 can be achieved). Consequently, NH_3 diffusing from the medullary interstitium into the collecting duct lumen (nonionic diffusion) is protonated to NH_4^+ by the acidic tubular fluid. Because the collecting duct is less permeable to NH_4^+ than to NH_3, NH_4^+ is trapped in the tubule lumen (diffusion trapping) and eliminated from the body in the urine.

Recently, two proteins (RhBG and RhCG), termed rhesus glycoproteins for their homology to the rhesus proteins found on the surface of erythrocytes that are responsible for hemolytic diseases and blood transfusion reactions, have been localized to the kidney and liver, where they are thought to be involved in the transport of NH_4^+. RhBG is localized to the basolateral membrane beginning in the late portion of the distal tubule and continuing throughout the collecting duct. The H^+-secreting intercalated cells in these segments appear to have very high levels of the protein; lesser amounts are found in the basolateral membrane of principal cells. RhCG is localized to the same nephron segments; however, it is found in the apical rather than the basolateral membrane. Although it is thought that these proteins may be involved with the transport of NH_4^+ across the distal tubule and collecting duct, their role relative to nonionic diffusion and diffusion trapping has not yet been elucidated.

H^+ secretion by the collecting duct is critical for the excretion of NH_4^+. If collecting duct H^+ secretion is inhibited, the NH_4^+ reabsorbed by the thick ascending limb of Henle's loop is not excreted in the urine. Instead, it is returned to the systemic circulation, where, as described previously, it is converted to urea by the liver, consuming HCO_3^- in the process. Thus, new HCO_3^- is produced during the metabolism of glutamine by cells of the proximal tubule. However, the overall process is not complete until the NH_4^+ is excreted (i.e., the production of urea from NH_4^+ by the liver is prevented). Thus, NH_4^+ excretion in the urine can be used as a "marker" of glutamine metabolism in the proximal tubule. In the net, one new HCO_3^- is returned to the systemic circulation for each NH_4^+ excreted in the urine.

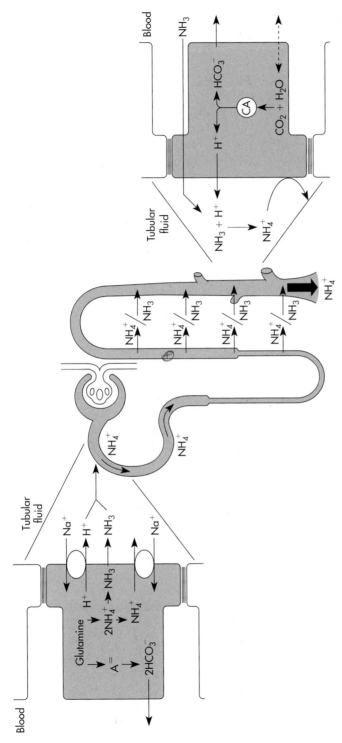

FIGURE 8-5 ■ Production, transport, and excretion of NH_4^+ by the nephron. Glutamine is metabolized to NH_4^+ and HCO_3^- in the proximal tubule. The NH_4^+ is secreted into the lumen, and the HCO_3^- enters the blood. The secreted NH_4^+ is reabsorbed in Henle's loop primarily by the thick ascending limb and accumulates in the medullary interstitium, where it exists as both NH_4^+ and NH_3 (pKa ≈ 9.0). NH_3 diffuses into the tubular fluid of the collecting duct, and H^+ secretion by the collecting duct leads to accumulation of NH_4^+ in the lumen by the processes of nonionic diffusion and diffusion trapping. For each molecule of NH_4^+ excreted in the urine, a molecule of "new" HCO_3^- is added back to the extracellular fluid. CA, carbonic anhydrase. Collecting duct NH_4^+ secretion via RhBG and RhCG is not depicted.

Assessing NH_4^+ excretion by the kidneys is done indirectly because assays of urine NH_4^+ are not routinely available. Consider, for example, the situation of metabolic acidosis. In metabolic acidosis, the appropriate renal response is to increase net acid excretion. Accordingly, little or no HCO_3^- appears in the urine, the urine is acidic, and NH_4^+ excretion is increased. To assess this, and especially the amount of NH_4^+ excreted, the "urinary net charge" or "urine anion gap" can be calculated by measuring the urinary concentrations of Na^+ K^+, and Cl^-.

$$\text{Urine anion gap} = [Na^+] + [K^+] - [Cl^-] \qquad (8\text{-}8)$$

The concept of urine anion gap during a metabolic acidosis assumes that the major cations in the urine are Na^+, K^+ and NH_4^+ and that the major anion is Cl^- (with urine pH less than 6.5, virtually no HCO_3^- is present). As a result, the urine anion gap yields a negative value when adequate amounts of NH_4^+ are being excreted. Indeed, the absence of a urine anion gap or the existence of a positive value indicates a renal defect in NH_4^+ production and excretion.

An important feature of the renal NH_4^+ system is that it can be regulated by systemic acid-base balance. Alterations in the pH of ECF, by affecting the pH of intracellular fluid, change glutamine metabolism in the cells of the proximal tubule. In addition, as already noted, cortisol levels increase during acidosis and cortisol stimulates ammoniagenesis (i.e., NH_4^+ production from glutamine). During systemic acidosis, the enzymes in the proximal tubule cell responsible for the metabolism of glutamine are stimulated. This involves the synthesis of new enzymes and requires several days for complete adaptation. With increased levels of these enzymes, NH_4^+ production is increased, allowing enhanced production of new HCO_3^-. Conversely, glutamine metabolism is reduced with alkalosis.

Other factors also regulate ammoniagenesis. Both angiotensin II and PTH stimulate ammoniagenesis, whereas ammoniagenesis is inhibited by prostaglandins. Because PTH levels are increased with acidosis, it may play a role in mediating the renal response, which, as noted, includes increased production and excretion of NH_4^+. Lastly, the $[K^+]$ of the ECF also alters NH_4^+ production. When hyperkalemia exists, NH_4^+ production is inhibited, whereas hypokalemia stimulates NH_4^+ production. The mechanism by which plasma $[K^+]$ alters NH_4^+ production is not fully understood. Alterations in the plasma $[K^+]$ may change the intracellular pH. The change in intracellular pH may then control glutamine metabolism. By this mechanism, hyperkalemia would raise intracellular pH and thereby inhibit glutamine metabolism. The opposite would occur during hypokalemia.

Renal tubule acidosis (RTA) refers to conditions in which net acid excretion by the kidneys is impaired. Under these conditions, the kidneys are unable to excrete a sufficient amount of net acid to balance nonvolatile acid production, and acidosis results. RTA can be caused by a defect in H^+ secretion in the proximal tubule **(proximal RTA)** or distal tubule **(distal RTA)** or by inadequate production and excretion of NH_4^+.

Proximal RTA can be caused by a variety of hereditary and acquired conditions (e.g., **cystinosis, Fanconi's syndrome,** administration of carbonic anhydrase inhibitors). The majority of cases of proximal RTA result from generalized tubule dysfunction rather than a selective defect in one of the proximal tubule acid-base transporters (e.g., Na^+-H^+ antiporter, Na-$3HCO_3^-$ symporter). Individuals who lack carbonic anhydrase (CA-II) present in the clinic with the features of proximal RTA, although distal H^+ secretion is also impaired. Regardless of the cause, if H^+ secretion by the cells of the proximal tubule is impaired, there is decreased reabsorption of the filtered load of HCO_3^-. Consequently, HCO_3^- is lost in the urine, the plasma $[HCO_3^-]$ decreases, and acidosis ensues.

Distal RTA also occurs in a number of hereditary and acquired conditions (e.g., **medullary sponge kidney,** certain drugs such as **amphotericin B,** and conditions secondary to urinary obstruction). Both autosomal dominant and autosomal recessive forms of distal RTA have been identified. An autosomal dominant form results from mutations in the gene coding for the Cl^- HCO_3^- antiporter (AE-1) in the basolateral membrane of the acid-secreting intercalated cell. Autosomal recessive forms are caused by mutations in various subunits of the H^+-ATPase. Some patients with Sjögren's syndrome, an autoimmune disease, develop distal RTA as a result of antibodies directed against the H^+-ATPase. Lastly, H^+ secretion by the distal tubule and the collecting duct may be normal, but the permeability of the cells to H$^+$ is increased. This occurs with the antifungal drug amphotericin B, the administration of which also leads to the development of distal RTA. Regardless of the cause of distal RTA, the ability to acidify the tubular fluid in the distal tubule and collecting duct is impaired. Consequently, titratable acid excretion is reduced, and nonionic diffusion and diffusion trapping of NH$_4^+$ are impaired. This, in turn, decreases net acid excretion, with the subsequent development of acidosis.

Failure to produce and excrete sufficient quantities of NH$_4^+$ can also reduce net acid excretion by the kidneys. This situation occurs as a result of generalized dysfunction of the distal tubule and collecting duct with impaired H$^+$, NH$_4^+$, and K$^+$ secretion. Generalized distal nephron dysfunction is seen in individuals with mutations in the Na$^+$ channel (ENaC), which are inherited in an autosomal recessive pattern. An autosomal dominant form is also seen with mutations in the mineralocorticoid receptor. More commonly, NH$_4^+$ production and excretion are impaired in patients with hyporeninemic hypoaldosteronism. These patients typically have moderate degrees of renal failure with reduced levels of renin and, thus, aldosterone. As a result, distal tubule and collecting duct function is impaired. Finally, a number of drugs can also result in distal tubule and collecting duct dysfunction. These include drugs that block the Na$^+$ channel (e.g., amiloride), block the production or action of angiotensin II (ACE inhibitor), or block the action of aldosterone (e.g., spironolactone). Regardless of the cause, the impaired function of the distal tubule and collecting duct results in the development of hyperkalemia, which in turn impairs ammoniagenesis by the proximal tubule. H$^+$ secretion by the distal tubule and collecting duct and thus NH$_4^+$ secretion are also impaired by these drugs. Thus, net acid excretion is less than net acid production, and metabolic acidosis develops.

If the acidosis that results from any of these forms of RTA is severe, individuals must ingest alkali (e.g., baking soda or a citrate-containing solution[6]) to maintain acid-base balance. In this way, the HCO$_3^-$ lost each day in the buffering of nonvolatile acid is replenished by the extra HCO$_3^-$ ingested in the diet.

---

[6]One of the byproducts of citrate metabolism is HCO$_3^-$. Ingestion of citrate-containing drinks is often more palatable to patients than ingesting baking soda.

RESPONSE TO ACID-BASE DISORDERS

The pH of the ECF is maintained within a very narrow range (7.35 to 7.45).[7] Inspection of equation 8-3 shows that the pH of the ECF varies when either the [HCO$_3^-$] or PCO$_2$ is altered. As already noted, disturbances of acid-base balance that result from a change in the [HCO$_3^-$] of the ECF are termed **metabolic acid-base disorders,** whereas those resulting from a change in the PCO$_2$ are termed **respiratory acid-base disorders.** The kidneys are primarily responsible for regulating the [HCO$_3^-$], whereas the lungs regulate the PCO$_2$.

When an acid-base disturbance develops, the body uses a series of mechanisms to defend against the change in the pH of the ECF. These defense mechanisms do not correct the acid-base disturbance but merely minimize the change in pH imposed by the disturbance. Restoration of the blood pH to its normal value requires correction of the underlying process or processes that produced the acid-base disorder. The body has three general mechanisms to compensate for, or defend against, changes in body fluid pH produced by acid-base disturbances: (1) extracellular and intracellular buffering, (2) adjustments in blood PCO$_2$ by alterations in the ventilatory rate of the lungs, and (3) adjustments in the renal net acid excretion.

Extracellular and Intracellular Buffers

The first line of defense against acid-base disorders is extracellular and intracellular buffering. The response of the extracellular buffers is virtually instantaneous, whereas the response to intracellular buffering is slower and can take several minutes.

Metabolic disorders that result from the addition of nonvolatile acid or alkali to the body fluids are buffered in both the extracellular and intracellular compartments. The HCO$_3^-$ buffer system is the principal

---

[7]For simplicity of presentation in this chapter, the value of 7.40 for body fluid pH is used as normal, even though the normal range is from 7.35 to 7.45. Similarly, the normal range for PCO$_2$ is 35 to 45 mm Hg. However, a PCO$_2$ of 40 mm Hg is used as the normal value. Finally, a value of 24 mEq/L is considered a normal ECF [HCO$_3^-$], even though the normal range is 22 to 28 mEq/L.

ECF buffer. When nonvolatile acid is added to the body fluids (or alkali is lost from the body), HCO_3^- is consumed during the process of neutralizing the acid load, and the $[HCO_3^-]$ of the ECF is reduced. Conversely, when nonvolatile alkali is added to the body fluids (or acid is lost from the body), H^+ is consumed, causing more HCO_3^- to be produced from the dissociation of H_2CO_3. Consequently, the $[HCO_3^-]$ increases.

Although the HCO_3^- buffer system is the principal ECF buffer, Pi and plasma proteins provide additional extracellular buffering. The combined action of the buffering processes for HCO_3^-, Pi, and plasma protein accounts for approximately 50% of the buffering of a nonvolatile acid load and 70% of that of a nonvolatile alkali load. The remainder of the buffering under these two conditions occurs intracellularly. Intracellular buffering involves the movement of H^+ into cells (during buffering of nonvolatile acid) or the movement of H^+ out of cells (during buffering of nonvolatile alkali). H^+ is titrated inside the cell by HCO_3^-, Pi, and the histidine groups on proteins.

Bone represents an additional source of extracellular buffering. With acidosis, buffering by bone results in its demineralization because Ca^{++} is released from bone as Ca^{++}-containing salts bind H^+ in exchange for Ca^{++}.

When respiratory acid-base disorders occur, the pH of body fluid changes as a result of alterations in the P_{CO_2}. Virtually all buffering in respiratory acid-base disorders occurs intracellularly. When the P_{CO_2} rises (respiratory acidosis), CO_2 moves into the cell, where it combines with H_2O to form H_2CO_3. H_2CO_3 then dissociates to H^+ and HCO_3^-. Some of the H^+ is buffered by cellular protein, and HCO_3^- exits the cell and raises the plasma $[HCO_3^-]$. This process is reversed when the P_{CO_2} is reduced (respiratory alkalosis). Under this condition, the hydration reaction ($H_2O + CO_2 \leftrightarrow H_2CO_3$) is shifted to the left by the decrease in P_{CO_2}. As a result, the dissociation reaction ($H_2CO_3 \leftrightarrow H^+ + HCO_3^-$) also shifts to the left, thereby reducing the plasma $[HCO_3^-]$.

Respiratory Compensation

The lungs are the second line of defense against acid-base disorders. As indicated by the Henderson-Hasselbalch equation (see equation 8-3), changes in the P_{CO_2} alter the blood pH: a rise decreases the pH, and a reduction increases the pH.

The ventilatory rate determines the P_{CO_2}. Increased ventilation decreases P_{CO_2}, whereas decreased ventilation increases it. The blood P_{CO_2} and pH are important regulators of the ventilatory rate. Chemoreceptors located in the brainstem (ventral surface of the medulla) and periphery (carotid and aortic bodies) sense changes in P_{CO_2} and $[H^+]$ and alter the ventilatory rate appropriately. Thus, when metabolic acidosis occurs, a rise in the $[H^+]$ (decrease in pH) increases the ventilatory rate. Conversely, during metabolic alkalosis, a decreased $[H^+]$ (increase in pH) leads to a reduced ventilatory rate. With maximal hyperventilation, the P_{CO_2} can be reduced to approximately 10 mm Hg. Because hypoxia, a potent stimulator of ventilation, also develops with hypoventilation, the degree to which the P_{CO_2} can be increased is limited. In an otherwise healthy individual, hypoventilation cannot raise the P_{CO_2} above 60 mm Hg. The respiratory response to metabolic acid-base disturbances may be initiated within minutes but may require several hours to complete.

Insulin-dependent diabetic patients can develop metabolic acidosis (secondary to the production of keto acids) if insulin dosages are not adequate. As a compensatory response to this acidosis, deep and rapid breathing develops. This breathing pattern is termed Kussmaul's respiration. With prolonged Kussmaul's respiration, the muscles involved can become fatigued. When this happens, respiratory compensation is impaired and the acidosis can become more severe.

Renal Compensation

The third and final line of defense against acid-base disorders is the kidneys. In response to an alteration in the plasma pH and P_{CO_2}, the kidneys make appropriate adjustments in the excretion of HCO_3^- and net acid. The renal response may require several days to reach completion because it takes hours to days to increase the synthesis and activity of the proximal tubule enzymes involved in NH_4^+ production. In the case of acidosis (increased $[H^+]$ or P_{CO_2}), the secretion of H^+ by the nephron is stimulated, and the entire filtered load of HCO_3^- is reabsorbed. Titratable acid excretion is increased, the production and excretion of NH_4^+ are also stimulated, and, thus, net acid excretion by the kidneys is increased (see equation 8-7).

The new HCO_3^- generated during the process of net acid excretion is added to the body, and the plasma $[HCO_3^-]$ increases.

When alkalosis exists (decreased $[H^+]$ or P_{CO_2}), the secretion of H^+ by the nephron is inhibited. As a result, HCO_3^- reabsorption is reduced, as is the excretion of both titratable acid and NH_4^+. Thus, net acid excretion is decreased and HCO_3^- appears in the urine. Also, some HCO_3^- is secreted into the urine by the HCO_3^-- secreting intercalated cells of the distal tubule and collecting duct. With enhanced excretion of HCO_3^-, the plasma $[HCO_3^-]$ decreases.

Loss of gastric contents from the body (i.e., vomiting, nasogastric suction) produces metabolic alkalosis secondary to the loss of HCl. If the loss of gastric fluid is significant, ECF volume contraction occurs. Under this condition, the kidneys cannot excrete sufficient quantities of HCO_3^- to compensate for the metabolic alkalosis. HCO_3^- is not excreted because the volume contraction enhances Na^+ reabsorption by the proximal tubule and increases aldosterone levels (see Chapter 6). These responses in turn limit HCO_3^- excretion because a significant amount of Na^+ reabsorption in the proximal tubule is coupled to H^+ secretion through the Na^+-H^+ antiporter. As a result, HCO_3^- is reabsorbed because of the need to reduce Na^+ excretion. In addition, the elevated aldosterone levels stimulate H^+ secretion by the distal tubule and collecting duct. Thus, in individuals who lose gastric contents, metabolic alkalosis and paradoxically acidic urine characteristically occur. Correction of the alkalosis occurs only when euvolemia is reestablished. With restoration of euvolemia, HCO_3^- reabsorption by the proximal tubule decreases, as does H^+ secretion by the distal tubule and collecting duct. As a result, HCO_3^- excretion increases, and the plasma $[HCO_3^-]$ returns to normal.

SIMPLE ACID-BASE DISORDERS

Table 8-2 summarizes the primary alterations and the subsequent compensatory or defense mechanisms of the various simple acid-base disorders. In all acid-base disorders the compensatory response does not correct the underlying disorder but simply reduces the magnitude of the change in pH. Correction of the acid-base disorder requires treatment of its cause.

When nonvolatile acid is added to the body fluids, as in **diabetic ketoacidosis,** the $[H^+]$ increases (pH decreases) and the $[HCO_3^-]$ decreases. In addition, the concentration of the anion associated with the nonvolatile acid increases. This change in the anion concentration provides a convenient way to analyze the cause of a metabolic acidosis by calculating what is termed the **anion gap.** The anion gap represents the difference between the concentration of the major ECF cation (Na^+) and the major ECF anions (Cl^- and HCO_3^-):

$$\text{Anion gap} = [Na^+] - ([Cl^-] + [HCO_3^-]) \quad \text{(8-9)}$$

Under normal conditions, the anion gap ranges from 8 to 16 mEq/L. It is important to recognize that an anion gap does not actually exist. All cations are balanced by anions. The gap simply reflects the parameters that are measured. In reality:

$$[Na^+] + [\text{unmeasured cations}] \quad \text{(8-10)}$$
$$= [Cl^-] + [HCO_3^-] + [\text{unmeasured anions}]$$

If the anion of the nonvolatile acid is Cl^-, the anion gap is normal. (That is, the decrease in the $[HCO_3^-]$ is matched by an increase in the $[Cl^-]$.) The metabolic acidosis associated with diarrhea or renal tubular acidosis has a normal anion gap. In contrast, if the anion of the nonvolatile acid is not Cl^- (e.g., lactate, β-hydroxybutyrate), the anion gap increases (i.e., the decrease in the $[HCO_3^-]$ is not matched by an increase in the $[Cl^-]$ but rather by an increase in the concentration of the unmeasured anion). The anion gap is increased in metabolic acidosis associated with renal failure, diabetes mellitus (ketoacidosis), lactic acidosis, and the ingestion of large quantities of aspirin. Thus, calculation of the anion gap is a useful way to identify the etiology of metabolic acidosis in the clinical setting.

Metabolic Acidosis

Metabolic acidosis is characterized by a decreased ECF $[HCO_3^-]$ and pH. It can develop through addition of nonvolatile acid to the body (e.g., diabetic ketoacidosis), loss of nonvolatile base (e.g., HCO_3^- loss caused by diarrhea), or failure of the kidneys to excrete sufficient net acid to replenish the HCO_3^- used to neutralize nonvolatile acids (e.g., renal tubular acidosis,

TABLE 8-2			
Characteristics of Simple Acid-Base Disorders			
DISORDER	PLASMA pH	PRIMARY ALTERATION	DEFENSE MECHANISMS
Metabolic acidosis	↓	↓ ECF[HCO_3^-]	ICF and ECF buffers Hyperventilation (↓ P_{CO_2}) Renal NAE
Metabolic alkalosis	↑	↑ ECF[HCO_3^-]	ICF and ECF buffers Hypoventilation (↑ P_{CO_2}) Renal NAE
Respiratory acidosis	↓	↑ P_{CO_2}	ICF buffers ↑ Renal NAE
Respiratory alkalosis	↑	↓ P_{CO_2}	ICF buffers ↓ Renal NAE

ECF, extracellular fluid; ICF, intracellular fluid; NAE, net acid excretion.

renal failure). As previously described, the buffering of H+ occurs in both the ECF and ICF compartments. When the pH falls, the respiratory centers are stimulated, and the ventilatory rate is increased (respiratory compensation). This reduces the P_{CO_2}, which further minimizes the fall in plasma pH. In general, there is a decrease of 1.2 mm Hg in the P_{CO_2} for every 1 mEq/L fall in ECF [HCO_3^-]. Thus, if the [HCO_3^-] was reduced to 14 mEq/L from a normal value of 24 mEq/L, the expected decrease in P_{CO_2} would be 12 mm Hg and the measured P_{CO_2} would fall to 28 mm Hg (normal P_{CO_2} = 40 mm Hg).

Finally, in metabolic acidosis, renal net acid excretion is increased. This occurs through the elimination of all HCO_3^- from the urine (enhanced reabsorption of filtered HCO_3^-) and through increased titratable acid and NH_4^+ excretion (enhanced production of new HCO_3^-). If the process that initiated the acid-base disturbance is corrected, the enhanced net acid excretion by the kidneys ultimately returns the pH and [HCO_3^-] to normal. After correction of the pH, the ventilatory rate also returns to normal.

Metabolic Alkalosis

Metabolic alkalosis is characterized by an increased ECF [HCO_3^-] and pH. It can occur through the addition of nonvolatile base to the body (e.g., ingestion of antacids), as a result of volume contraction (e.g., hemorrhage), or, more commonly, from the loss of

nonvolatile acid (e.g., loss of gastric HCl because of prolonged vomiting). Buffering occurs predominantly in the ECF compartment and to a lesser degree in the ICF compartment. The increase in the pH inhibits the respiratory centers, the ventilatory rate is reduced, and thus the P_{CO_2} is elevated (respiratory compensation). With appropriate respiratory compensation, a 0.7 mm Hg increase in P_{CO_2} is expected for every 1 mEq/L rise in ECF [HCO_3^-].

The renal compensatory response to metabolic alkalosis is to increase the excretion of HCO_3^- by reducing its reabsorption along the nephron. Normally, this occurs quite rapidly (minutes to hours) and effectively. However, as already noted, when alkalosis occurs with ECF volume contraction (e.g., vomiting in which fluid loss occurs with H+ loss), HCO_3^- is not excreted. In volume-depleted individuals, renal excretion of HCO_3^- is enhanced, and alkalosis is corrected, only with restoration of euvolemia. Enhanced renal excretion of HCO_3^- eventually returns the pH and [HCO_3^-] to normal, provided that the underlying cause of the initial acid-base disturbance is corrected. When the pH is corrected, the ventilatory rate also returns to normal.

Respiratory Acidosis

Respiratory acidosis is characterized by an elevated P_{CO_2} and reduced ECF pH. It results from decreased gas exchange across the alveoli as a result of either inadequate ventilation (e.g., drug-induced depression of the respiratory centers) or impaired gas diffusion (e.g., pulmonary edema, such as that which occurs in cardiovascular or lung disease). In contrast to the metabolic disorders, buffering during respiratory acidosis occurs almost entirely in the ICF compartment. The increase in the P_{CO_2} and the decrease in pH stimulate both HCO_3^- reabsorption by the nephron and titratable acid and NH_4^+ excretion (renal compensation). Together, these responses increase net acid excretion and generate new HCO_3^-. The renal compensatory response takes several days to occur. Consequently, respiratory acid-base disorders are commonly divided into acute and chronic phases. In the acute phase, the time for the renal compensatory response is not sufficient, and the body relies on ICF buffering to minimize the change in pH. During this phase, and because of the buffering, there is a 1 mEq/L increase in ECF [HCO_3^-] for every 10 mm Hg rise in P_{CO_2}.

In the chronic phase, renal compensation occurs, and there is a 3.5 mEq/L increase in ECF [HCO_3^-] for each 10 mm Hg rise in Pco_2. Correction of the underlying disorder returns the Pco_2 to normal, and renal net acid excretion decreases to its initial level.

Respiratory Alkalosis

Respiratory alkalosis is characterized by a reduced Pco_2 and an increased ECF pH. It results from increased gas exchange in the lungs, usually caused by increased ventilation from stimulation of the respiratory centers (e.g., by drugs or disorders of the central nervous system). Hyperventilation also occurs at high altitude and as a result of anxiety, pain, or fear. As noted, buffering is primarily in the ICF compartment. As with respiratory acidosis, respiratory alkalosis has both acute and chronic phases reflecting the time required for renal compensation to occur. In the acute phase of respiratory alkalosis, which reflects intracellular buffering, the ECF [HCO_3^-] decreases 2 mEq/L for every 10 mm Hg fall in Pco_2. With renal compensation, the elevated pH and reduced Pco_2 inhibit HCO_3^- reabsorption by the nephron and reduce titratable acid and NH_4^+ excretion. As a result of these two effects, net acid excretion is reduced. With complete renal compensation there is an expected 5 mEq/L decrease in ECF [HCO_3^-] for every 10 mm Hg reduction in Pco_2. Correction of the underlying disorder returns the Pco_2 to normal, and renal excretion of acid then increases to its initial level.

ANALYSIS OF ACID-BASE DISORDERS

The analysis of an acid-base disorder is directed at identifying the underlying cause so that appropriate therapy can be initiated. The patient's medical history and associated physical findings often provide valuable clues about the nature and origin of an acid-base disorder. In addition, the analysis of an arterial blood sample is frequently required. Such an analysis is straightforward if approached systematically. For example, consider the following data:

pH	7.35
[HCO_3^-]	16 mEq/L
Pco_2	30 mm Hg

The acid-base disorder represented by these values, or any other set of values, can be determined using the following three-step approach (Figure 8-6):

1. *Examination of the pH*: When the pH is considered first, the underlying disorder can be classified as either an acidosis or an alkalosis. The defense mechanisms of the body cannot correct an acid-base disorder by themselves. Thus, even if the defense mechanisms are completely operative, the change in pH indicates the acid-base disorder. In the example provided, the pH of 7.35 indicates acidosis.

2. *Determination of metabolic versus respiratory disorder*: Simple acid-base disorders are either metabolic or respiratory. To determine which disorder is present, the clinician must next examine the ECF [HCO_3^-] and Pco_2. As previously discussed, acidosis could be the result of a decrease in the [HCO_3^-] (metabolic) or an increase in the Pco_2 (respiratory). Alternatively, alkalosis could be the result of an increase in the ECF [HCO_3^-] (metabolic) or a decrease in the Pco_2 (respiratory). For the example provided, the ECF [HCO_3^-] is reduced from normal (normal = 24 mEq/L), as is the Pco_2 (normal = 40 mm Hg). The disorder must therefore be metabolic acidosis; it cannot be a respiratory acidosis because the Pco_2 is reduced.

3. *Analysis of a compensatory response*: Metabolic disorders result in compensatory changes in ventilation and thus in the Pco_2, whereas respiratory disorders result in compensatory changes in renal net acid excretion and thus in the ECF [HCO_3^-]. In an appropriately compensated metabolic acidosis, the Pco_2 is decreased, whereas it is elevated in compensated metabolic alkalosis. With respiratory acidosis, complete compensation results in an elevation of the [HCO_3^-]. Conversely, the ECF [HCO_3^-] is reduced in response to respiratory alkalosis. In this example, the Pco_2 is reduced from normal, and the magnitude of this reduction (10 mm Hg decrease in Pco_2 for an 8 mEq/L increase in ECF [HCO_3^-]) is as expected (see Figure 8-6). Therefore, the acid-base disorder is a simple metabolic acidosis with appropriate respiratory compensation.

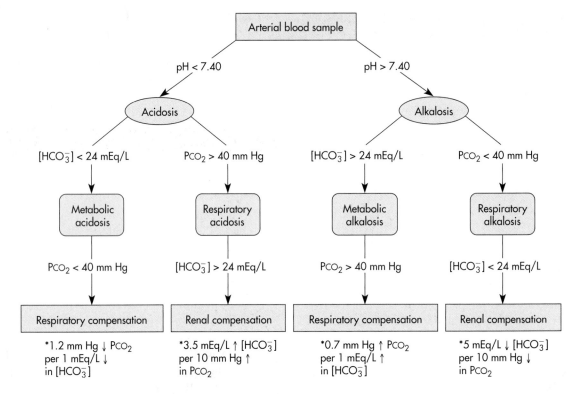

FIGURE 8-6 ■ Approach for the analysis of simple acid-base disorders.

If the appropriate compensatory response is not present, a **mixed acid-base disorder** should be suspected. Such a disorder reflects the presence of two or more underlying causes for the acid-base disturbance. A mixed disorder should be suspected when analysis of the arterial blood gas indicates that appropriate compensation has not occurred. For example, consider the following data:

pH   6.96
[HCO_3^-]   12 mEq/L
P_{CO_2} 55 mm Hg

When the three-step approach is followed, it is evident that the disturbance is an acidosis that has both a metabolic component (ECF [HCO_3^-] < 24 mEq/L) and a respiratory component (P_{CO_2} > 40 mm Hg). Thus, this disorder is mixed. Mixed acid-base disorders can occur, for example, in an individual who

has a history of a chronic pulmonary disease such as emphysema (i.e., chronic respiratory acidosis) and who develops an acute gastrointestinal illness with diarrhea. Because diarrhea fluid contains HCO_3^-, its loss from the body results in the development of metabolic acidosis.

A mixed acid-base disorder is also indicated when a patient has abnormal P_{CO_2} and ECF [HCO_3^-] values but the pH is normal. Such a condition can develop in a patient who has ingested a large quantity of aspirin. The salicylic acid (active ingredient in aspirin) produces metabolic acidosis, and at the same time it stimulates the respiratory centers, causing hyperventilation and respiratory alkalosis. Thus, the patient has a reduced ECF [HCO_3^-] and a reduced P_{CO_2}. (*Note:* The P_{CO_2} is lower than would occur with normal respiratory compensation of a metabolic acidosis.)

SUMMARY

1. The pH of the body fluids is maintained within a narrow range by the coordinated function of the lungs, liver, and kidneys. These organs maintain acid-base balance by balancing the excretion of acid and alkali with the amounts ingested in the diet and produced by metabolism.

2. The kidneys maintain acid-base balance through the excretion of an amount of acid equal to the amount of nonvolatile acid produced by metabolism and the quantity ingested in the diet. The kidneys also prevent the loss of HCO_3^- in the urine by reabsorbing virtually all the HCO_3^- filtered at the glomeruli. Both the reabsorption of filtered HCO_3^- and the excretion of acid are accomplished by the secretion of H^+ by the nephrons.

3. Renal net acid excretion (NAE) is quantitated as:

$$NAE = [(U_{NH_4^+} \times \dot{V}) + (U_{TA} \times \dot{V})] - (U_{HCO_3^-} \times \dot{V})$$

4. The primary urinary buffer is Pi (titratable acid). The excretion of titratable acid together with the production (from glutamine metabolism) and excretion of NH_4^+ are critical to the generation of new HCO_3^- by the kidneys.

5. The body uses three lines of defense to minimize the impact of acid-base disorders on body fluid pH: (1) ECF and ICF buffering, (2) respiratory compensation, and (3) renal compensation.

6. Metabolic acid-base disorders result from primary alterations in the ECF $[HCO_3^-]$, which in turn results from the addition of acid to or loss of alkali from the body. In response to metabolic acidosis, pulmonary ventilation is increased, which decreases the P_{CO_2}, and renal net acid excretion is increased. An increase in the ECF $[HCO_3^-]$ causes alkalosis. This decreases pulmonary ventilation, which elevates the P_{CO_2}. The pulmonary response to metabolic acid-base disorders occurs in a matter of minutes. Renal net acid excretion is also decreased. This response may take several days.

7. Respiratory acid-base disorders result from primary alterations in the P_{CO_2}. Elevation of the P_{CO_2} produces acidosis, and the kidneys respond with an increase in net acid excretion. Conversely, reduction of the P_{CO_2} produces alkalosis, and renal net acid excretion is reduced. The kidneys respond to respiratory acid-base disorders over several hours to days.

KEY WORDS AND CONCEPTS

- Acid
- Alkali
- HCO_3^- buffer system
- Carbonic anhydrase (CA)
- Henderson-Hasselbalch equation
- Acidosis
- Alkalosis
- Volatile acid
- Nonvolatile acid
- Diabetes mellitus
- Hypoxia
- Intercalated cell
- Titratable acids
- Ammonium (NH_4^+)
- Net acid excretion (NAE)
- Formation of new HCO_3^-
- Nonionic diffusion
- Diffusion trapping (of ammonia)
- Metabolic acid-base disorder
- Respiratory acid-base disorder
- Chemoreceptors
- ECF and ICF buffering
- Respiratory compensation
- Plasma anion gap
- Urinary net charge (urine anion gap)
- Renal compensation
- Simple acid-base disorders
- Mixed acid-base disorder

SELF-STUDY PROBLEMS

1. If there were no urinary buffers, how much urine (L/day) would the kidneys have to produce to excrete net acid equal to the amount of nonvolatile acid produced from metabolism? Assume that nonvolatile acid production is 70 mEq/day and the minimum urine pH is 4.0.

2. In the accompanying table, indicate the simple acid-base disorder that exists for the laboratory data given. Use the following as normal values: pH = 7.40; $[HCO_3^-]$ = 24 mEq/L; P_{CO_2} = 40 mm Hg.

pH	$[HCO_3^-]$ (mEq/L)	P_{CO_2} (mm Hg)	Disorder
7.23	10	25	
7.46	30	44	
7.37	28	50	
7.66	22	20	
7.34	26	50	
7.54	18	22	

3. A previously healthy individual develops a gastrointestinal illness with nausea and vomiting. The following laboratory data are obtained after 12 hours of this illness:

Body weight	70 kg
Blood pressure	120/80 mm Hg
Plasma pH	7.48
P_{CO_2}	44 mm Hg
Plasma $[HCO_3^-]$	32 mEq/L
Urine pH	7.5

a. What is the acid-base disorder of this individual? What was its origin? The illness continues, and 48 hours later the following laboratory data are obtained:

Body weight	68 kg
Blood pressure	80/40 mm Hg
Plasma pH	7.50
P_{CO_2}	48 mm Hg
Plasma $[HCO_3^-]$	36 mEq/L
Urine pH	6.0

b. Has the acid-base disturbance changed? How do you explain the paradoxical decrease in urine pH?

4. What would happen to urinary HCO_3^- excretion if a drug that inhibits carbonic anhydrase is administered, and by what mechanism would this effect occur? What type of acid-base disorder could result from the use of this drug?

5. A previously healthy 28-year-old man is seen in the emergency room with severe right flank pain. Shortly after arrival, he passes a kidney stone. He reports that several people in his family have also had kidney stones. The following laboratory data are obtained (see Appendix B for normal values):

Serum $[Na^+]$	137 mEq/L
Serum $[K^+]$	3.1 mEq/L
Serum $[Cl^-]$	111 mEq/L
Serum $[HCO_3^-]$	13 mEq/L
Arterial pH	7.28
Arterial P_{CO_2}	28 mm Hg
Urine pH	7.10

a. What is the acid-base disorder, and what is the plasma anion gap?
b. How do you explain his urine pH value, and how did this contribute to the formation of his kidney stone?

REGULATION OF CALCIUM AND PHOSPHATE HOMEOSTASIS

■ ■ ■ ■ ■ ■ ■ ■ ■ ■ ■ ■ ■ ■

OBJECTIVES

Upon completion of this chapter, the student should be able to answer the following questions:

1. What is the physiologic importance of calcium (Ca^{++}) and phosphate (Pi)?

2. How does the body maintain Ca^{++} and Pi homeostasis?

3. What is the relative importance of the kidneys versus the gastrointestinal tract and bone in maintaining plasma Ca^{++} and Pi levels?

4. What hormones and factors regulate plasma Ca^{++} and Pi levels?

5. What are the cellular mechanisms responsible for Ca^{++} and Pi reabsorption along the nephron?

6. What hormones regulate renal Ca^{++} and Pi excretion?

7. What is the role of the calcium-sensing receptor?

Ca^{++} and inorganic phosphate (Pi)[1] are multivalent ions that subserve many complex and vital functions. Ca^{++} is an important cofactor in many enzymatic reactions; it is a key second messenger in numerous signaling pathways; it plays an important role in neural transduction, blood clotting, and muscle contraction; and it is a critical component of the extracellular matrix, cartilage, teeth, and bone. Pi, like Ca^{++}, is a key component of bone. Pi is important for metabolic processes, including formation of ATP, and it is an important component of nucleic acids. Phosphorylation of proteins is an important mechanism of cellular signaling, and Pi is an important buffer in cells, plasma, and urine.

In a normal adult, the renal excretion of Ca^{++} and Pi is balanced by gastrointestinal absorption. If the plasma concentrations of Ca^{++} and Pi decline substantially, gastrointestinal absorption, bone resorption (i.e., the loss of Ca^{++} and Pi from bone), and renal tubular reabsorption increase and return plasma concentrations of Ca^{++} and Pi to normal levels. During growth and pregnancy, intestinal absorption exceeds urinary excretion, and these ions accumulate in newly formed fetal tissue and bone. In contrast, bone disease (e.g., osteoporosis) or a decline in lean body mass increases urinary multivalent ion loss without a change in intestinal absorption. These conditions produce a net loss of Ca^{++} and Pi from the body.

This brief introduction reveals that the kidneys, in conjunction with the gastrointestinal tract and bone, play a major role in maintaining plasma Ca^{++} and Pi levels as well as Ca^{++} and Pi balance. Accordingly, this chapter discusses Ca^{++} and Pi handling by the kidneys with an emphasis on the hormones and factors that regulate urinary excretion.

---

[1]At physiologic pH, inorganic phosphate exists as HPO_4^{-2} and $H_2PO_4^-$ (pK = 6.8). For simplicity, we collectively refer to these ion species as Pi.

CALCIUM

Cellular processes in which Ca^{++} plays a part include bone formation, cell division and growth, blood coagulation, hormone-response coupling, and electrical stimulus-response coupling (e.g., muscle contraction, neurotransmitter release). A total of 99% of Ca^{++} is stored in bone, approximately 1% is found in the intracellular fluid (ICF), and 0.1% is located in the ECF (Table 9-1). The total Ca^{++} concentration ($[Ca^{++}]$) in plasma is 10 mg/dL (2.5 mM or 5 mEq/L), and its concentration is normally maintained within very narrow limits. A low ionized plasma $[Ca^{++}]$ (**hypocalcemia**) increases the excitability of nerve and muscle cells and can lead to hypocalcemic **tetany,** which is characterized by skeletal muscle spasms. Tetany associated with hypocalcemia occurs because hypocalcemia causes the threshold potential to shift to more negative values (i.e., closer to the resting membrane voltage; see Figure 7-1). An elevated ionized plasma $[Ca^{++}]$ (**hypercalcemia**) may decrease neuromuscular excitability or produce cardiac arrhythmias, lethargy, disorientation, and even death. This effect of hypercalcemia occurs because hypercalcemia causes the threshold potential to shift to less negative values (i.e., further from the resting membrane voltage). Within cells, Ca^{++} is sequestered in the endoplasmic reticulum and mitochondria, or it is bound to proteins. Thus, the free

intracellular $[Ca^{++}]$ is very low (~100 nM). The large concentration gradient for $[Ca^{++}]$ across cell membranes is maintained by a Ca^{++}-ATPase pump (PMCa1b) in all cells and by a $3Na^+$-Ca^{++} exchanger (NCX1) in some cells.

Overview of Ca^{++} Homeostasis

Ca^{++} homeostasis depends on two factors: (1) the total amount of Ca^{++} in the body and (2) the distribution of Ca^{++} between bone and the ECF. The total body Ca^{++} level is determined by the relative amounts of Ca^{++} absorbed by the gastrointestinal tract and excreted by the kidneys (Figure 9-1). The gastrointestinal tract absorbs Ca^{++} through an active, carrier-mediated transport mechanism that is stimulated by **calcitriol,** a metabolite of vitamin D_3. Net Ca^{++} absorption is normally 200 mg/day, but it can increase to 600 mg/day

			COMPARTMENT	
TABLE 9-1				
Body Content and Distribution of Ca^{++} and Pi				
Ion	Body Content	Bone	Intracellular	Extracellular
Ca^{++}	1300 g	99%	1%	0.10%
Pi	700 g	86%	14%	0.03%

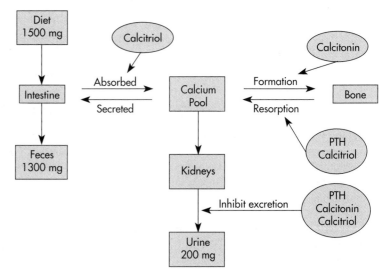

FIGURE 9-1 ■ Overview of Ca^{++} homeostasis. See text for details. PTH, parathyroid hormone.

when calcitriol levels rise. In adults, Ca^{++} excretion by the kidneys equals the amount absorbed by the gastrointestinal tract (200 mg/day), and it changes in parallel with the reabsorption of Ca^{++} by the gastrointestinal tract. Thus, in adults, Ca^{++} balance is maintained because the amount of Ca^{++} ingested in an average diet (1500 mg/day) equals the amount lost in the feces (1300 mg/day, the amount that escapes absorption by the gastrointestinal tract) plus the amount excreted in the urine (200 mg/day).

The second factor that controls Ca^{++} homeostasis is the distribution of Ca^{++} between bone and the ECF. Three hormones (**parathyroid hormone [PTH]**, **calcitriol,** and **calcitonin**) regulate the distribution of Ca^{++} between bone and the ECF and thereby regulate the plasma $[Ca^{++}]$. PTH is secreted by the parathyroid glands, and its secretion is stimulated by a decline in the plasma $[Ca^{++}]$ (i.e., hypocalcemia). Hypocalcemia stimulates the **calcium-sensing receptor (CaSR)** in the plasma membrane of chief cells in parathyroid glands, which in turn increases PTH gene expression and release. PTH increases the plasma $[Ca^{++}]$ by (1) stimulating bone resorption, (2) increasing Ca^{++} reabsorption by the kidneys, and (3) stimulating the production of calcitriol, which in turn increases Ca^{++} absorption by the gastrointestinal tract and facilitates PTH-mediated bone resorption. The production of calcitriol, a metabolite of vitamin D_3 produced in the kidney proximal tubule, is stimulated by hypocalcemia and hypophosphatemia. In addition, hypocalcemia stimulates PTH secretion, which also stimulates vitamin D_3 production by the proximal tubule cells. Calcitriol increases the plasma $[Ca^{++}]$ primarily by stimulating Ca^{++} absorption from the gastrointestinal tract. It also facilitates the action of PTH on bone and increases the expression of key Ca^{++} transport and binding proteins in the kidneys. Calcitonin is secreted by thyroid C cells (also known as parafollicular cells), and its secretion is stimulated by hypercalcemia. Calcitonin decreases the plasma $[Ca^{++}]$ mainly by stimulating bone formation (i.e., deposition of Ca^{++} in bone). Figure 9-2 illustrates the relationship between the plasma $[Ca^{++}]$ and plasma levels of PTH and calcitonin. Although calcitonin plays an important role in Ca^{++} homeostasis in lower vertebrates, it plays only a minor role in normal Ca^{++} homeostasis in humans.

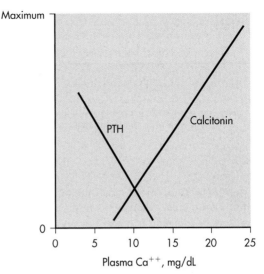

FIGURE 9-2 ■ Effect of the plasma $[Ca^{++}]$ on plasma levels of PTH and calcitonin. *(Modified from Azria M: The calcitonins: physiology and pharmacology. Basel, Switzerland, 1989, Karger.)*

Conditions that lower PTH levels (i.e., hypoparathyroidism after parathyroidectomy for an adenoma) reduce the plasma $[Ca^{++}]$, which can cause hypocalcemic tetany (intermittent muscular contractions). In severe cases, **hypocalcemic tetany** can cause death by asphyxiation. Hypercalcemia can also cause lethal cardiac arrhythmias and decreased neuromuscular excitability. Clinically, the most common causes of hypercalcemia are primary hyperparathyroidism and malignancy-associated hypercalcemia. Primary hyperparathyroidism results from the overproduction of PTH caused by a tumor of the parathyroid glands. In contrast, malignancy-associated hypercalcemia, which occurs in 10% to 20% of all patients with cancer, is caused by the secretion of **parathyroid hormone-related peptide (PTHRP)**, a PTH-like hormone secreted by carcinomas in various organs. Increased levels of PTH and PTHRP cause hypercalcemia and hypercalciuria.

Approximately 50% of the Ca^{++} in plasma is ionized, 45% is bound to plasma proteins (mainly albumin), and 5% is complexed to several anions, including HCO_3^-, citrate, Pi, and $SO_4^=$ (Table 9-2). The pH of plasma influences this distribution. Acidosis increases

TABLE 9-2			
Forms of Ca^{++} and Pi in Plasma			
ION	mg/dL	IONIZED	PROTEIN BOUND	COMPLEXED
Ca^{++}	10 mg/dL	50%	45%	5%
Pi	4 mg/dL	84%	10%	6%

Ca^{++} is bound (i.e., complexed) to various anions in the plasma, including HCO$_3^-$, citrate, Pi, and So$_4^=$. Pi is complexed to various cations, including Na$^+$ and K$^+$.

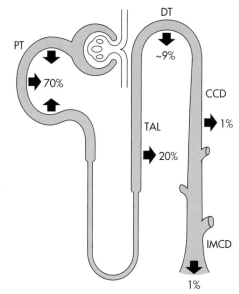

FIGURE 9-3 ■ Ca^{++} transport along the nephron. Percentages refer to the amount of the filtered Ca^{++} reabsorbed by each segment. Approximately 1% of the filtered Ca^{++} is excreted. CCD, cortical collecting duct; DT, distal tubule; IMCD, inner medullary collecting duct; PT, proximal tubule; TAL, thick ascending limb.

the percentage of ionized Ca^{++} at the expense of Ca^{++} bound to proteins, whereas alkalosis decreases the percentage of ionized Ca^{++}, again by altering the Ca^{++} bound to proteins. Individuals with alkalosis are susceptible to tetany, whereas individuals with acidosis are less susceptible to tetany, even when total plasma Ca^{++} levels are reduced. The increase in the [H$^+$] in patients with metabolic acidosis causes more H$^+$ to bind to plasma proteins, HCO$_3^-$, citrate, Pi, and SO$_4^=$, thereby displacing Ca^{++}. This displacement increases the plasma concentration of ionized Ca^{++}. In alkalosis the [H$^+$] of plasma decreases. Some H$^+$ ions dissociate from plasma proteins, HCO$_3^-$, citrate, Pi, and SO$_4^=$ in exchange for Ca^{++}, thereby decreasing the plasma concentration of ionized Ca^{++}. In addition, the plasma albumin concentration affects ionized plasma [Ca^{++}]. Hypoalbuminemia increases the ionized [Ca^{++}], whereas hyperalbuminemia decreases ionized plasma [Ca^{++}]. Under both conditions the total plasma [Ca^{++}] may not reflect the total ionized [Ca^{++}], which is the physiologic relevant measure of Ca^{++} homeostasis. The Ca^{++} available for glomerular filtration consists of the ionized fraction and the amount complexed with anions. Thus, about 55% of the Ca^{++} in the plasma is available for glomerular filtration.

Ca^{++} Transport along the Nephron

Normally, 99% of the filtered Ca^{++} (i.e., ionized and complexed) is reabsorbed by the nephron. The proximal tubule reabsorbs about 70% of the filtered Ca^{++}. Another 20% is reabsorbed in the loop of Henle (mainly the cortical portion of the thick ascending limb), about 9% is reabsorbed by the distal tubule, and less than 1% is reabsorbed by the collecting duct. About 1% (200 mg/day) is excreted in the urine. This fraction is equal to the net amount absorbed daily

by the gastrointestinal tract. Figure 9-3 summarizes the handling of Ca^{++} by the different portions of the nephron.

Ca^{++} reabsorption by the proximal tubule occurs by two pathways: transcellular and paracellular (Figure 9-4). Ca^{++} reabsorption across the cellular pathway accounts for 20% of proximal reabsorption. Ca^{++} reabsorption through the cell is an active process that occurs in two steps. First, Ca^{++} diffuses down its electrochemical gradient across the apical membrane through Ca^{++} channels and into the cell. Second, at the basolateral membrane, Ca^{++} is extruded from the cell against its electrochemical gradient by a Ca^{++}-ATPase. A total of 80% of Ca^{++} is reabsorbed between cells across the tight junctions (i.e., paracellular pathway). This passive, paracellular reabsorption of Ca^{++} occurs by solvent drag along the entire length of the proximal tubule and is also driven by the positive luminal voltage in the second half of the proximal tubule (i.e., diffusion). Thus, approximately 80% of Ca^{++} reabsorption is paracellular, and approximately 20% is transcellular in the proximal tubule.

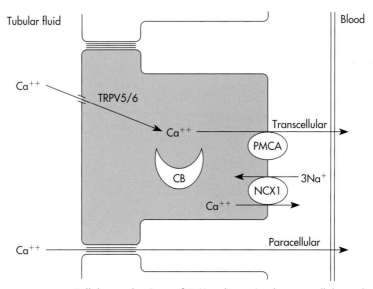

Tubular fluid

Blood

Ca^{++}

TRPV5/6

Ca^{++}

Transcellular

PMCA

CB

3Na$^+$

NCX1

Ca^{++}

Ca^{++}

Paracellular

FIGURE 9-4 ■ Cellular mechanisms of Ca^{++} reabsorption by transcellular and cellular pathways. Note that not all transport mechanisms are expressed in every nephron segment. In distal tubule cells, Ca^{++} enters cells across the apical membrane through Ca^{++}-permeable ion channels (TRPV5 and TRPV6). Inside distal tubule cells, Ca^{++} binds to calbindin (calbindin-D$_{28K}$ and calbindin-D$_{9K}$ [CB]), and the Ca^{++}-calbindin complex diffuses across the cell to deliver Ca^{++} to the basolateral membrane. Ca^{++} is transported across the basolateral membrane by a 3Na$^+$-Ca^{++} antiporter (NCX1) and the Ca^{++}-ATPase (PMCa1b). In the proximal tubule Ca^{++} reabsorption involves uptake across the brush border membrane through a Ca^{++}-permeable ion channel and exit across the basolateral membrane through the Ca^{++}-ATPase. A large portion of proximal tubule Ca^{++} reabsorption occurs by the paracellular pathway. This component of proximal tubule Ca^{++} reabsorption is driven by solvent drag. Reabsorption of Ca^{++} by the paracellular pathway in the TAL is driven by the transepithelial electrochemical gradient for Ca^{++}. Two proteins, claudin-16 and paracellin (PCLN-1), that contribute to tight junctions regulate the paracellular diffusion of Ca^{++} (see Box pg. 154). Ca^{++} reabsorption in the distal tubule occurs exclusively by the transcellular pathway.

Ca^{++} reabsorption by the loop of Henle is restricted to the cortical portion of the thick ascending limb (see Figure 9-4). Ca^{++} is reabsorbed by cellular and paracellular routes through mechanisms similar to those described for the proximal tubule but with one difference. Ca^{++} is not reabsorbed by solvent drag in this segment. (The thick ascending limb is impermeable to water.) In the thick ascending limb, Ca^{++} and Na$^+$ reabsorption parallel each other. These processes are parallel because of the significant component of Ca^{++} reabsorption that occurs by passive paracellular mechanisms secondary to Na$^+$ reabsorption and by

the generation of the lumen-positive transepithelial voltage. Loop diuretics inhibit Na$^+$ reabsorption by the thick ascending limb of the loop of Henle and in so doing reduce the magnitude of the lumen-positive transepithelial voltage (see Chapter 10). This action in turn inhibits the reabsorption of Ca^{++} by the paracellular pathway. Thus, loop diuretics are used to increase renal Ca^{++} excretion in patients with hypercalcemia. Therefore, Na$^+$ reabsorption also changes in parallel with Ca^{++} reabsorption by both the proximal tubule and the thick ascending limb of the loop of Henle.

Mutations in two tight junction proteins, **claudin-16** and **paracellin 1** (PCLN-1), alter the diffusive movement of Ca^{++} across tight junctions in the thick ascending limb of Henle's loop. Familial hypomagnesemic hypercalcemia is caused by mutations in claudin-16, a protein that is a component of the tight junctions in thick ascending limb cells. This disorder is characterized by enhanced excretion of Ca^{++} and magnesium (Mg^{++}) because of a fall in the passive reabsorption of these ions across the paracellular pathway in the TAL. The mutation in the claudin-16 gene reduces the permeability of the paracellular pathway to Ca^{++} and Mg^{++}, thereby reducing passive, paracellular reabsorption of both ions. Mutations in paracellin1 are present in patients with the hypomagnesemia, hypercalciuria syndrome (HHS). In these patients, Ca^{++} excretion is impaired because the mutation in paracellin 1 impairs the paracellular reabsorption of Ca^{++} in the thick ascending limb.

In the distal tubule, where the voltage in the tubule lumen is electrically negative with respect to the blood, Ca^{++} reabsorption is entirely active because Ca^{++} is reabsorbed against its electrochemical gradient (see Figure 9-4). Ca^{++} reabsorption by the distal tubule is exclusively transcellular. Calcium enters the cell across the apical membrane by the Ca^{++}-permeable epithelial ion channels (TRPV5/TRPV6). Inside the cell, Ca^{++} binds to calbindin. The calbindin-Ca^{++} complex carries Ca^{++} across the cell and delivers Ca^{++} to the basolateral membrane, where it is extruded from the cell by either the Ca^{++}-ATPase (PMCA1b) or the $3Na^+/Ca^{++}$ antiporter (NCX1). Urinary Na^+ excretion and Ca^{++} excretion usually change in parallel. However, excretion of these ions does not always change in parallel because the reabsorption of Ca^{++} and Na^+ by the distal tubule is independent and is differentially regulated. For example, **thiazide diuretics** inhibit Na^+ reabsorption by the distal tubule and stimulate Ca^{++} reabsorption by this segment. Accordingly, the net effects of thiazide diuretics are to increase urinary Na^+ excretion and to reduce urinary Ca^{++} excretion (see Chapter 10).

Regulation of Urinary Ca^{++} Excretion

Several hormones and factors influence urinary Ca^{++} excretion (Table 9-3). Of these, PTH exerts the most powerful control on renal Ca^{++} excretion, and it is

TABLE 9-3

Summary of Hormones and Factors Affecting Ca^{++} Reabsorption

	NEPHRON LOCATION		
Factor/Hormone	Proximal Tubule	TAL	Distal Tubule
Volume expansion	Decrease	No change	Decrease
Hypercalcemia	Decrease	Decrease (CaSR & PTH)	Decrease (CaSR & PTH)
Hypocalcemia	Increase	Increase (CaSR & PTH)	Increase (CaSR & PTH)
Phosphate loading			Increase (PTH)
Phosphate depletion			Decrease (PTH)
Acidosis			Decrease
Alkalosis			Increase
PTH	Decrease	Increase	Increase
Vitamin D			Increase
Calcitonin		Increase	Increase

CaSR, calcium-sensing receptor; PTH, parathyroid hormone; TAL, thick ascending limb.
Modified from Yu A: Renal transport of calcium, magnesium, and phosphate. In Brenner BM, editor: *Brenner and Rector's the kidney*, ed 7, Philadelphia, 2004, WB Saunders.

responsible for maintaining Ca^{++} homeostasis. Overall, this hormone stimulates Ca^{++} reabsorption by the kidneys (i.e., reduces Ca^{++} excretion). Although PTH inhibits the reabsorption of NaCl and fluid and therefore Ca^{++} reabsorption by the proximal tubule, PTH stimulates Ca^{++} reabsorption by the thick ascending limb of the loop of Henle and the distal tubule. In humans this effect is greater in the distal tubule. Changes in the ECF [Ca^{++}] also regulate urinary Ca^{++} excretion, with hypercalcemia increasing excretion and hypocalcemia decreasing excretion. Hypercalcemia increases urinary Ca^{++} excretion by (1) reducing proximal tubule Ca^{++} reabsorption (reduced paracellular reabsorption related to increased interstitial fluid [Ca^{++}]), (2) inhibiting Ca^{++} reabsorption by the thick ascending limb of the loop of Henle by activation of the CaSR located in the basolateral membrane of these cells (the activity of the Na^+-K^+-$2Cl^-$ symporter is decreased, thereby reducing the magnitude of the lumen-positive transepithelial voltage), and (3) suppressing Ca^{++} reabsorption by the distal tubule by reducing PTH levels. As a result, urinary Ca^{++} excretion increases.

Calcitonin stimulates Ca^{++} reabsorption by the thick ascending limb and distal tubule, but it is less effective than PTH, and it is not known how important this effect is in humans. Calcitriol either directly or indirectly enhances Ca^{++} reabsorption by the distal tubule, but it is also less effective than PTH.

Several factors disturb Ca^{++} excretion. An increase in the plasma [Pi] concentration (e.g., caused by an increased dietary intake of Pi) elevates PTH levels and thereby decreases Ca^{++} excretion. A decline in the plasma [Pi] (e.g., caused by dietary Pi depletion) has the opposite effect. Changes in the ECF volume alter Ca^{++} excretion mainly by affecting NaCl and fluid reabsorption in the proximal tubule. Volume contraction increases NaCl and water reabsorption by the proximal tubule and thereby enhances Ca^{++} reabsorption. Accordingly, urinary Ca^{++} excretion declines. Volume expansion has the opposite effect. Acidosis increases Ca^{++} excretion, whereas alkalosis decreases excretion. The regulation of Ca^{++} reabsorption by pH occurs in the distal tubule. Alkalosis stimulates the apical membrane Ca^{++} channel (TRPV5), thereby increasing Ca^{++} reabsorption. By contrast, acidosis inhibits the same channel, thereby reducing Ca^{++} reabsorption.

Calcium-Sensing Receptor

The CaSR is a receptor expressed in the plasma membrane of cells involved in regulating Ca^{++} homeostasis. The CaSR senses small changes in extracellular $[Ca^{++}]$. Ca^{++} binds to CaSR receptors in PTH-secreting cells of the parathyroid gland, calcitonin-secreting parafollicular cells in the thyroid gland, and calcitriol-producing cells of the proximal tubule. Activation of the receptor by an increase in plasma $[Ca^{++}]$ results in inhibition of PTH secretion and the production of calcitriol and stimulation of calcitonin secretion. Moreover, the reduction in PTH secretion also contributes to decreased production of calcitriol because PTH is a potent stimulus of calcitriol synthesis. By contrast, a fall in plasma $[Ca^{++}]$ has the opposite effect on PTH, calcitriol, and calcitonin secretion. These three hormones act on the kidneys, intestine, and bone to regulate plasma $[Ca^{++}]$ by mechanisms described elsewhere in this chapter.

The CaSR also maintains Ca^{++} homeostasis by directly regulating Ca^{++} excretion by the kidneys. CaSRs in the thick ascending limb and distal tubule respond directly to changes in plasma $[Ca^{++}]$ and regulate Ca^{++} absorption by these nephron segments. An increase in plasma $[Ca^{++}]$ activates CaSR in the thick ascending limb and distal tubule and inhibits Ca^{++} absorption in these nephron segments, thereby stimulating urinary Ca^{++} excretion. By contrast, a fall in plasma $[Ca^{++}]$ leads to an increase in Ca^{++} absorption by the thick ascending limb and distal tubule and a corresponding decrease in urinary Ca^{++} excretion. Thus, the direct effect of plasma $[Ca^{++}]$ on CaSRs in the thick ascending limb and distal tubule acts in concert with changes in PTH to regulate urinary Ca^{++} excretion and thereby maintain Ca^{++} homeostasis.

Mutations in the gene coding for the **CaSR** cause disorders in Ca^{++} homeostasis. **Familial hypocalciuric hypercalcemia (FHH)** is an autosomal dominant disease caused by an inactivating mutation of CaSR. The hypercalcemia is caused by deranged Ca^{++}-regulated PTH secretion (i.e., PTH levels are elevated at any level of plasma $[Ca^{++}]$) The hypocalciuria is caused by enhanced Ca^{++} reabsorption in the thick ascending limb and distal tubule owing to elevated PTH levels and defective CaSR regulation of Ca^{++} transport in the kidneys. **Autosomal dominant hypocalcemia** is caused by an activating mutation in CaSR. Activation of CaSRs causes deranged Ca^{++}-regulated PTH secretion (i.e., PTH levels are decreased at any level of plasma $[Ca^{++}]$). Hypercalciuria results and is caused by decreased PTH levels and defective CaSR-regulated Ca^{++} transport in the kidneys.

PHOSPHATE

Pi is an important component of many organic molecules, including DNA, RNA, ATP, and intermediates of metabolic pathways. It is also a major constituent of bone. Its concentration in plasma is an important determinant of bone formation and resorption. In addition, urinary Pi is an important buffer (titratable acid) for the maintenance of acid-base balance (see Chapter 8). A total of 86% of Pi is located in bone, approximately 14% is located in the ICF, and 0.03% is located in the ECF (see Table 9-1). The normal plasma [Pi] is 4 mg/dL. Approximately 10% of the Pi in the plasma is protein bound and is therefore unavailable for ultrafiltration by the glomerulus (see Table 9-2). Accordingly, the [Pi] in the ultrafiltrate is 10% less than that in plasma.

Overview of Pi Homeostasis

A general scheme of Pi homeostasis is shown in Figure 9-5. The maintenance of Pi homeostasis depends on two factors: (1) the amount of Pi in the body and (2) the distribution of Pi between the ICF and ECF compartments. Total body Pi levels are determined by the relative amount of Pi absorbed by the gastrointestinal tract versus the amount excreted by the kidneys. Pi absorption by the gastrointestinal tract occurs by active and passive mechanisms; Pi absorption increases as dietary Pi rises, and it is stimulated by calcitriol. Despite variations in Pi intake between 800 and 1500 mg/day, the kidneys keep the total body Pi balance constant by excreting an amount of Pi in the urine equal to the amount absorbed by the gastrointestinal tract. Thus, renal Pi excretion is the primary mechanism by which the body regulates Pi balance and thereby Pi homeostasis.

The second factor that maintains Pi homeostasis is the distribution of Pi among bone and the ICF and ECF compartments. PTH, calcitriol, and calcitonin regulate the distribution of Pi between bone and the ECF. As with Ca^{++} homeostasis, calcitonin is the least important of the hormones involved in Pi homeostasis in humans. The release of Pi from bone is stimulated by the same hormones (i.e., PTH, calcitriol) that release Ca^{++} from this pool. Thus, the release of Pi is always accompanied by a release of Ca^{++}. In contrast, calcitonin increases bone formation and thereby decreases the plasma [Pi].

The kidneys also make an important contribution to the regulation of the plasma [Pi]. A small rise in the plasma [Pi] increases the amount of Pi filtered by the glomerulus. Because the kidneys normally reabsorb Pi at a maximum rate, any increase in the amount filtered leads to a rise in urinary Pi excretion. In fact, an increase in the amount of Pi filtered enhances urinary Pi excretion to a value greater than the rate of Pi absorption by the gastrointestinal tract. This process results in a net loss of Pi from the body and decreases plasma [Pi]. In this way, the kidneys regulate the plasma [Pi]. The maximum reabsorptive rate for Pi varies and is regulated by dietary Pi intake. A high-Pi diet decreases the maximum reabsorptive rate of Pi by the kidneys, and a low-Pi diet increases it. This effect is independent of changes in PTH levels.

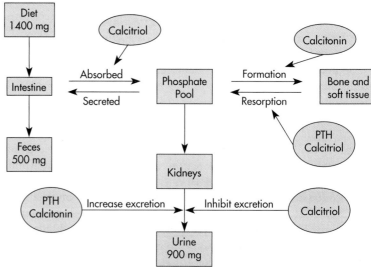
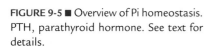

FIGURE 9-5 ■ Overview of Pi homeostasis. PTH, parathyroid hormone. See text for details.

In patients with **chronic renal failure,** the kidneys cannot excrete Pi. Because of continued Pi absorption by the gastrointestinal tract, Pi accumulates in the body, and the plasma [Pi] rises. The excess Pi complexes with Ca^{++} and reduces the plasma [Ca^{++}]. Pi accumulation also decreases the production of calcitriol. This response reduces Ca^{++} absorption by the intestine, an effect that further reduces the plasma [Ca^{++}]. This reduction in plasma [Ca^{++}] increases PTH secretion and Ca^{++} release from bone. These actions result in **osteitis fibrosa cystica** (i.e., increased bone resorption with replacement by fibrous tissue, which renders bone more susceptible to fracture). Chronic hyperparathyroidism (i.e., elevated PTH levels related to the fall in plasma [Ca^{++}]) during chronic renal failure can lead to metastatic calcifications in which Ca^{++} and Pi precipitate in arteries, soft tissues, and viscera. The deposition of Ca^{++} and Pi in heart and lung tissue may cause myocardial failure and pulmonary insufficiency, respectively. The prevention and treatment of hyperparathyroidism and Pi retention include a low-Pi diet or the administration of a "phosphate binder" (i.e., an agent that forms insoluble Pi salts and thereby renders Pi unavailable for absorption by the gastrointestinal tract). Supplemental Ca^{++} and calcitriol are also prescribed.

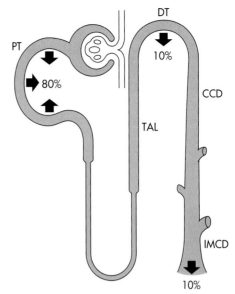

FIGURE 9-6 ■ Pi transport along the nephron. Pi is reabsorbed primarily by the proximal tubule. Percentages refer to the amount of the filtered Pi reabsorbed by each nephron segment. Approximately 10% of the filtered Pi is excreted. CCD, cortical collecting duct; DT, distal tubule; IMCD, inner medullary collecting duct; PT, proximal tubule; TAL, thick ascending limb.

Pi Transport along the Nephron

Figure 9-6 summarizes Pi transport by the various portions of the nephron. The proximal tubule reabsorbs 80% of the Pi filtered by the glomerulus, and the distal tubule reabsorbs 10%. In contrast, the loop of Henle and the collecting duct reabsorb negligible amounts of Pi. Therefore about 10% of the filtered load of Pi is excreted.

Pi reabsorption by the proximal tubule occurs mainly, if not exclusively, by a transcellular route. Pi uptake across the apical membrane occurs through Na^+-Pi symport mechanisms (NPT). Three symporters have been identified; one transports $2Na^+$ with each Pi (NPT1), and the other two transport $3Na^+$ with each Pi (NPT2 and NPT3). NPT2 is the most important symporter involved in Pi reabsorption by the proximal tubule (Figure 9-7). Pi exits across the basolateral membrane by a Pi-inorganic anion antiporter.

The cellular mechanism of Pi reabsorption by the distal tubule has not been characterized.

Regulation of Urinary Pi Excretion

Several hormones and factors regulate urinary Pi excretion (Table 9-4). PTH, the most important hormone that controls Pi excretion, inhibits Pi reabsorption by the proximal tubule and thereby increases Pi excretion. PTH reduces Pi reabsorption by stimulating the endocytic removal of NPT2 from the brush border membrane of the proximal tubule. Dietary Pi intake also regulates Pi excretion by mechanisms unrelated to changes in PTH levels. Pi loading increases excretion, whereas Pi depletion decreases it. Changes in dietary Pi intake modulate Pi transport by altering the transport rate of each NPT2 symporter and by altering the number of transporters.

ECF volume also affects Pi excretion. Volume expansion increases excretion, and volume contraction

FIGURE 9-7 ■ Cellular mechanisms of Pi reabsorption by the proximal tubule. The apical transport pathway operates primarily as a 3Na⁺-Pi symporter (NPT2). Pi leaves the cell across the basolateral membrane by a Pi-anion antiporter. A⁻ indicates an anion. ATP, adenosine triphosphate.

decreases it. The effect of ECF volume on Pi excretion is indirect and may involve changes in the levels of hormones other than PTH. Acid-base balance also influences Pi excretion; acidosis increases Pi excretion, and alkalosis decreases it. Glucocorticoids increase the excretion of Pi. Glucocorticoids increase the delivery of Pi to the distal tubule and collecting duct by inhibiting Pi reabsorption by the proximal tubule. This inhibition enables the distal tubule and collecting duct to secrete more H^+ and to generate more HCO_3^- because Pi is an important urinary buffer (see Chapter 8). Finally, growth hormone decreases Pi excretion. Several phosphaturic factors, also called phosphatonins, including **fibroblast growth factor 23 (FGF-23)** and **frizzeled-related protein 4 (FRP-4),** are hormones produced by tumors in patients with osteomalacia that inhibit renal Pi reabsorption. An increase in dietary Pi enhances plasma FGF-23 levels, which by reducing NPT2 expression in the apical membrane of the proximal tubule, enhances urinary Pi excretion and also decreases calcitriol levels. Prolonged increases in plasma [Pi] are associated with increased tissue calcification and reduced life span.

TABLE 9-4	
Summary of Hormones and Factors Affecting Pi Reabsorption by the Proximal Tubule	
FACTOR/HORMONE	**PROXIMAL TUBULE REABSORPTION**
Volume expansion	Decrease
Hypercalcemia: acute	Increase
Hypercalcemia: chronic	Decrease
Phosphate loading	Decrease
Phosphate depletion	Increase
Metabolic acidosis: chronic	Decrease
Metabolic alkalosis: chronic	Increase
PTH	Decrease
Vitamin D: acute	Increase
Vitamin D: chronic	Decrease
Growth hormone	Increase
FGF-23/GGF-24	Decrease
Glucocorticoids	Decrease

FGF-23, fibroblast growth factor 23; PTH, parathyroid hormone.

In the absence of glucocorticoids (e.g., in **Addison's disease**), Pi excretion is depressed, as is the ability of the kidneys to excrete titratable acid and to generate new HCO_3^-. Growth hormone also has an important effect on Pi homeostasis. Growth hormone increases the reabsorption of Pi by the proximal tubule. As a result, growing children have a higher plasma [Pi] than adults, and this elevated [Pi] is important for the formation of bone.

INTEGRATIVE REVIEW OF PARATHYROID HORMONE, CALCITRIOL, AND CALCITONIN ON Ca⁺⁺ AND Pi HOMEOSTASIS

Hypocalcemia is the major stimulus of PTH secretion. As summarized in Figure 9-8, PTH has numerous effects on Ca^{++} and Pi homeostasis. PTH stimulates bone resorption, increases urinary Pi excretion, decreases urinary Ca^{++} excretion, and stimulates the production of calcitriol, which stimulates Ca^{++} and Pi absorption by the intestine. Because changes in Pi handling in bone, the intestines, and the kidneys tend to balance out, PTH increases the plasma $[Ca^{++}]$ while having little effect on the plasma [Pi]. Overall, a rise in the plasma PTH levels increases the plasma $[Ca^{++}]$ and decreases the plasma [Pi]. A decline in plasma PTH levels has the opposite effect.

Calcitriol also plays an important role in Ca^{++} and Pi homeostasis (Figure 9-9). The primary action of calcitriol is to stimulate Ca^{++} and Pi absorption by the intestine. To a lesser degree it acts with PTH to release Ca^{++} and Pi from the bone and decreases Ca^{++} excretion by the kidneys. The net effect of calcitriol is to increase the plasma $[Ca^{++}]$ and [Pi]. Thus, the major stimuli of calcitriol production are hypocalcemia through PTH and hypophosphatemia (i.e., a low plasma [Pi]).

Although calcitriol does not play a major role in Ca^{++} and Pi homeostasis in humans, it does act, especially in lower mammals to block bone resorption and stimulate Ca^{++} deposition in bone (Figure 9-10). Also, calcitonin has a modest direct effect to decrease urinary Ca^{++} excretion. The major stimulus of calcitonin secretion is an increase in the plasma $[Ca^{++}]$. Because changes in Pi handling in bone, the intestines, and the kidneys tend to balance out, calcitonin decreases the plasma $[Ca^{++}]$ while having little effect on the plasma [Pi].

Estrogens defend against PTH-mediated resorption of bone. In estrogen-deficient conditions, most prominently those following menopause, the unabated effect of PTH on bone contributes significantly to the development of osteoporosis.

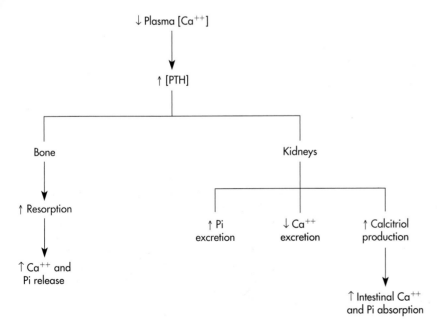

FIGURE 9-8 ■ Effects of parathyroid hormone (PTH) on Ca^{++} and Pi homeostasis. The major stimulus of PTH secretion is hypocalcemia. *(Modified from Rose BD, Rennke HG, editors: Renal pathophysiology: the essentials. Baltimore, 1994, Williams & Wilkins.)*

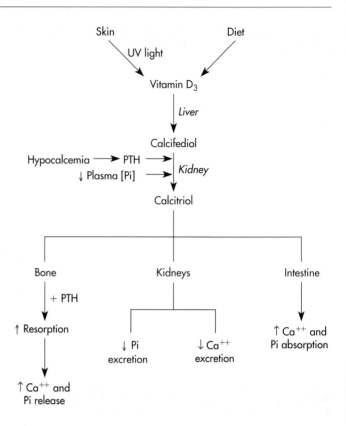

FIGURE 9-9 ■ Activation of vitamin D_3 and its effect on Ca^{++} and Pi metabolism. Hypocalcemia, through PTH, and hypophosphatemia are the major stimuli of the metabolism of calcifediol to calcitriol in the kidneys. The net effect of calcitriol is to increase the plasma $[Ca^{++}]$ and $[Pi]$. *(Modified from Rose BD, Rennke HG, editors: Renal pathophysiology: the essentials. Baltimore, 1994, Williams & Wilkins.)*

FIGURE 9-10 ■ Effect of calcitonin on Ca^{++} and Pi homeostasis. The major stimulus of calcitonin secretion is hypercalcemia. The net effect of calcitonin is to reduce the plasma $[Ca^{++}]$. Quantitatively, therefore, the most important effects of calcitonin are to stimulate bone formation and to decrease bone resorption. Although calcitonin reduces urinary Ca^{++} excretion and intestinal Ca^{++} absorption, these effects are relatively minor and have little effect on the plasma $[Ca^{++}]$. The effects of calcitonin on the kidneys and calcitriol production are relatively minor compared with its effect on bone. *(Modified from Rose BD, Rennke HG, editors: Renal pathophysiology: the essentials. Baltimore, 1994, Williams & Wilkins.)*

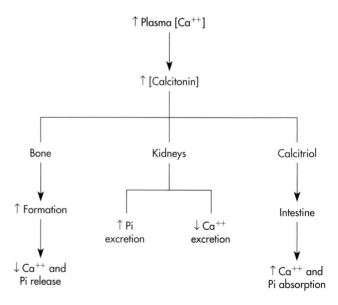

SUMMARY

1. The kidneys, in conjunction with the gastrointestinal tract and bone, play a vital role in regulating the plasmas [Ca^{++}] and [Pi].
2. Plasma Ca^{++} is regulated by PTH and calcitriol. Calcitonin is not a major regulatory hormone in humans. Ca^{++} excretion by the kidneys is determined by (1) the net rate of intestinal Ca^{++} absorption, (2) the balance between bone formation and resorption, and (3) the net rate of Ca^{++} reabsorption by the distal tubule and thick ascending limb of the loop of Henle.
3. Ca^{++} reabsorption by the thick ascending limb is regulated by PTH and calcitriol, both of which stimulate Ca^{++} reabsorption.
4. The plasma [Pi] is regulated by the maximal reabsorptive capacity of Pi by the kidneys.
5. A fall in the [Pi] stimulates the production of calcitriol, which releases Pi from bone into the ECF and increases Pi absorption by the intestine.

KEY WORDS AND CONCEPTS

- Hypocalcemia
- Hypercalcemia
- Calcitriol
- Vitamin D$_3$
- Calcium-sensing receptor (CaSR)
- 3Na$^+$-Pi symporter (NPT2)
- Calcitonin
- Parathyroid hormone (PTH)
- Fibroblast growth factor 23 (FGF-23)
- Parathyroid hormone–related peptide (PTHRP)
- Claudin-16
- Paracellin 1

SELF-STUDY PROBLEMS

1. How is Ca^{++} reabsorption in the proximal tubule dependent on Na$^+$ reabsorption? What would happen to Ca^{++} excretion if a subject was given a diuretic, such as mannitol, that inhibits sodium and water reabsorption by the proximal tubule?
2. What effect would furosemide, an inhibitor of Na$^+$ reabsorption by the thick ascending limb of Henle's loop, have on urinary Ca^{++} excretion?
3. What would happen to Pi excretion if plasma [Pi] was increased from 4 to 6 mg/dL?

PHYSIOLOGY OF DIURETIC ACTION

OBJECTIVES

Upon completion of this chapter, the student should be able to answer the following questions:

1. What effects do diuretics have on Na⁺ handling by the kidneys?

2. What effects do aquaretics have on water handling by the kidneys?

3. Why do diuretics decrease the volume of the extracellular fluid (ECF)?

4. What mechanisms are involved in delivering diuretics to their sites of action along the nephron?

5. What is the primary nephron site where each class of diuretics acts, and what is the specific membrane transport protein affected?

6. How do nephrons alter their function in response to diuretics, and how does this affect the action of diuretics?

7. What are the effects of the various classes of diuretics on the renal handling of K^+, Ca^{++}, HCO_3^-, Pi, and solute-free water?

$\mathbf{D}$iuretics, as the name implies, are drugs that cause an increase in urine output. It is important, however, to distinguish this diuresis from that which occurs following the ingestion of large volumes of water. In the latter case, the urine is primarily made up of water, and solute excretion is not increased. In contrast, diuretics result in the enhanced excretion of both solute and water.

All diuretics have as their common mode of action the inhibition of Na⁺ reabsorption by the nephron. Consequently, they cause an increase in the excretion of Na⁺, termed **natriuresis.** However, the effects of diuretics are not limited to Na⁺ handling. The renal handling of many other solutes is also influenced, usually as a consequence of alterations in Na⁺ transport. Recently, drugs have been developed that block the action of ADH on the distal tubule and collecting duct. These drugs, called **aquaretics,** cause a water diuresis.

This chapter reviews the various diuretics' cellular mechanisms of action and the nephron sites at which these diuretics act. In addition to their effects on Na⁺ handling by the nephron, their effects on the renal handling of other solutes (K^+, Ca^{++}, Pi, and HCO_3^-) and water are considered. Aquaretics are briefly presented.

GENERAL PRINCIPLES OF DIURETIC ACTION

The primary action of diuretics is to increase the excretion of Na⁺. As described in Chapter 6, alterations in Na⁺ excretion by the kidneys result in alterations in

163

the volume of the extracellular fluid (ECF) compartment. Consequently, diuretics decrease the volume of the ECF. Indeed, diuretics are commonly given in clinical situations when the ECF compartment is expanded, with the intent of reducing its volume. Because the ECF volume also determines blood volume and pressure, diuretics are commonly used in the therapy of hypertension.

Although generally predictable for a particular class of diuretics, the effects of diuretic administration can be quite variable. Several factors are important in determining the overall effect of a particular diuretic:

1. The nephron segment where the diuretic acts
2. The response of nephron segments not affected by the diuretic
3. The delivery of sufficient quantities of the diuretic to its site of action
4. The volume of the ECF

Sites of Action of Diuretics

Figure 10-1 depicts the nephron sites at which the different classes of diuretics act. The osmotic diuretics act along the proximal tubule and thin descending limb of Henle's loop. The carbonic anhydrase inhibitors act primarily in the proximal tubule. The thick ascending limb of Henle's loop is the site of action of the loop diuretics. The early portion of the distal tubule is the site of action of the thiazide diuretics, and the K+-sparing diuretics act on the late portion of the distal tubule and the cortical portion of the collecting duct.

The site of action of a diuretic in turn determines the magnitude of the associated natriuresis. The effect diuretics have on the handling of solutes other than Na+ also depends on the site of action. Examples illustrating this point are given in subsequent sections.

Response of Other Nephron Segments

When a diuretic inhibits Na+ reabsorption at one nephron site, it causes increased delivery of Na+ and water to more distal segments. The functions of these more distal segments and their ability or inability to handle this increased load ultimately determine the overall effect of the diuretic on urinary solute and water excretion. Examples of this are considered in

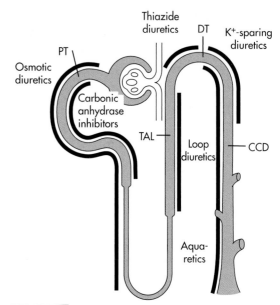

FIGURE 10-1 ■ Sites of action of diuretics and aquaretics along the nephron. CCD, cortical collecting duct; DT, distal tubule; PT, proximal tubule; TAL, thick ascending limb.

detail with discussion of each of the various diuretics. In addition, diuretic-induced changes in ECF volume (see later) may modulate Na+ transport in segments of the nephron not affected by the diuretic and thereby influence the degree of natriuresis.

Adequate Delivery of Diuretics to Their Site of Action

The effect of a diuretic on Na+ excretion also depends on the delivery of adequate quantities of the drug to its site of action. With the exception of the aldosterone antagonists, which act intracellularly, diuretics act from the lumen of the nephron (carbonic anhydrase inhibitors have both a luminal and intracellular site of action). Diuretics gain access to the lumen by glomerular filtration and through secretion by the organic anion and organic cation secretory systems located in the proximal tubule (see Chapter 4). Because some diuretics are largely bound to plasma proteins (e.g., loop diuretics), their secretion by the proximal tubule is the primary mechanism for delivery of the diuretic to its site of action in the lumen of the nephron. Thus, the effect of a diuretic can be blunted if, for example, it is administered with another drug that competes for the same organic anion and organic cation secretory mechanism.

Volume of the Extracellular Fluid

The effect of a diuretic also depends on the volume of the ECF. As described in Chapter 6, when the volume of the ECF is decreased, the GFR is reduced, thereby reducing the filtered load of Na^+. In addition, Na^+ reabsorption by the nephron is enhanced. Thus, the effect of a diuretic that acts on the distal tubule would be blunted if administered in the setting of a reduced ECF volume. Under this condition, the decreased GFR (i.e., decreased filtered load of Na^+), together with enhanced Na^+ reabsorption by the proximal tubule, would result in the delivery of a smaller quantity of Na^+ to the distal tubule. Thus, even if the diuretic completely inhibited Na^+ reabsorption in the distal tubule, the associated natriuresis would be less than would occur if the ECF volume were normal.

DIURETIC BRAKING PHENOMENON

As illustrated in Figure 10-2, administration of a diuretic to an individual with fixed Na^+ intake results in a short-lived natriuresis. The transient response, called the **diuretic braking phenomenon,** reflects several changes in renal function that are both a direct effect of the diuretic and secondary to changes in the volume of the ECF. One component of this response is that diuretic-induced inhibition of Na^+ reabsorption in one nephron segment, with the resultant delivery of excess Na^+ to more distal nephron segments, simulates the reabsorption of Na^+ at these sites. A second important component of this response is that loss of NaCl and water from the body, as a result of diuretic action, results in a decrease in the volume of the ECF. This in turn is sensed by the body's vascular baroreceptors and effector mechanisms to increase NaCl and water conservation by the kidneys (see Chapter 6 for details).

Studies in experimental animals have shown that loop and thiazide diuretics increase the abundance of the transporters they inhibit. For example, loop diuretics, which inhibit the Na^+-K^+-2Cl^- symporter in the apical membrane of the cells of the thick ascending limb of Henle's loop, also increase the abundance of the transporter in this segment. Similarly, thiazide diuretics, which inhibit the Na^+-Cl^- symporter in the apical membrane of the early portion of the distal tubule, also increase the abundance of these transporters in this segment. In addition, both loop and thiazide diuretics increase the abundance of the Na^+ channel (ENaC) in the late portion of the distal tubule and collecting duct. These effects are independent of

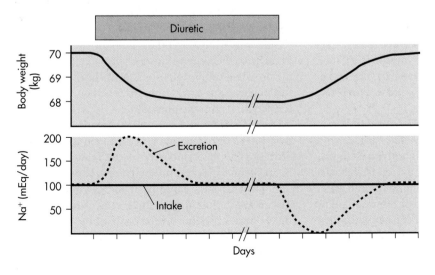

FIGURE 10-2 ■ Effect of long-term diuretic therapy on renal Na^+ excretion. Because diuretics induce a natriuresis, extracellular fluid volume is reduced. This is detected as a decrease in body weight.

changes in aldosterone levels and presumably are mediated in some manner by the increased delivery of Na⁺ from the upstream segments. Thiazide diuretics also increase the abundance of aquaporin-2 in the principal cells of the late portion of the distal tubule and the collecting duct. Whether this is a direct or indirect effect (i.e., related to changes in ECF volume) is uncertain. Regardless of the mechanism, the increased expression of aquaporin-2 is expected to increase water reabsorption by the ADH-sensitive nephron segments.

With the diuretic-induced decrease in the ECF volume, the renin-angiotensin-aldosterone system is activated, renal sympathetic nerve activity is increased, and ADH secretion is stimulated; all of which act to reduce urinary NaCl and water excretion (see Chapter 6 for details). At the cellular level, aldosterone increases the abundance of the Na^+-Cl^- symporter in the early portion of the distal tubule as well as ENaC in the late distal tubule and collecting duct. ADH also increases the abundance of key transporters. Specifically, ADH increases the abundance of Na^+-K^+-$2Cl^-$ in the thick ascending limb of Henle's loop, Na^+-Cl^- symporter in the early portion of the distal tubule, and ENaC in the late distal tubule and collecting duct. Finally, angiotensin II increases the abundance of the Na^+-H^+ antiporter (NHE-3) in the proximal tubule.

As a result of the braking phenomenon, a new steady state is reached where even with continued administration of the diuretic urinary Na⁺ excretion once again equals intake. However, this occurs at a reduced ECF volume, which is detected as a decrease in body weight. When diuretic therapy is discontinued, renal Na⁺ excretion is reduced. After a period of positive Na⁺ balance, during which the ECV returns to normal (i.e., return of body weight to its original value), a new steady state is again achieved.

The concept of steady state deserves special emphasis. Normally, individuals are in steady-state balance with regard to solute (e.g., Na⁺) and water, with intake equaling excretion. Administration of a diuretic temporarily disrupts this balance by increasing solute and water excretion, and a negative balance exists. However, solute and water excretion cannot exceed intake indefinitely, and a new steady state is eventually achieved. In this new steady state, intake and excretion are again balanced,

but the ECF volume is reduced as a result of diuretic-induced excretion of NaCl and water. In general, when an individual has been taking a diuretic for several days or longer, a new steady state is achieved. If Na⁺ intake is not increased, the ECF volume is decreased in proportion to the degree of negative Na⁺ balance.

MECHANISMS OF ACTION OF DIURETICS

Osmotic Diuretics

Osmotic diuretics, as the name implies, are agents that inhibit the reabsorption of solute and water by altering osmotic driving forces along the nephron. Unlike the other classes of diuretics, osmotic diuretics do not inhibit a specific membrane transport protein. They simply affect water transport across the cells of the nephron through the generation of an osmotic pressure gradient. The best example of an exogenous osmotic diuretic is the sugar mannitol. When present in abnormally high concentrations, endogenous substances such as glucose (i.e., in patients with diabetes mellitus) and urea (i.e., in patients with renal disease whose plasma urea levels are elevated) can also act as osmotic diuretics.

Osmotic diuretics (e.g., mannitol) gain access to the tubular fluid by glomerular filtration. Because they are not reabsorbed or only poorly reabsorbed, they remain within the lumen, where they can exert an osmotic pressure inhibiting tubular fluid reabsorption. Osmotic diuretics affect fluid reabsorption in the segments that have high permeability to water (i.e., the proximal tubule and thin descending limb of Henle's loop). Because of the large volumes of filtrate reabsorbed in the proximal tubule (60% to 70% of the filtered load), this nephron site is most important when considering the action of osmotic diuretics.

As described in Chapter 4, reabsorption of tubular fluid by the proximal tubule is essentially an isosmotic process (i.e., the osmolality of the reabsorbed fluid is only slightly hyperosmotic compared with that of tubular fluid). Solute (primarily NaCl) is actively reabsorbed by the proximal tubule cells. This sets up a small osmotic pressure difference across the tubule, with the lumen being 3 to 5 mOsm/kg H_2O hypo-osmotic with respect to the interstitial fluid. Given the fact that water is readily able to cross the proximal tubule, this small osmotic pressure gradient is sufficient to cause water reabsorption. Also, as water flows from the lumen to the interstitium, it brings additional solute with it by solvent drag.

When an osmotic diuretic is present in the tubular fluid, its concentration increases progressively as a result of NaCl and water reabsorption by the nephron. With this increase in concentration, an osmotic gradient develops opposite to the normal gradient generated by NaCl reabsorption. As a result, both NaCl (solvent drag component) and water reabsorption are reduced. With an osmotic diuresis there is also an increase in blood flow to the medulla of the kidney. This dissipates the standing interstitial osmotic gradient (see Chapter 5) and thus also impairs water reabsorption by the thin descending limb of Henle's loop.

Some of the Na$^+$ that is not reabsorbed by the proximal tubule is reabsorbed downstream by the thick ascending limb, distal tubule, and collecting duct. Thus, the degree of natriuresis seen with osmotic diuretics is less than expected on the basis of the magnitude of proximal tubule reabsorption. Although Na$^+$ excretion rates as high as 60% of the filtered load have been seen in experimental situations, the usual natriuresis seen in individuals treated with osmotic diuretics is only about 10% of the filtered load.

Carbonic Anhydrase Inhibitors

Carbonic anhydrase inhibitors (e.g., acetazolamide) reduce Na$^+$ reabsorption by their effect on carbonic anhydrase. This enzyme is abundant in the proximal tubule and therefore represents the major site of action of these diuretics. Carbonic anhydrase is also present in other cells along the nephron (e.g., thick ascending limb of Henle's loop and intercalated cells of the collecting duct), and administration of carbonic anhydrase inhibitors affects the activity of the enzyme at these sites as well. However, the effects of these diuretics are almost entirely attributed to their inhibition of the enzyme in the proximal tubule. This reflects the fact that approximately one third of proximal tubule Na$^+$ reabsorption occurs in exchange for H$^+$ (through the Na$^+$-H$^+$ antiporter) and thus is dependent upon the activity of carbonic anhydrase (see Chapter 8).

Even though one third of proximal tubule Na$^+$ reabsorption is coupled to the secretion of H$^+$, inhibition of this process by the carbonic anhydrase inhibitors does not result in a large natriuresis. The reason for this is the same as that described for the osmotic diuretics and is related to the ability of the thick ascending limb, distal tubule and collecting duct to increase their reabsorptive rates when Na$^+$ delivery is increased. Typically, administration of carbonic anhydrase inhibitors results in Na$^+$ excretion rates that are 5% to 10% of the filtered load.

Loop Diuretics

Loop diuretics (e.g., furosemide, bumetanide, torsemide, and ethacrynic acid) are organic anions that enter the tubular lumen primarily through secretion by the organic anion secretory system of the proximal tubule. They inhibit Na$^+$ reabsorption by the thick ascending limb of Henle's loop by blocking the Na$^+$-K$^+$-2Cl$^-$ symporter located in the apical membrane of these cells (see Chapter 4). By this action, they not only inhibit Na$^+$ reabsorption but also disrupt the process of countercurrent multiplication and the kidneys' ability to dilute and concentrate the urine. Dilution is impaired because solute (NaCl) reabsorption by the water-impermeable thick ascending limb of Henle's loop is inhibited. NaCl reabsorption by the medullary portion of the thick ascending limb is also critical for the generation and maintenance of an elevated medullary interstitial fluid osmolality. Therefore, inhibition of transport by the loop diuretics results in a decrease in the osmolality of the medullary interstitial fluid. With a decrease in medullary interstitial fluid osmolality, water reabsorption from the collecting duct is impaired, and the concentrating ability of the kidneys is reduced. Water reabsorption from the thin descending limb of Henle's loop is also impaired by loop diuretics, again because of the decrease in medullary interstitial fluid osmolality. This decrease in thin descending limb reabsorption accounts in part for the increase in water excretion seen with loop diuretics.

Loop diuretics are the most potent diuretics available, increasing the excretion of Na$^+$ to as much as 25% of the filtered load. This large natriuresis reflects the fact that the thick ascending limb normally reabsorbs approximately 20% to 25% of the filtered load of Na^+, and the downstream segments (distal tubule and collecting duct) have a limited capacity to reabsorb the increased NaCl they receive in this situation. Some of the loop diuretics (e.g., furosemide) are weak inhibitors of carbonic anhydrase, and this action may contribute to the natriuresis under certain conditions.

Thiazide Diuretics

Like the loop diuretics, thiazide diuretics (e.g., chlorothi-azide, metolazone)[1] are organic anions. Because they are largely bound to plasma proteins, they gain access to the tubular lumen primarily by secretion in the proximal tubule. They act to inhibit Na^+ reabsorption in the early portion of the distal tubule by blocking the Na^+-Cl^- symporter in the apical membrane of these cells (see Chapter 4). Because water cannot cross this portion of the nephron, it is a site where the urine is diluted. Therefore, thiazides reduce the ability to dilute the urine maximally by inhibiting NaCl reabsorption. Because thiazide diuretics act in the cortex and not the medulla, they do not affect the ability of the kidneys to concentrate the urine maximally. Like the loop diuretics, some of the thiazide diuretics are also weak carbonic anhydrase inhibitors. Natriuresis with thiazide diuretics is 5% to 10% of the filtered load.

K+-Sparing Diuretics

The K^+-sparing diuretics act on the region of the nephron where K^+ secretion occurs (late portion of the distal tubule and cortical collecting duct). They produce a small natriuresis (3% to 5% of the filtered load), reflecting the amount of Na^+ reabsorbed by this region of the nephron. As the name implies, their utility lies in their ability to inhibit K^+ secretion by this region of the nephron.

There are two classes of K^+-sparing diuretics: one acts by antagonizing aldosterone's action on the principal cell (e.g., spironolactone and eplerenone), whereas the other class blocks the entry of Na^+ into the same

cells through the Na^+-selective channels (ENaC) in the apical membrane (e.g., amiloride, triamterene). Amiloride and triamterene are organic cations that enter the tubular lumen primarily by secretion by the organic cation secretory system of the proximal tubule.

As described in detail in Chapters 6 and 9, aldosterone stimulates both Na^+ reabsorption and K^+ secretion by the principal cells of the late distal tubule and collecting duct. Thus, in the presence of an aldosterone antagonist, these effects are reversed and both Na^+ reabsorption and K^+ secretion are reduced.

As discussed in Chapter 6, **congestive heart failure** is associated with stimulation of the renin-angiotensin-aldosterone system, which enhances the reabsorption of NaCl and water by the kidneys and thereby increases the ECF volume, resulting in the formation of edema. As a result, standard care for patients with moderate or severe congestive heart failure includes an angiotensin-converting enzyme (ACE) inhibitor (or an angiotensin II receptor antagonist) and a diuretic to increase renal salt and water excretion. Although ACE inhibitors and angiotensin II receptor antagonists inhibit aldosterone secretion, this effect is not complete. In addition, other factors can cause aldosterone secretion (e.g., an increase in ECF [K^+]), and aldosterone is produced locally in the heart. Recently, it has been shown that aldosterone can induce myocardial fibrosis by autocrine and paracrine mechanisms. Clinical studies have shown that administration of an aldosterone antagonist in combination with standard therapies reduces the risk of death in patients with heart failure. This beneficial effect of aldosterone antagonists is distinct from their effect on the kidney.

The ability of the Na^+ channel blockers amiloride and triamterene to inhibit Na^+ reabsorption and K^+ secretion is similar to that of spironolactone, but the cellular mechanism is different. Amiloride and triamterene block the entry of Na^+ into the principal cell by inhibiting the Na^+ channel (ENaC) in the apical membrane. With decreased Na^+ entry, there is reduced Na^+ extrusion across the basolateral membrane through the Na^+,K^+-ATPase. This in turn reduces cellular K^+ uptake and ultimately its secretion into the tubular fluid. Inhibition of apical membrane Na^+ channels

---

[1]Metolazone is not in the same chemical class of drugs as the thiazides. However, because its site of action is the same, it is grouped with this class of drugs.

also alters the electrical profile across the luminal membrane, with the voltage across this membrane increasing in magnitude. Because of this voltage change, the electrochemical gradient for K^+ movement out of the cell is reduced. This membrane voltage effect also contributes to the inhibition of K^+ secretion.

Trimethoprim is an antibiotic used to treat *Pneumocystis carinii* infections. *P. carinii* infections are commonly seen in individuals whose immune systems are compromised (e.g., individuals with acquired immunodeficiency syndrome [AIDS]). Hyperkalemia may occur in individuals treated with trimethoprim and as a result of reduced renal K^+ excretion. K^+ excretion is reduced because trimethoprim inhibits K^+ secretion by the principal cells of the late distal tubule and cortical collecting duct. The mechanism for this inhibition of K^+ secretion is similar to that of amiloride and triamterene (i.e., inhibition of the Na^+ channel [ENaC] in the apical membrane of the cell).

Aquaretics

In recent years, drugs that are antagonists of the ADH receptor (V_2) have been developed. They act on the late portion of the distal tubule and the collecting duct to block the action of ADH. As a result of their action, the urine cannot be concentrated and dilute urine is excreted, reflecting the fact that tubular fluid reaching these ADH-sensitive segments of the nephron is hypo-osmotic to the ECF (see Chapter 5). These drugs are particularly helpful in treating patients whose ECF is hypo-osmotic owing to the failure of the kidneys to excrete solute-free water because ADH levels are elevated by nonosmotic and nonhemodynamic mechanisms (e.g., syndrome of inappropriate ADH secretion [SIADH]).

EFFECT OF DIURETICS ON THE EXCRETION OF WATER AND OTHER SOLUTES

Through their effects on Na^+ handling along the nephron, diuretics also influence the handling of water and other solutes. Table 10-1 summarizes the effects of the various diuretics on the handling of some of these solutes and the ability of the kidneys to excrete (C_{H_2O}) and reabsorb ($T^C_{H_2O}$) solute-free water.

Solute-Free Water

As discussed in Chapter 5, the kidneys' ability to excrete or reabsorb solute-free water depends on several factors. With regard to the action of diuretic agents, the factors of concern are as follows:

1. The normal function of the nephron segments (particularly the thick ascending limb)
2. The delivery of adequate solute to Henle's loop
3. The maintenance of a hyperosmotic medullary interstitium (reabsorption of solute-free water only)

			HCO$_3^-$	Ca^{++}	FREE-WATER	FREE-WATER
DIURETIC	**Na$^+$ EXCRETION (%)***	**K$^+$**	**EXCRETION**	**EXCRETION**	**EXCRETION**	**REABSORPTION**
Osmotic diuretic	10	↑	↑	↑	↑	↑
CAI	5-10	↑	↑	↑	↑	↑
Loop diuretic	25	↑	↓	↑	↓	↓
Thiazide diuretic	5-10	↑	↓	↓	↓	NC
K$^+$-sparing diuretic	3-5	↓	↑	NC	NC	NC
Aquaretics	0	NC	NC	NC	↑	↓

*Percentage of filtered load excreted into the urine.
All the effects (except HCO$_3^-$ excretion) reflect the initial effect of the diuretic. The effects of loop and thiazide diuretics on HCO$_3^-$ excretion occur with prolonged use of these drugs and are secondary to the diuretic-induced decrease in extracellular fluid volume.
CAI, carbonic anhydrase inhibitor; NA, not applicable; NC, no change.

The thick ascending limb of Henle's loop is the most important site for the separation of solute and water. As noted, this separation not only dilutes the tubular fluid but also, by establishing a hyperosmotic medullary interstitium, allows water reabsorption from the collecting duct and thus concentration of the urine. Inhibition of thick ascending limb Na^+ reabsorption by loop diuretics therefore results in inhibition of both solute-free water excretion (C_{H_2O}) and solute-free water reabsorption ($T^C_{H_2O}$).

The early portion of the distal tubule is also a site of solute and water separation and thus tubular fluid dilution. Accordingly, inhibition of Na^+ reabsorption by the thiazide diuretics impairs dilution of the urine. However, thiazide diuretics impair urine dilution to a lesser degree than do loop diuretics, reflecting the difference in the NaCl reabsorptive capacity between the distal tubule (5% of the filtered load) and the thick ascending limb (25% of the filtered load). In contrast to the loop diuretics, thiazide diuretics do not significantly impair the kidneys' ability to concentrate the urine. As already noted, concentration of the urine requires a hyperosmotic medullary interstitium so that water can be reabsorbed from the collecting duct in the presence of ADH. Because thiazide diuretics act on distal tubules that are located in the cortex, their action at this site does not appreciably alter the medullary interstitial osmotic gradient. Consequently, urine-concentrating ability is unaffected by thiazide diuretics.

The action of diuretics in the proximal tubule (osmotic diuretics and carbonic anhydrase inhibitors) results in an increase in the delivery of NaCl and water to Henle's loop. In view of the thick ascending limb's ability to increase its transport rate in response to an increased delivered load of NaCl, the separation of solute and water increases. As a result, these diuretic agents increase the kidneys' ability to excrete solute-free water as well as reabsorb solute-free water.

Although the late portion of the distal tubule and the collecting duct are able to dilute the luminal fluid in the absence of ADH, Na^+ transport in these segments is not of sufficient magnitude to contribute significantly to the excretion of solute-free water. Consequently, the K^+-sparing diuretics do not appreciably alter free-water excretion. Like thiazide diuretics, K^+-sparing diuretics do not alter solute-free water

reabsorption because the nephron sites of action are located in the cortex.

Aquaretics increase solute-free water excretion and impair solute-free water reabsorption.

K^+ Excretion

One of the major consequences of diuretic use (excluding the K^+-sparing diuretics) is increased excretion of K^+. This can be of sufficient magnitude to result in hypokalemia. The basis for this diuretic-induced increase in renal K^+ excretion lies in the fact that when a diuretic inhibits Na^+ and water reabsorption in segments upstream from the late portion of the distal tubule and cortical collecting duct (K^+ secretory site of the nephron), tubular fluid flow rate increases. The increased tubular fluid flow rate stimulates K^+ secretion at this site (see Chapter 7 for details). In addition, by their action on Na^+ balance, diuretics decrease the ECF volume. This, in turn, leads to increased secretion of aldosterone by the adrenal cortex (see Chapter 6), which acts at this site to stimulate K^+ secretion.

The decrease in ECF volume also stimulates ADH secretion. As described in Chapter 7, ADH stimulates K^+ secretion by the principal cells of the late distal tubule and collecting duct. This stimulatory effect is normally offset by the inhibitory effect of the reduced tubular flow rate also induced by ADH. As a result, ADH does not normally alter renal K^+ excretion. However, in the presence of a diuretic that is acting upstream to the late portion of the distal tubule and the collecting duct, ADH does increase renal K^+ excretion because in this setting tubular fluid flow is elevated by the action of the diuretics.

The K^+-sparing diuretics prevent the increase in K^+ excretion caused by the other diuretics; therefore, they are usually given in combination with these other diuretics to prevent or at least minimize the development of hypokalemia.

HCO_3^- Excretion

By inhibiting H^+ secretion in the proximal tubule and thereby increasing HCO_3^- excretion, carbonic anhydrase inhibitors can result in the development of a metabolic acidosis.

Although only carbonic anhydrase inhibitors directly alter H+ secretion by the nephron, all diuretics can secondarily affect systemic acid-base balance. Both loop and thiazide diuretics can induce a metabolic alkalosis, which is a consequence of the decrease in ECF volume that accompanies their use. With a decrease in the ECF volume, Na+ is more avidly reabsorbed by the nephron. In the proximal tubule, this enhanced Na+ reabsorption results in enhanced H+ secretion through the Na+-H+ antiporter. Thus, a greater fraction of the filtered load of HCO₃⁻ is reabsorbed. In addition, the reduction in ECF volume stimulates aldosterone secretion by the adrenal cortex. As discussed in Chapter 8, aldosterone stimulates H+ secretion by intercalated cells of the distal tubule and collecting duct. Because, as noted, proximal tubule HCO₃⁻ reabsorption is increased, virtually none of the filtered load of HCO₃⁻ reaches the distal tubule. Therefore, the increased H+ secretion that occurs in the distal tubule and collecting duct results in the production of new HCO₃⁻ as the H+ is excreted with non-HCO₃⁻ urinary buffers (i.e., titratable acid). The increased secretion of H+ in the distal tubule and collecting duct also enhances the excretion of ammonium, which results in the addition of new HCO₃⁻ to the ECF. As a result, net acid excretion by the kidneys is increased and metabolic alkalosis develops.

By inhibiting Na+ reabsorption in the late portion of the distal tubule and cortical collecting duct, K+-sparing diuretics secondarily inhibit H+ secretion and thus can lead to the development of a metabolic acidosis. H+ secretion by these nephron segments is facilitated by the lumen-negative transepithelial voltage. Normally, Na+ reabsorption in these nephron segments results in the generation of such a voltage. By inhibiting Na+ reabsorption and thus the negative luminal voltage, K+-sparing diuretics reduce H+ secretion. With reduced H+ secretion, insufficient quantities of net acid are excreted and a metabolic acidosis ensues.

Ca++ and Pi Excretion

With the exception of K+-sparing diuretics, all the diuretics can significantly alter Ca++ excretion by the kidney. With inhibition of proximal tubule solute and water reabsorption (osmotic diuretics and carbonic anhydrase inhibitors), there is reduced reabsorption of

Ca++ and thus increased excretion. The amount of Ca++ excreted is less than expected from inhibition of proximal tubule transport. This again reflects the ability of the downstream segments (particularly the thick ascending limb of Henle's loop) to increase reabsorption following an increased delivered load. The mechanism by which these diuretics inhibit proximal tubule Ca++ reabsorption is related to their ability to reduce solvent drag (see Chapter 9). With the use of carbonic anhydrase inhibitors, increased Ca++ excretion occurs in the setting of an alkaline urine (increased urinary [HCO₃⁻]). Because Ca++ is less soluble in alkaline urine, the potential exists for the formation of Ca++-containing renal stones.

Loop diuretics also increase Ca++ excretion, an action explained by the effect of these diuretics on the transepithelial voltage of the thick ascending limb of Henle's loop. Normally, the transepithelial voltage of this segment is oriented lumen positive (see Chapter 4), providing a driving force for the movement of Ca++ from the lumen to blood through the paracellular pathway (see Chapter 9). When transport of NaCl by Henle's loop is blocked by loop diuretics, this lumen-positive voltage is abolished and thus the driving force for Ca++ reabsorption is reduced. Normally, Henle's loop reabsorbs about 20% of the filtered load of Ca++ (see Chapter 9). Inhibition of Ca++ reabsorption by loop diuretics can therefore have a significant effect on Ca++ excretion. For this reason, loop diuretics are often used to treat hypercalcemia. Despite this action of loop diuretics, hypercalcemia can occur with their long-term use. The mechanism responsible for this effect is related to the diuretic-induced decrease in the ECF volume. When the ECF volume is decreased, proximal tubule reabsorption is enhanced, which increases Ca++ reabsorption at this site and therefore decreases urinary Ca++ excretion.

Thiazide diuretics stimulate Ca++ reabsorption by the cells of the distal tubule and thus reduce Ca++ excretion. The distal tubule normally reabsorbs approximately 9% of the filtered load of Ca++ (see Chapter 9). The reabsorption of Ca++ at this site is an active, transcellular process involving entry of Ca++ into the cell through channels in the apical membrane and extrusion from the cell across the basolateral membrane by the Ca++-ATPase and 3Na+-Ca++ antiporter. The thiazide diuretics, by inhibiting the entry of NaCl into the cell, cause the membrane potential to hyperpolarize (i.e., the cell interior becomes more electrically negative).[2] This hyperpolarization in turn activates a Ca^{++} channel in the apical membrane of the cell and increases the electrochemical gradient for Ca^{++} entry into the cell. The increased entry of Ca^{++} into the cell is matched by increased extrusion across the basolateral membrane by the Ca^{++}-ATPase and $3Na^+$-Ca^{++} antiporter. The net effect is an increase in Ca^{++} reabsorption. Because thiazides reduce urinary Ca^{++} excretion, they are sometimes used to lower the incidence of Ca^{++}-containing stone formation in individuals who normally excrete high levels of Ca^{++} in their urine.

With the exception of the K^+-sparing diuretics, all diuretics acutely increase Pi excretion. However, the cellular mechanisms for this effect are not completely understood. The effect is modified, however, with long-term diuretic therapy. With the decrease in ECF volume that accompanies long-term diuretic use, proximal tubule Na^+ reabsorption is stimulated. Because the proximal tubule reabsorbs the largest portion of the filtered load of Pi and because this reabsorptive process is coupled with Na^+ (see Chapters 4 and 9), Pi excretion is reduced in this setting.

SUMMARY

1. Diuretics inhibit solute (primarily NaCl) transport at various sites along the nephron. As a result of their action, the excretion of solute and water by the kidneys increases.

2. By increasing the excretion of NaCl by the kidneys, diuretics cause a decrease in the volume of the ECF. This decreased ECF volume results in a loss of body weight because 1 L of ECF fluid weighs 1 kg.

3. The ability of a particular diuretic to increase solute and water excretion depends on several factors, including the nephron segment where the diuretic acts, the ability of other nephron segments not affected by the diuretic to increase their reabsorption of solute and water, the delivery of sufficient quantities of the diuretic to its site of action, and diuretic-induced changes in ECF volume that may affect renal solute and water transport.

4. Osmotic diuretics inhibit solute and water reabsorption in the proximal tubule and descending thin limb of Henle's loop. Quantitatively, the proximal tubule is the more important site of action.

5. Carbonic anhydrase inhibitors act primarily in the proximal tubule to inhibit Na^+, HCO_3^-, and water reabsorption.

6. Loop diuretics inhibit NaCl reabsorption by the thick ascending limb of Henle's loop. They are the most potent diuretics and can increase Na^+ excretion to as much as 25% of the filtered load.

7. Thiazide diuretics inhibit NaCl reabsorption in the early portion of the distal tubule.

8. K^+-sparing diuretics act at the late portion of the distal tubule and the cortical collecting duct. They inhibit Na^+ reabsorption and in doing so inhibit K^+ secretion. Their most important use is related to their ability to reduce renal K^+ excretion.

9. Aquaretics block the ADH receptor (V_2) in the late portion of the distal tubule and the collecting duct. They impair the ability of the kidneys to concentrate the urine leading to the excretion of solute-free water.

10. Osmotic diuretics and carbonic anhydrase inhibitors increase the kidneys' ability to excrete and reabsorb solute-free water. The loop diuretics impair both solute-free water reabsorption and excretion, whereas the thiazide diuretics impair only solute-free water excretion. The K^+-sparing diuretics do not have a significant effect on solute-free water excretion. Aquaretics increase solute-free water excretion and impair solute-free water reabsorption.

---

[2]Hyperpolarization of the membrane potential occurs as a result of a decrease in the intracellular [Cl^-]. The basolateral membrane of the distal tubule cell contains Cl^- channels; thus, the membrane potential is determined in part by the Cl^- equilibrium potential. A decrease in the intracellular [Cl^-] therefore increases the magnitude of this equilibrium potential (i.e., it becomes more negative).

11. All diuretics, with the exception of the K^+-sparing diuretics, increase the renal excretion of K^+. This effect is in response to increased delivery of tubular fluid to the K^+ secretory portion of the nephron (distal tubule and cortical collecting duct) and increased aldosterone and ADH levels secondary to the diuretic-induced decrease in ECF volume.

12. The carbonic anhydrase inhibitors and K^+-sparing diuretics can induce a metabolic acidosis. The loop diuretics and thiazide diuretics can cause a metabolic alkalosis.

13. Acutely, loop diuretics increase Ca^{++} excretion. By reducing the ECF volume, chronic administration of loop diuretics can decrease Ca^{++} excretion. Thiazide diuretics decrease Ca^{++} excretion.

14. With the exception of K^+-sparing diuretics, all diuretics acutely increase Pi excretion. When the ECF volume is decreased by chronic diuretic use, Pi excretion is reduced.

KEY WORDS AND CONCEPTS

- Organic anion secretory system
- Organic cation secretory system
- Steady state
- Diuretic braking phenomenon
- Osmotic diuretics
- Carbonic anhydrase inhibitors
- Loop diuretics
- Thiazide diuretics
- K^+-sparing diuretics
- Aquaretics

SELF-STUDY PROBLEMS

1. Patients with nephrogenic diabetes insipidus can obtain symptomatic relief from their polyuria with long-term use of a thiazide diuretic. What are the mechanisms by which long-term thiazide therapy produces a decrease in urine volume in these patients?

2. An individual takes a thiazide diuretic as partial therapy for hypertension. Before therapy, plasma $[K^+]$ is 4 mEq/L. After several months of therapy, the individual's blood pressure is reduced and plasma $[K^+]$ is 3 mEq/L.
   a. By what mechanism could the diuretic lead to a decrease in blood pressure?
   b. By what mechanism did the plasma $[K^+]$ fall? What other classes of diuretics would produce this effect?
   c. What can be done to increase the plasma $[K^+]$ to the level it was at before diuretic therapy was initiated?

3. The antibiotic penicillin is secreted into the urine by the organic anion secretory system of the proximal tubule. If an individual taking a thiazide diuretic for hypertension develops an infection requiring penicillin, what effect, if any, could this have on the action of the diuretic?

4. Two individuals are administered a diuretic for several weeks. Individual A receives a loop diuretic and individual B a thiazide diuretic. Both ingest a diet that contains 100 mEq/day of Na^+. After these individuals have taken their respective diuretics for 2 weeks, consider the following questions:
   a. How much Na^+ does each of these individuals excrete in a day and why?
   b. Both individuals are deprived of water. Individual A is able to concentrate the urine to 400 mOsm/kg H_2O. Individual B is able to concentrate the urine to 1000 mOsm/kg H_2O. How do you explain the difference in response of these two individuals to water deprivation?
   c. Both individuals are water loaded. Individual A is able to dilute his urine to 300 mOsm/kg H_2O. Individual B is able to dilute his urine to 250 mOsm/kg H_2O. How do you explain the inability of these individuals to dilute their urine maximally?

ADDITIONAL READING

The following resources are offered as suggestions for students who wish to learn more about the kidney and the urinary tract and build upon the foundation laid out in this book. Where appropriate, we have provided sources that explore in more depth some of the molecular advances that have been made. Sources that are more clinically oriented are also included.

GENERAL

Brenner BM, editor: *Brenner and Rector's the kidney,* ed 7. Philadelphia, 2004, Saunders. (A two-volume, comprehensive text on the kidney. Includes sections on normal physiology, pathophysiology, and clinical nephrology. Each chapter is written by experts in the field and includes an extensive list of references.)

Johnson RY, Freehally J, editors: *Comprehensive clinical nephrology,* ed 2. Philadelphia, 2003, Mosby. (A clinically oriented textbook of nephrology, which has overviews of normal physiology and pathophysiology.)

Massry SG, Glassock RJ, editors: *Textbook of nephrology,* ed 4. Philadelphia, 2001, Lippincott Williams & Wilkins. (A clinically oriented textbook of nephrology, which has overviews of normal physiology and pathophysiology.)

Rose BD: *Clinical physiology of acid-base and electrolyte disorders,* ed 5. New York, 2001, McGraw-Hill. (A clearly written book that discusses fluid and electrolyte disorders from basic physiologic principles. A good next book for those who want to explore the material presented in this book in greater detail.)

Schrier RW, editor: *Diseases of the kidney and urinary tract,* ed 7. Philadelphia, 2001, Lippincott Williams & Wilkins. (A three-volume, comprehensive text on pathophysiology and clinical nephrology. Each chapter is written by experts in the field and includes an extensive list of references.)

Seldin DW, Giebisch G, editors: *The kidney: physiology and pathophysiology,* ed 3. Philadelphia, 2000, Lippincott Williams & Wilkins. (A two-volume, comprehensive text on the kidney, similar in many ways to the Brenner text. Includes sections on normal physiology, pathophysiology, and clinical nephrology. Each chapter is written by experts in the field and includes an extensive list of references.)

CHAPTER 1

King LS, Kozono D, Agre P: From structure to disease: the evolving tale of aquaporin biology. *Nat Rev Mol Cell Biol* 5:687-698, 2004. (An up-to-date review of the aquaporin protein family and the role aquaporins play in tissues throughout the body under both normal and disease conditions. The senior author, Peter Agre, received a Nobel Prize in 2003 for the discovery of aquaporins.)

Nolan J: Fluid replacement. *Br Med Bull* 55:821-843, 1999. (Very clinically oriented review of principles and practice of intravenous fluid therapy.)

Rose BD: *Clinical physiology of acid-base and electrolyte disorders,* ed 5. New York, 2001, McGraw-Hill. (Chapter 1 discusses the basic principles of ions in solution. Chapter 7 describes the exchange of water across cell membranes and capillaries.)

Taylor AE, Moore TM: Capillary fluid exchange. *Adv Physiol Educ* 22:s203-s210, 1999. (A clear and concisely written review of the physiology of the movement of fluid across the capillary wall. A summary of the Starling forces across specific capillary beds is included.)

CHAPTER 2

Anyatonwu GI, Ehrlich BE: Calcium signaling and polycystin-2. *Biochem Biophys Res Commun* 322:1364-1373, 2004. (An overview of polycystin 1 and polycystin 2 function with regard to Ca^{++} signaling.)

Huber TB, Benzing T: The slit diaphragm: a signaling platform to regulate podocyte function. *Curr Opin Nephrol Hypertens* 14:211-216, 2005. (An overview of podocytes and the slit diaphragm and the role that slit diaphragm proteins play in cell signaling.)

Kriz W, Bankir L: A standard nomenclature for structures of the kidney. *Am J Physiol* 254:F1, 1988. (A complete review of renal nomenclature, providing most synonyms for each structure. Does not, however, contain any references.)

Ly J, Alexander M, Quaggin SE: A podocentric view of nephrology. *Curr Opin Nephrol Hypertens* 13:299-305, 2004. (A review of the podocyte structure and function and a discussion of diseases that affect podocyte structure and function.)

Madsen K, Tisher CC: Anatomy of the kidney. In Brenner BM, editor: *Brenner and Rector's the kidney*, ed 7. Philadelphia, 2004, WB Saunders. (A complete and detailed review of renal structure and ultrastructure. Superb electron micrographs.)

Pirson Y: Making the diagnosis in Alport's syndrome. *Kidney Int* 56:760, 1999. (A case presentation of a child with Alport's syndrome. Included are a discussion of the differential diagnosis and a review of the genetics and pathophysiology.)

Praetorius HA, Spring KR: A physiological view of the primary cilium. *Annu Rev Physiol* 67:515-529, 2005. (A detailed overview of the primary cilium, with an emphasis on its mechanosensory and chemosensory functions.)

Wilson PD: Polycystic kidney disease. *N Engl J Med* 350:151-164, 2004. (A comprehensive and nicely illustrated review of PKD.)

CHAPTER 3

Arendshorst WJ, Navar LG: Renal circulation and glomerular hemodynamics. In Schrier RW, editor: *Diseases of the kidney and urinary tract*, ed 7. Philadelphia, 2001, Lippincott Williams & Wilkins. (A comprehensive review of renal hemodynamics and its regulation.)

Dworkin LD, Sun AM, Brenner BM: The renal circulations. In Brenner BM, editor: *Brenner and Rector's the kidney*, ed 7. Philadelphia, 2004, WB Saunders. (Superb illustrations of the renal circulatory system. A very detailed review of the anatomy of the vasculature.)

Komlosi P, Fintha A, Bell PD: Current mechanisms of macula densa signaling. *Acta Physiol Scand* 181:463-469, 2004. (An excellent short summary of the physiology of the macula densa.)

Lafayette RA, Perrone RD, Levey AS: Laboratory evaluation of renal function. In Schrier RW, editor: *Diseases of the kidney and urinary tract*, ed 7. Philadelphia, 2001, Lippincott Williams & Wilkins. (Describes the general approach for the clinical evaluation of renal function. The use of creatinine clearance for the measurement of glomerular filtration rate is discussed.)

Maddox DA, Brenner BM: Glomerular ultrafiltration. In Brenner BM, editor: *Brenner and Rector's the kidney*, ed 7. Philadelphia, 2004, WB Saunders (An advanced review of glomerular ultrafiltration with complete presentations of hormonal regulation of GFR and RBF, autoregulation of GFR, and tubuloglomerular feedback.)

Persson AEG, Ollerstam A, Liu R, Brown R: Mechanisms for the macula densa release of renin. *Acta Physiol Scand* 181:471-474, 2004. (An excellent short summary of the physiology of the macula densa.)

CHAPTER 4

Burton DC, Petrie MC, Hillier C, et al: The clinical relevance of adrenomedullin: a promising profile? *Pharmacol Ther* 103:179-201, 2004. (An excellent summary of the clinical relevance of adrenomedullin.)

Forte JLF Jr: Uroguanylin and guanylin peptides: pharmacology and experimental therapeutics. *Pharmacol Ther* 104:137-162, 2004. (A very detailed review of uroguanylin and guanylin.)

Guay-Woodford LM: Overview: the genetics of renal disease. *Semin Nephrol* 19:312, 1999. (A compilation of genes and genetic diseases of the kidneys.)

King LS, Kozono D, Agre P: From structure to disease: the evolving tale of aquaporin biology. *Nat Rev Mol Cell Biol* 5:687-698, 2004. (An overview of aquaporins, coauthored by Dr. Peter Agre, recipient of the Noble Prize in Physiology in 2003 for his studies on aquaporins.)

Kuhn M: Molecular physiology of natriuretic peptide signaling. *Basic Res Cardiol* 99:76-82, 2004. (An excellent summary of the physiology of natriuretic peptides.)

McCormick JA, Bhalla V, Pao AC, Pearce D: SGK1: a rapid aldosterone-induced regulator of renal sodium reabsorption. *Physiology (Bethesda)* 20:134-139, 2005. (A short overview on SGK and its role in regulating sodium excretion.)

Moe OW, Baum M, Berry C, Rector FC Jr: Renal transport of glucose, amino acids, sodium, chloride, and water. In Brenner BM, editor: *Brenner and Rector's the kidney*, ed 7. Philadelphia, 2004, WB Saunders. (A complete and up-to-date review of solute transport along the nephron.)

Wright SH, Dantzler WH: Molecular and cellular physiology of renal organic anion transport. *Physiol Rev* 84:987-1049, 2004. (A complete and up-to-date review of organic anion transport in the proximal tubule.)

CHAPTER 5

Antunes-Rodrigues J, De Castro M, Elias LL, et al: Neuroendocrine control of body fluid metabolism. *Physiol Rev* 84:169-208, 2004. (An in-depth and comprehensive review with a focus on the neurobiologic aspects of the ADH and thirst systems.)

Berl T, Verbalis J: Pathophysiology of water metabolism. In Brenner BM, editor: *Brenner and Rector's the kidney*, ed 7. Philadelphia, 2004, WB Saunders. (An excellent review on the control of ADH secretion and disorders of the urine concentration and dilution process.)

Brown D, Nielsen S: The cell biology of vasopressin action. In Brenner BM, editor: *Brenner and Rector's the kidney*, ed 7. Philadelphia, 2004, WB Saunders. (A clearly written and detailed review of the molecular and cell biology of ADH action.)

Feldman BJ, Rosenthal SM, Vargas GA, et al: Nephrogenic syndrome of inappropriate antidiuresis. *N Engl J Med* 352:1884-1890, 2005. (The first report of two infants with activating mutations in the V_2 receptor gene.)

King LS, Kozono D, Agre P: From structure to disease: the evolving tale of aquaporin biology. *Nat Rev Mol Cell Biol* 5:687-698, 2004. (An up-to-date review of the aquaporin protein family and the role aquaporins play in tissues throughout the body under both normal and disease conditions. The senior author, Peter Agre, received a Nobel Prize in 2003 for the discovery of aquaporins.)

Knepper MA, Gamba G: Urine concentration and dilution. In Brenner BM, editor: *Brenner and Rector's the kidney*, ed 7. Philadelphia, 2004, WB Saunders. (A comprehensive review of current understanding of how the kidney excretes both dilute and concentrated urine.)

Nguyen MK, Nielsen S, Kurtz I: Molecular pathogenesis of nephrogenic diabetes insipidus. *Clin Exp Nephrol* 7: 9-17, 2003. (This review discusses both acquired and inherited forms of nephrogenic diabetes insipidus.)

Sands JM: Mammalian urea transporters. *Annu Rev Physiol* 65: 543-566, 2003. (This review covers not only the distribution of various urea transporters in the kidney but also how expression of the transporters might be regulated and how defects in the transporters affect the ability of the kidney to concentrate and dilute the urine.)

Verbalis JG: Diabetes insipidus. *Rev Endocr Metab Disord* 4:177-185, 2003. (Clear and concise review focused primarily on central diabetes insipidus.)

Verbalis JG: Disorders of body water homeostasis. *Best Pract Res Clin Endocrinol Metab* 17:471-503, 2003. (A thorough review of the physiology of body fluids, the control of ADH secretion, and disorders of water balance.)

CHAPTER 6

Abassi ZA, Winaver J, Skorecki KL: Control of extracellular fluid volume and the pathophysiology of edema formation. In Brenner BM, editor: *Brenner and Rector's the kidney*, ed 7. Philadelphia, 2004, WB Saunders. (A comprehensive review of Na^+ handling by the kidney from the perspective of maintenance of ECF volume.)

Antunes-Rodrigues J, De Castro M, Elias LL, et al: Neuroendocrine control of body fluid metabolism. *Physiol Rev* 84:169-208, 2004. (An in-depth and comprehensive review with a focus on the neurobiologic aspects of the ADH and thirst systems. It also discusses the neuroendocrine control of ANP secretion.)

Baxter GF: The natriuretic peptides. *Basic Res Cardiol* 99:71-75, 2004. (A clear and concise review discovery, synthesis, secretion, and action of ANP and BNP.)

Biner HL, Arpin-Bott MP, Loffing J, et al: Human cortical distal nephron: distribution of electrolyte and water transport pathways. *J Am Soc Nephrol* 13:836-847, 2002. (An elegant and detailed study of the localization of key Na^+ transporters and aquaporins along the human distal tubule and cortical portion of the collecting duct.)

Charles CJ, Lainchbury JG, Nicholls MG, et al: Adrenomedullin and the renin-angiotensin-aldosterone system. *Regul Pept* 112:41-49, 2003. (A review of the actions of adrenomedullin, with a focus on interactions with the renin-angiotensin-aldosterone system.)

Forte LR: A novel role for uroguanylin in the regulation of sodium balance. *J Clin Invest* 112:1138-1141, 2003. (A concise review that describes the role uroguanylin plays in the regulation of renal NaCl excretion in response to ingested NaCl.)

Knepper MA, Kim G-H, Masilamani S: Renal tubule sodium transporter abundance profiling in the kidney: response to aldosterone and variations in NaCl intake. *Ann NY Acad Sci* 986:562-569, 2003. (A review of how aldosterone and alterations in NaCl intake regulate the abundance of Na^+ transporters along the length of the nephron.)

Loffing J, Kaissling B: Sodium and calcium transport pathways along the mammalian distal nephron: from rabbit to human. *Am J Physiol* 284:F628-F643, 2002. (An elegant study, which highlights species differences in the localization of Na^+ and Ca^{++} transporters in the distal tubule and cortical portion of the collecting duct.)

Meneton P, Loffing J, Warnock DG: Sodium and potassium handling by the aldosterone-sensitive distal nephron: the pivotal role of the distal and connecting tubule. *Am J Physiol* 287:F593-F601, 2003. (A clear and comprehensive review of Na^+ transport in the distal tubule and collecting duct, with a focus on the relative role of the various segments that constitute this portion of the nephron.)

Persson AEG, Ollerstam A, Liu R, Brown R: Mechanisms for macula densa cell release of renin. *Acta Scand Physiol* 181:471-474, 2004. (A concise review of current evidence for how the macula densa controls renin secretion.)

Persson PB: Renin: origin, secretion and synthesis. *J Physiol* 552: 667-671, 2003. (A concise review on the mechanisms of renin secretion by the juxtaglomerular cells.)

Schweda F, Kurtz A: Cellular mechanism of renin release. *Acta Physiol Scand* 181:383-390, 2004. (A concise review on the mechanisms of renin secretion by the juxtaglomerular cells.)

Xu J: Renalase is a novel, soluble monoamine oxidase that regulates cardiac function and blood pressure. *J Clin Invest* 115: 1275-1280, 2005. (An elegant study that provides evidence that the kidney secretes a monoamine oxidase that metabolizes catecholamines.)

CHAPTER 7

Hebert SC, Desir G, Giebisch G, Wang W: Molecular diversity and regulation of renal potassium channels. *Physiol Rev* 85:319-371, 2005. (An overview of K^+ channels and their regulation.)

Malnic G, Bailey MA, Giebisch G: Control of renal potassium excretion. In Brenner BM, editor: *Brenner and Rector's the kidney*, ed 7. Philadelphia, 2004, WB Saunders. (A detailed review of the cellular mechanisms of K^+ transport and the factors and hormones regulating urinary potassium excretion.)

CHAPTER 8

Breton S: The cellular physiology of carbonic anhydrase. *J Pancreas* (Online) 2:159-164, 2001. (A concise review of carbonic anhydrase.)

DuBose TD Jr: Acid-base disorders. In Brenner BM, editor: *Brenner and Rector's the kidney*, ed 7. Philadelphia, 2004, WB Saunders. (Detailed review of acid-base disorders, with discussions of the causes, pathophysiology, and treatment.)

Goldfarb S: Renal tubular acidosis. *Hosp Phys* 6:2-12, 2003. (Case-based review of renal acidification and renal tubular acidosis.)

Hamm LL: Renal acidification mechanisms. In Brenner BM, editor: *Brenner and Rector's the kidney*, ed 7. Philadelphia, 2004, WB Saunders. (A complete and comprehensive review of the cellular and molecular mechanisms of H^+ and HCO_3^- transport by the various segments of the nephron and how these mechanisms are regulated.)

Moe OW, Fuster D: Clinical acid-base pathophysiology: disorders of plasma anion gap. *Best Pract Res Clin Endocrinol Metab* 17:559-574, 2003. (In-depth review of metabolic acidosis and the use of the anion gap in diagnosis.)

Nakhoul NL, Hamm LL: Non-erythroid Rh glycoproteins: a putative new family of mammalian ammonium transporters. *Pflugers Arch Eur J Physiol* 447:807-812, 2004. (A review of the history of Rh glycoproteins and their potential role as ammonium transporters in the kidneys.)

Nicoletta JA, Schwartz GJ: Distal renal tubular acidosis. *Curr Opin Pediatr* 16:194-198, 2004. (A concise review of the various causes of distal renal tubular acidosis.)

Wagner CA, Finberg KE, Breton S, et al: Renal vacuolar H^+-ATPase. *Physiol Rev* 84:1263-1314, 2004. (A comprehensive and in-depth review of molecular biology and function of the H^+-ATPase in the kidneys.)

Weiner ID, Verlander D: Renal and hepatic expression of the ammonium transporter proteins, Rh B glycoprotein and Rh C glycoprotein. *Acta Physiol Scand* 179:331-338, 2003. (A study that details the localization of these Rh glycoproteins along the nephron.)

CHAPTER 9

Ba J, Friedman PA: Calcium-sensing receptor regulation of renal mineral ion transport. *Cell Calcium* 35:229-237, 2004. (A short review of the calcium-sensing receptor.)

Chang W, Shoback D: Extracellular Ca^{++}-sensing receptors: an overview. *Cell Calcium* 35:183-196, 2004. (A short overview of the calcium-sensing receptor.)

Friedman PA: Renal calcium metabolism. In Seldin DW, Giebisch G, editors: *The kidney: physiology and pathophysiology*, ed 3. Philadelphia, 2000, Lippincott Williams & Wilkins. (A thorough review of calcium metabolism.)

Hoenderop JGJ, Nilius B, Bindels RJM: Calcium absorption across epithelia. *Physiol Rev* 85:373-422, 2005. (A very complete review of calcium transport across the kidney and other epithelia.)

Murer H, Kaissling B, Forster I, Biber J: Cellular mechanisms in proximal tubular handling of phosphate. In Seldin DW, Giebisch G, editors: *The kidney: physiology and pathophysiology*, ed 3. Philadelphia, 2000, Lippincott Williams & Wilkins. (A thorough review of Pi transport by the proximal tubule.)

Pollack MR, Yu ASL: Clinical disturbances of calcium, magnesium and phosphate metabolism. In Brenner BM, editor: *Brenner and Rector's the kidney*, ed 7. Philadelphia, 2004, WB Saunders. (A detailed review of the pathophysiology of Ca^{++} and Pi homeostasis.)

Yu ASL: Renal transport of calcium, magnesium, and phosphate. In Brenner BM, editor: *Brenner and Rector's the kidney*, ed 7. Philadelphia, 2004, WB Saunders. (A detailed review of renal transport of Ca^{++} and Pi.)

CHAPTER 10

Costello-Boerrigter LC, Boerrigter G, Burnett JC Jr: Revisiting salt and water retention: new diuretics, aquaretics, and natriuretics. *Med Clin North Am* 87:475-491, 2003. (Review of the use of diuretics in treatment of Na^+ retention states. Congestive heart failure is emphasized.)

Ecelbarger CA, Kim GH, Wade JB, Knepper MA: Regulation of the abundance of renal sodium transporters and channels by vasopressin. *Exp Neurol* 171:227-234, 2001. (Review of the effects of ADH on increasing the abundance of Na^+ transporters in various segments of the nephron. A response that contributes to the diuretic braking phenomenon.)

Kim GH, Lee JW, Oh YK, et al: Antidiuretic effect of hydrochlorothiazide in lithium-induced nephrogenic diabetes insipidus is associated with upregulation of aquaporin-2, Na-Cl co-transporter, and epithelial sodium channel. *J Am Soc Nephrol* 15:2836-2843, 2004. (Study done in rats in which diabetes insipidus was induced by Li^+ ingestion. It shows that thiazide diuretics increase the abundance of Na^+ transporters and aquaporin-2 in these animals, leading to improvement in polyuria.)

Na KY, Oh YK, Han JS, et al: Upregulation of Na^+ transporter abundances in response to chronic thiazide or loop diuretic treatment in rats. *Am J Physiol* 284:F133-F143, 2003. (Study done in rats showing that chronic thiazide therapy increases the abundance of specific Na^+ transporters along the nephron. This response contributes to the diuretic braking phenomenon.)

Shankar SS, Brater DC: Loop diuretics: from the Na-K-2Cl transporter to clinical use. *Am J Physiol* 284:11-21, 2003. (Comprehensive review of the physiology and clinical use of loop diuretics.)

Sica DA: Diuretic-related side effects: development and treatment. *J Clin Hypertens* 6:532-540, 2004. (Clinically oriented review of the side effects that result from use of diuretics.)

Wilcox CS: Diuretics. In Brenner BM, editor: *Brenner and Rector's the kidney*, ed 7. Philadelphia, 2004, WB Saunders. (A complete and comprehensive review of the physiology, pharmacology, and clinical use of diuretics.)

APPENDIX A

INTEGRATIVE CASE STUDIES

CASE 1

A 65-year-old man has congestive heart failure. He is seen by his physician because he has run out of his medications. He presents with easy fatigability, shortness of breath, and swelling of his ankles. On physical examination he is found to have distended neck veins and pitting edema of the ankles. His breathing is rapid (20/min), and rales (i.e., fluid in the lungs) are heard bilaterally at the bases of the lungs. He is afebrile, with a pulse rate of 110 beats/min and a blood pressure of 110/70. A blood sample is obtained, and the following abnormalities are noted:

Serum $[Na^+]$ = 130 mEq/L
Serum $[K^+]$ = 3.0 mEq/L
Serum [creatinine] = 1.4 mg/dL

Questions

1a. Is the extracellular fluid (ECF) volume in this man increased or decreased from normal? What evidence in the physical examination supports your conclusion?

1b. Is the effective circulating volume (ECV) in this man increased or decreased from normal?

1c. What would you predict to be the levels (activities) of ANP, ADH, renin-angiotensin-aldosterone, and the sympathetic nervous system in this man, and why?

1d. How would you characterize renal Na^+ handling in this man? What evidence in the physical examination supports this conclusion?

1e. What is the mechanism for the development of hyponatremia in this man?

1f. What is the mechanism for the development of hypokalemia in this man?

1g. The physician treating this man prescribes a loop diuretic in order to reduce Na^+ retention and reduce his edema. It is known that patients with congestive heart failure do not respond as well to loop diuretics as healthy patients would (i.e., the degree of natriuresis is less). What explains the decreased effect of the loop diuretic in a patient with congestive heart failure?

1h. What effect will the loop diuretic have on this man's ECF volume and ECV?

1i. While he is taking the loop diuretic, the serum $[K^+]$ of this man decreases from 3.0 to 2.5 mEq/L. What is the mechanism for this diuretic-induced hypokalemia?

1j. After administration of the diuretic, the serum [creatinine] increases from 1.4 to 1.8 mg/dL. Why was the serum [creatinine] elevated, and why did it increase further after treatment with the loop diuretic?

CASE 2

A 49-year-old woman sees her physician because of weakness, easy fatigability, and loss of appetite. During the past month she has lost 7 kg (15 lb). On physical examination she is found to have hyperpigmentation especially of the oral mucosa and gums. She is hypotensive, and her blood pressure falls when she assumes an upright posture (BP = 100/60 mm Hg supine and

80/50 mm Hg erect). The following laboratory data are obtained.

Serum [Na$^+$] = 132 mEq/L
Serum [K$^+$] = 6.5 mEq/L
Serum [HCO$_3^-$] = 20 mEq/L
Urine [Na$^+$] = 20 mEq/L

Questions

2a. The plasma level of what hormone(s) would be expected to be below normal in this woman?

2b. How do you explain the urine [Na$^+$] of 20 mEq/L in this woman? What would you expect the urine [Na$^+$] to be in an individual who is volume depleted? What relationship does this have to the hypotension in this woman?

2c. What is the mechanism for development of hyponatremia in this woman?

2d. Why does this woman have hyperkalemia?

2e. What is the acid-base disturbance in this woman, and what is its cause?

CASE 3

A 70-year-old man with lung cancer develops the syndrome of inappropriate antidiuretic hormone secretion (SIADH). He is admitted to the hospital, and the following data are obtained. His vital signs are normal, as is the physical examination. There is no evidence of ECF volume contraction or ECF volume expansion.

Body weight = 70 kg
Serum [Na$^+$] = 120 mEq/L (normal = 135-147 mEq/L)
Urine osmolality = 600 mOsm/kg H$_2$O
Urine [Na$^+$] excretion = 80 mEq/day

Questions

3a. What determines the amount of Na$^+$ that is excreted in the urine, and is Na$^+$ excretion in this patient normal (assume that he ingests approximately 80 mEq/day of Na$^+$)?

3b. 1 L of isotonic saline is administered intravenously with the goal of raising the serum [Na$^+$]. How much of the infused NaCl will be excreted in the urine (for simplicity, assume that 1 L of isotonic saline contains 150 mmol/L of NaCl)? What effect will this infusion have on the plasma [Na$^+$]?

3c. What effect would the administration of 1 L of hypertonic saline (3% NaCl solution) have on the plasma [Na$^+$]?

3d. What other therapies could be used to treat this man's hyponatremia?

CASE 4

An 18-year-old man with insulin-dependent (type 1) diabetes mellitus is seen in the emergency department. He reports not taking his insulin during the previous 24 hours because he did not feel well and was not eating. He now has weakness, nausea, thirst, and frequent urination. His blood pressure is 100/60 mm Hg supine and 80/50 erect. His pulse rate increases from 100/min supine to 110/min when erect. On physical examination he is found to have deep and rapid respiration (Kussmaul's respiration). At 1:00 AM the following laboratory data are obtained:

Plasma [Na$^+$] = 140 mEq/L
Serum [Cl$^-$] = 95 mEq/L
Plasma [K$^+$] = 6.5 mEq/L
Plasma [HCO$_3^-$] = 7 mEq/L
Blood pH = 6.99
Arterial P$_{CO_2}$ = 18 mm Hg
Plasma [glucose] = 600 mg/dl
Urine contains glucose and ketones

The diagnosis of diabetic ketoacidosis is made, and the man is admitted to the hospital. Saline is administered intravenously and insulin therapy begun. The results of therapy are illustrated in the following table.

Time	Serum [K$^+$] (mEq/L)	Plasma pH	Serum [HCO$_3^-$] (mEq/L)	Serum [Glucose] (mg/dl)
1:00 AM	6.5	6.99	7	600
3:00 AM	4.5	7.10	12	400
4:00 AM	4.0	7.16	14	300
5:00 AM	3.5	7.20	16	250
7:00 AM	3.2	7.24	18	200

Questions

4a. What type of acid-base disorder does this man have? What is the plasma anion gap, and what is its significance?

4b. What can you conclude about K$^+$ balance in this man?

4c. Explain why the serum [K$^+$] fell during the first hour of treatment.

CASE 5

A previously healthy 28-year-old man is seen in the emergency department with right side flank pain. Shortly after arrival, he passes a small kidney stone. He denies any significant previous renal or gastrointestinal problems. There is a family history of kidney stones. The results of laboratory tests done in the emergency department include the following:

Serum $[Na^+]$ = 137 mEq/L
Serum $[K^+]$ = 3.1 mEq/L
Serum $[Cl^-]$ = 111 mEq/L
Serum $[HCO_3^-]$ = 13 mEq/L
Arterial pH = 7.28
Arterial P_{CO_2} = 28 mm Hg
Urine pH = 6.4

Questions

5a. What is the acid-base disorder? What is the anion gap, and what does it tell you about this man's acid-base disorder?

5b. How do you explain the urine pH of 6.4 when his plasma $[HCO_3^-]$ is 13 mEq/L and the plasma pH is 7.28?

5c. The man's "urinary net charge" is calculated, and a value of +13 is obtained. What information does this give you regarding renal acid-base transport, and how does this help you to determine the cause of his acid-base disorder?

CASE 6

Paramedics bring a 16-year-old asthmatic to the emergency department. History obtained from the parents indicates that she has had asthma for 4 years, which is induced by exercise and is exacerbated during upper respiratory infections. She currently uses an inhaler (β-adrenergic agonist) before exercise. Four days ago she developed symptoms of an upper respiratory infection, and she increased the use of her inhaler. This morning she had acute shortness of breath and her parents called 911. When the paramedics arrived she was cyanotic, and epinephrine was administered with some improvement.

On physical examination she appears anxious and in moderate distress. On auscultation of the chest, wheezes are heard throughout both lung fields. The following laboratory data are obtained.

Serum $[Na^+]$ = 140 mEq/L
Serum $[K^+]$ = 3.3 mEq/L
Serum $[Cl^-]$ = 105 mEq/L
Serum $[HCO_3^-]$ = 15 mEq/L
Serum [creatinine] = 1.0 mg/dL
Arterial pH = 7.0
Arterial P_{CO_2} = 60 mm Hg
Arterial P_{O_2} = 40 mmHg

Questions

6a. What is the acid-base disorder in this girl?

6b. What is the most likely cause for her hypokalemia?

APPENDIX B

NORMAL LABORATORY VALUES

	TRADITIONAL UNITS	SI UNITS
Arterial Blood Gases		
P_{CO_2}	33-44 mm Hg	4.4-5.9 kPa
P_{CO_2}	75-105 mm Hg	10.0-14.0 kPa
pH	7.35-7.45	$[H^+]$ 36-44 nmol/L
Serum Electrolytes*		
Na^+	135-147 mEq/L	135-147 mmol/L
Cl^-	95-105 mEq/L	95-105 mmol/L
K^+	3.5-5.0 mEq/L	3.5-5.0 mmol/L
HCO_3^-	22-28 mEq/L	22-28 mmol/L
Ca^{++}	8.4-10.0 mg/dL	2.1-2.8 mmol/L
Pi	3.0-4.5 mg/dL	1.0-1.5 mmol/L
Anion Gap	8-16 mEq/L	8-16 mmol/L
Serum Proteins		
Total	6.0-7.8 g/dL	60-78 g/L
Albumin	3.5-5.5 g/dL	35-55 g/L
Globulin	2.3-3.5 g/dL	23-35 g/L
Other Serum Constituents		
Creatinine	0.6-1.2 mg/dL	53-106 mmol/L
Glucose (fasting)	70-110 mg/dL	3.8-6.1 mmol/L
Urea nitrogen (BUN)	7-18 mg/dL	1.2-3.0 mmol/L
Serum osmolality	285-295 mOsm/kg H_2O	285-295 mOsm/kg H_2O
Creatinine Clearance		
Male	90-140 ml/min	90-140 ml/min
	130-200 L/day	130-200 L/day
Female	80-125 ml/min	80-125 ml/min
	115-180 L/day	115-180 L/day

*Serum is derived from clotted blood (devoid of clotting factors), whereas plasma is derived from unclotted blood (contains clotting factors). However, concentrations of most substances are the same whether determined on a sample of plasma or serum. Most clinical chemistry laboratories determine concentrations of serum samples.

BUN, blood urea nitrogen.

APPENDIX C

■ ■ ■ ■ ■ ■ ■ ■ ■ ■ ■

N E P H R O N   F U N C T I O N

SUMMARY BY TRANSPORT PROCESS

TABLE C-1		
Na^+ and Cl^- Reabsorption		
NEPHRON SEGMENT	**MECHANISM**	**REGULATION**
Proximal tubule	Na^+-H^+ antiport	↓ECF volume (+)
	Na^+-solute symport	↑ECF volume (−)
	Cl^--anion exchange	Angiotensin II (+)
	Paracellular	Sympathetic nerves (+)
		Epinephrine (+)
		Dopamine (−)
		Starling forces (+)
Henle's loop		
Thin descending limb	None	Aldosterone (+)
Thin ascending limb	Paracellular	Sympathetic nerves (+)
Thick ascending limb	$1Na^+$-$1K^+$-$2Cl^-$ symport	
	Paracellular	
Early distal tubule	Na^+-Cl^- symport	Aldosterone (+)
		Sympathetic nerves (+)
		Angiotensin II (+)
Late distal tubule and collecting duct	Na^+ channel	Aldosterone (+)
		Sympathetic nerves (+)
		Angiotensin II (+)
		ANP, BNP, urodilatin (−)
		Uroguanylin, guanylin (−)

(+), Stimulation; (−), inhibition.

TABLE C-2
K^+ Reabsorption

NEPHRON SEGMENT	MECHANISM	REGULATION
Proximal tubule	Paracellular	↓ECF volume (+)
		↑ECF volume (−)
Henle's loop		
Thin descending limb	None	Aldosterone (+)
Thin ascending limb	None	
Thick ascending limb	$1Na^+$-$1K^+$-$2Cl^-$ symport	
	Paracellular	
Early distal tubule	None	
Late distal tubule and collecting duct	H^+,K^+-ATPase	Dietary K^+ depletion (+)

(+), Stimulation; (−), inhibition.

TABLE C-3
K^+ Secretion

NEPHRON SEGMENT	MECHANISM	REGULATION
Proximal tubule	None	
Henle's loop		
Thin descending limb	None	
Thin ascending limb	None	
Thick ascending limb	None	
Early distal tubule	None	
Late distal tubule and collecting duct	K^+ channel	Plasma $[K^+]$ (+)
		Aldosterone (+)
		ADH (+)
		Flow rate (+)
		Acid-base balance (+/−)
		Glucocorticoids (+)

(+), Stimulation; (−), inhibition.

TABLE C-4
H^+ Secretion (HCO_3^- Reabsorption)

NEPHRON SEGMENT	MECHANISM	REGULATION
Proximal tubule	Na^+-H^+ antiport	↑Filtered load of HCO_3^- (+)
	H^+-ATPase	↓ECF volume (+)
		↑P_{CO_2} (+)
		↓Plasma $[HCO_3^-]$ (+)
		Endothelin (+)
		Glucocorticoid (+)
		Acute PTH (−)
Henle's loop		
Thin descending limb	None	↑P_{CO_2} (+)
Thin ascending limb	None	↓Plasma $[HCO_3^-]$ (+)
Thick ascending limb	Na^+-H^+ antiport	Chronic PTH (+)
	H^+-ATPase	
Early distal tubule	H^+-ATPase	↑P_{CO_2} (+)
	Na^+-H^+ antiport	↓Plasma $[HCO_3^-]$ (+)
Late distal tubule and collecting duct	H^+-ATPase	↑P_{CO_2} (+)
	H^+-K^+-ATPase	↓Plasma $[HCO_3^-]$ (+)
		Aldosterone (+)

(+), Stimulation; (−), inhibition.

TABLE C-5
HCO₃⁻ Secretion

NEPHRON SEGMENT	MECHANISM	REGULATION
Proximal tubule	None	
Henle's loop		
Thin descending limb	None	
Thin ascending limb	None	
Thick ascending limb	None	
Early distal tubule	None	
Late distal tubule and collecting duct	H^+-ATPase Cl^--HCO_3^- antiport	Metabolic alkalosis (+)

(+), Stimulation; (−), inhibition.

TABLE C-6
Water Reabsorption

NEPHRON SEGMENT	MECHANISM	REGULATION
Proximal tubule	AQP water channel	Starling forces
Henle's loop		
Thin descending limb	AQP water channel	
Thin ascending limb	None	
Thick ascending limb	None	
Early distal tubule	None	
Late distal tubule and collecting duct	AQP water channel	ADH (+) ANP, BNP, urodilatin, uroguanylin, guanylin (−)

(+), Stimulation; (−), inhibition.

TABLE C-7
Pi Reabsorption

NEPHRON SEGMENT	MECHANISM	REGULATION
Proximal tubule	$3Na^+$-Pi symport	PTH (+) Pi depletion (+) ↓ECF volume (+) Acidosis (−) Glucocorticoids (−) FGF-23 (−) FRP-4 (−)
Henle's loop		
Thin descending limb	None	
Thin ascending limb	None	
Thick ascending limb	None	
	None	
Early distal tubule	None	
Late distal tubule and collecting duct	None	

(+), Stimulation; (−), inhibition.

TABLE C-8
Ca⁺⁺ Reabsorption

NEPHRON SEGMENT	MECHANISM	REGULATION
Proximal tubule	Ca^{++} channel Paracellular	PTH (−) ↓ECF volume (+) ↓Plasma [Pi] (+)
Henle's loop		
Thin descending limb	None	
Thin ascending limb	None	
Thick ascending limb	Paracellular	PTH (+) ↓Plasma [Pi] (+) CaSR (−)
Early distal tubule	Ca^{++} channel	PTH (+) Calcitonin (+) Calcitriol (+) ↓Plasma [Pi] (+) Acidosis (−) CaSR (−)
Late distal tuble and collecting duct	None	

(+), Stimulation; (−), inhibition.

SUMMARY BY NEPHRON SEGMENT

Proximal Tubule

Reabsorption

Water	67% of the filtered load
NaCl	67% of the filtered load
K^+	67% of the filtered load
Ca^{++}	70% of the filtered load
Pi	80% of the filtered load
HCO_3^-	80% of the filtered load
Protein	100% of the filtered load
Urea	67% of the filtered load

Secretion

NH_4^+	Variable
Organic anions	Variable
Organic cations	Variable

Henle's Loop (Thick Ascending Limb)

Reabsorption

Water	15% of the filtered load (thin descending limb only)
NaCl	25% of the filtered load
K^+	20% of the filtered load
Ca^{++}	20% of the filtered load
HCO_3^-	10% of the filtered load
NH_4^+	Variable

Secretion

Urea (thin descending limb only)

Distal Tubule

Reabsorption

NaCl	5% of the filtered load
Ca^{++}	9% of the filtered load
HCO_3^-	6% of the filtered load
Pi	10% of the filtered load
Water	Variable in the late portion depending on ADH, ANP, BNP, uroguanylin, and guanylin levels

Collecting Duct

Reabsorption

Water	Variable depending on ADH, ANP, BNP, uroguanylin and guanylin levels
NaCl	3% of the filtered load
K^+	Normally zero
HCO_3^-	4% of the filtered load
Urea	Variable in medullary collecting duct depending on ADH levels

Secretion

K^+	0%-70% of the filtered load
NH_4^+	Variable
Urea	Variable (medullary portion only)

APPENDIX D

ANSWERS TO SELF-STUDY PROBLEMS

CHAPTER 1

1.

		Molarity (mmol/L)	Osmolality (mOsm/kg H₂O)
9 g	NaCl	154	308
72 g	Glucose	400	400
22.2 g	CaCl₂	200	600
3 g	Urea	50	50
8.4 g	NaHCO₃	100	200

2. The cell will swell when placed in the solution because the solute is only a partially effective osmole (i.e., this is a hypotonic solution). Because the reflection coefficient (σ) is 0.5, the effective osmolality of the solution is only 150 mOsm/kg H_2O. The solution would have to contain 600 mmol/L of this solute to be isotonic.

3. Na^+, with its anions Cl^- and HCO_3^-, constitutes the majority of particles in the ECF and is therefore the major determinant of plasma osmolality. Consequently, plasma osmolality can be estimated by simply doubling the plasma $[Na^+]$. Thus, the estimated plasma osmolality in this individual is as follows:

$$P_{osm} = 2(130) = 260 \text{ mOsm/kg } H_2O$$

This value is well below the normal range of 285 to 295 mOsm/kg H_2O and will result in movement of water from the ECF into the ICF. Because ions move freely across the capillary wall, the $[Na^+]$ (and osmolality) of the plasma and interstitial fluid will be the same. Therefore, water movement across the capillary endothelium will not be affected.

4. The increase in venous pressure causes increased movement of fluid out of the capillary. As a result, fluid accumulates in the interstitial space. Some of this fluid will be taken up by the lymphatics, and lymphatic flow will increase. However, when

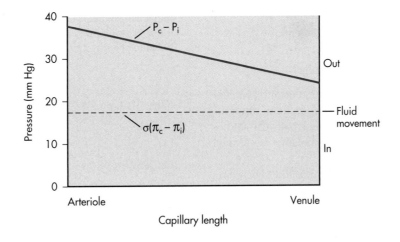

the capacity of the lymphatics to remove this fluid is exceeded, the volume of the interstitial space increases, and edema forms (see also Chapter 6).

5. This is an isotonic solution and will therefore remain confined initially to the ECF. The ECF volume will increase by 1 L, and ICF volume will be unchanged (initial volumes being 10 L [ECF] and 20 L [ICF], respectively). Plasma [Na$^+$] will decrease because of the addition of 1 L of Na$^+$-free solution to the ECF. The new plasma [Na$^+$] is calculated by:

Initial ECF Na$^+$ content = 145 mEq/L × 10 L
                            = 1450 mEq
New [Na$^+$]   = 1450 mEq/11 L
                            = 132 mEq/L

Therefore the immediate effect is:

ECF volume: _11_   L
ICF volume: _20_   L
Plasma [Na$^+$]:   _132_   mEq/L

In the long term, the dextrose will be metabolized to CO_2 and H_2O. Thus, infusion of a dextrose solution is equivalent to infusion of solute-free water. After metabolism and equilibration over several hours, the 1 L of infused fluid will distribute into both the ICF and ECF in proportion to the ratio of their volumes (two thirds into the ICF and one third into the ECF).

ICF volume   = 20 L + 0.67 L = 20.67 L
ECF volume   = 10 L + 0.3 L = 10.3 L
New [Na$^+$]   = 1,450 mEq/10.3 L = 141 mEq/L

Therefore the long-term effect is:

ECF volume: _10.3_   L
ICF volume: _20.7_   L
Plasma [Na$^+$]:   _141_   mEq/L

As noted previously, a dextrose solution is equivalent to solute-free water. Therefore, these solutions would be used when the patient had lost solute-free water and body fluid osmolality is elevated (i.e., hypernatremia).

6. A 0.9% NaCl solution is isotonic saline. Therefore, the entire infused volume will remain in the ECF. In this example, the ECF will increase by 1 L and the ICF will not change. One approach to this problem is to calculate the amount of Na$^+$ in the infused volume and then determine the effect on the plasma [Na$^+$]. For example:

0.9% NaCl   = 154 mEq/L
Amount of infused Na$^+$ = 1 L × 154 mEq/L
                         = 154 mEq
New ECF Na$^+$ content   = 1450 mEq + 154 mEq
                         = 1604 mEq
New plasma [Na$^+$]   = 1604 mEq/11 L
                         = 146 mEq/L

Therefore the immediate effect is:

ECF volume: _11_   L
ICF volume: _20_   L
Plasma [Na$^+$]:   _146_   mEq/L

The long-term effect of this infusion is identical to that seen immediately. Thus, the long-term effect is:

ECF volume: _11_   L
ICF volume: _20_   L
Plasma [Na$^+$]:   _146_   mEq/L

From this it is apparent that infusion of isotonic saline into an individual with a normal serum [Na$^+$] will result in an increase in the volume of the ECF, equal to the entire infused volume, with no appreciable change in the serum [Na$^+$].

7. The initial volumes of the body fluid compartments and the osmoles in these compartments are calculated as follows (osmolality is estimated as $2 \times [Na^+] = 280$ mOsm/kg H_2O):

Initial total body water   = 0.6(60 kg) = 36 L
Initial ICF volume   = 0.4(60 kg) = 24 L
Initial ECF volume   = 0.2(60 kg) = 12 L
Initial total body osmoles = (total body water)(body fluid osmolality)
                            = (36 L)(280 mOsm/kg H_2O)
                            = 10,080 mOsm
Initial ICF osmoles   = (ICF volume)(body fluid osmolality)
                            = (24 L)(280 mOsm/kg H_2O)
                            = 6720 mOsm
Initial ECF osmoles   = Total body osmoles − ICF osmoles
                            = 10,080 mOsm − 6720 mOsm
                            = 3360 mOsm

Four kilograms of body weight are lost. It is assumed that this entire weight reduction reflects fluids lost through vomiting and diarrhea. Thus, 4 L of fluid are lost. Because the plasma [Na$^+$] is unchanged, a proportional amount of solute was also lost (isotonic loss of fluid). No fluid shifts occur between the ECF and ICF because of the absence of an osmotic gradient between these compartments. Therefore, the ECF loses 4 L of volume, and $4 \times 280 = 1120$ mOsm of solute.

New total body water	= 36 L − 4 L = 32 L
New ICF volume	= 24 L (unchanged)
New ECF volume	= 12 L − 4 L = 8 L
New total body osmoles	= 10,080 mOsm − 1120 mOsm = 8960 mOsm
New ICF osmoles	= 6720 mOsm (unchanged)
New ECF osmoles	= 3360 mOsm − 1120 mOsm = 2240 mOsm

8. The initial volumes of the body fluid compartments and the osmoles in these compartments are calculated as in problem 7:

Initial total body water	= 0.6(50 kg) = 30 L
Initial ICF volume	= 0.4(50 kg) = 20 L
Initial ECF volume	= 0.2(50 kg) = 10 L
Initial total body osmoles	= (total body water) × (body fluid osmolality) = (30 L)(290 mOsm/kg H$_2$O) = 8700 mOsm
Initial ICF osmoles	= (ICF volume)(body fluid osmolality) = (20 L)(290 mOsm/kg H$_2$O) = 5800 mOsm
Initial ECF osmoles	= Total body osmoles − ICF osmoles = 8700 mOsm − 5800 mOsm = 2900 mOsm

The total amount of mannitol added to the ECF must be calculated to determine its effect on body fluids. At 5 g/kg, a total of 250 g was added to the ECF (1.374 moles of mannitol). Because mannitol is a single particle in solution, this adds 1374 mOsm to the ECF. The mannitol will raise ECF osmolality and result in the shift of fluid from the ICF into the ECF.

New total body water	= 30 L (unchanged)
New total body osmoles	= 8700 mOsm +1374 mOsm = 10,074 mOsm
New ICF osmoles	= 5800 mOsm (unchanged)
New ECF osmoles	= 2900 mOsm +1374 mOsm = 4274 mOsm
New plasma osmolality	= $\dfrac{\text{New total osmoles}}{\text{Total body water}}$ = $\dfrac{10,074 \text{ mOsm}}{30 \text{ L}}$ = 336 mOsm/kg H$_2$O
New ICF volume	= $\dfrac{\text{ICF osmoles}}{\text{New P}_{osm}}$ = $\dfrac{5800 \text{ mOsm}}{336 \text{ mOsm/kg H}_2\text{O}}$ = 17.3 L
New ECF volume	= total body water − ICF volume = 30 L − 17.3 L = 12.7 L

Because mannitol increases the osmolality of the ECF, 2.7 L of fluid shifts from the ICF into the ECF. To calculate the new plasma [Na$^+$], assume that the amount of Na$^+$ in the ECF is unchanged after mannitol infusion. Originally, there were 2900 mOsm attributable to Na$^+$ ($2 \times$ [Na$^+$] × ECF volume) in the ECF. Because the Na$^+$ osmoles are unchanged but are now present in a larger volume, the new plasma [Na$^+$] is calculated as follows:

New plasma Na$^+$ osmoles	= $\dfrac{2900 \text{ mOsm from Na}^+}{12.7 \text{ L}}$ = 228 mOsm/L
New plasma [Na$^+$]	= $\dfrac{\text{Na}^+ \text{ osmoles}}{2}$ = $\dfrac{228 \text{ mOsm/L}}{2}$ = 114 mEq/L

9. Both individuals start out with the same total body water (36 L) and total body osmoles (10,440 mOsm) assuming a plasma [Na$^+$] of 145 mEq/L and a plasma osmolality of 290 mOsm/kg H$_2$O. Subject A loses 1 L of total body water and 1000 osmoles of

total body solute, resulting in a new plasma osmolality of

$$P_{osm} = (10,440 \text{ mOsm} - 1000 \text{ mOsm})/35 \text{ L}$$
$$= 270 \text{ mOsm/kg } H_2O$$

Subject B loses 4 L of total body water and 1600 mOsm of total body osmoles, resulting in a new plasma osmolality of

$$P_{osm} = (10,440 \text{ mOsm} - 1600 \text{ mOsm})/32 \text{ L}$$
$$= 276 \text{ mOsm/kg } H_2O$$

CHAPTER 2

1. The gross anatomic features of the kidney include the cortex, medulla, nephrons, blood vessels, lymphatics, nerves, renal pyramids, papilla, minor calyx, major calyces, and pelvis.
2. The nephron consists of a renal corpuscle, proximal tubule, loop of Henle, distal tubule, and collecting duct system.
3. The renal artery branches progressively to form the interlobar artery, the arcuate artery, the interlobular artery, and the afferent arteriole, which leads into the glomerular capillaries (i.e., glomerulus). The glomerular capillaries come together to form the efferent arteriole, which leads into a second capillary network, the peritubular capillaries, which supply blood to the nephron. The vessels of the venous system run parallel to the arterial vessels and progressively form the interlobular vein, arcuate vein, interlobar vein, and renal vein, which courses beside the ureter.
4. The renal corpuscle is the first part of the nephron and is composed of glomerular capillaries and Bowman's capsule.
5. The glomerular capillaries have a fenestrated endothelium that prevents the filtration of cells. The capillaries are surrounded by a basement membrane composed of three layers: lamina rara interna, lamina densa, and lamina rara externa. The basement membrane is an important filtration barrier to plasma proteins. Filtration slits of the podocytes, which encircle the glomerular capillaries, are also a filtration barrier for proteins. Proteins are filtered on the basis of size and charge.

6. Structures that compose the juxtaglomerular apparatus include the macula densa of the thick ascending limb, extraglomerular mesangial cells, and the renin-producing granular cells of the afferent arterioles.
7. The juxtaglomerular apparatus is one component of a feedback mechanism (i.e., tubuloglomerular feedback) that regulates renal blood flow and glomerular filtration rate. It also regulates renin secretion by the granular cells of the afferent arteriole.
8. The mesangium consists of mesangial cells and the mesangial matrix. Mesangial cells, which possess many properties of smooth muscles cells, surround the glomerular capillaries, provide structural support for the glomerular capillaries, secrete the extracellular matrix, exhibit phagocytic activity that removes macromolecules from the mesangium, and secrete prostaglandins and proinflammatory cytokines. Because they also contract and are adjacent to glomerular capillaries, mesangial cells may influence the GFR by regulating blood flow through the glomerular capillaries or by altering the capillary surface area. Mesangial cells located outside the glomerulus (between the afferent and efferent arterioles) are called extraglomerular mesangial cells.
9. Renal nerves regulate renal blood flow, glomerular filtration rate, and salt and water reabsorption by the nephron. The nerve supply to the kidneys consists of sympathetic nerve fibers that originate in the celiac plexus. There is no parasympathetic innervation. Adrenergic fibers that innervate the kidneys release norepinephrine and dopamine. The adrenergic fibers lie adjacent to the smooth muscle cells of the major branches of the renal artery (interlobar, arcuate, and interlobular arteries) and the afferent and efferent arterioles. Moreover, sympathetic nerves innervate the renin-producing granular cells of the afferent arterioles. Renin secretion is stimulated by increased sympathetic activity. Nerve fibers also innervate the proximal tubule, loop of Henle, distal tubule, and collecting duct; activation of these nerves enhances Na^+ reabsorption by these nephron segments.

CHAPTER 3

1. Before phlorhizin administration
   Serum [inulin]:   1 mg/ml
   Serum [glucose]:   1 mg/ml
   Inulin excretion rate: 100 mg/min
   Glucose excretion rate: 0 mg/min
   Inulin clearance: 100 ml/min
   Glucose clearance: 0 ml/min

   After phlorhizin administration
   Serum [inulin]:   1 mg/ml
   Serum [glucose]:   1 mg/ml
   Inulin excretion rate: 100 mg/min
   Glucose excretion rate: 100 mg/min
   Inulin clearance: 100 ml/min
   Glucose clearance: 100 ml/min

   Before treatment with phlorhizin, the filtered load of glucose (GFR [glucose]) is 100 mg/min (GFR calculated from inulin clearance). With this filtered load of glucose, all the glucose is reabsorbed and none is excreted. Thus, the clearance of glucose is zero. After phlorhizin the filtered load is unchanged, but there is no glucose reabsorption. Therefore, all the glucose that is filtered is excreted, and the clearance of glucose equals that of inulin.

2. a. Although the appearance of red cells in the urine can result from damage to the glomerular filtration barrier, red cells can also appear in the urine for other reasons. For example, they can appear as a result of bleeding in any part of the lower urinary tract. Such bleeding is seen with kidney stones and occasionally as a result of a bacterial infection of the lower urinary tract, which causes bleeding. Thus, the appearance of blood in the urine does not necessarily mean the glomerular filtration barrier is damaged.
   b. Because glucose is filtered and completely reabsorbed by the proximal tubule, it is not normally found in the urine. Its presence in the urine indicates an elevated plasma glucose level such that the filtered load (i.e., GFR × plasma [glucose]) is greater than the ability of the proximal tubule to reabsorb glucose. Because glucose is freely filtered by the normal glomerulus, damage to the ultrafiltration barrier would not increase its filtration.
   c. In healthy individuals, Na^+ normally appears in the urine. Like glucose, Na^+ is freely filtered by the normal glomerulus. Therefore, damage to the filtration barrier does not increase the rate of Na^+ excretion.
   d. This is the correct answer. Normally, the urine contains essentially no protein. The glomerulus prevents the filtration of plasma proteins. However, when the glomerulus is damaged, large amounts of plasma proteins are filtered. If the amount filtered overwhelms the reabsorptive capacity of the proximal tubule, protein appears in the urine (proteinuria).

3. The equation for blood flow through an organ is $Q = \Delta P/R$. Sympathetic agonists, angiotensin II, and prostaglandins change blood flow by altering the resistance (R). Whereas sympathetic agonists and angiotensin II increase R and thereby decrease renal blood flow (RBF), prostaglandins decrease R and thereby increase RBF.

4. Normally, renal prostaglandin production is low, and nonsteroidal anti-inflammatory drugs (NSAIDs) do not have an appreciable effect on prostaglandin production. However, during reductions in GFR and RBF, elevated prostaglandin levels cause vasodilation of the afferent and efferent arterioles. This effect prevents excessive decreases in RBF and GFR. Administration of NSAIDs to patients with low GFR and RBF inhibits prostaglandin production and further reduces GFR and RBF.

CHAPTER 4

1. The glomeruli filter 25,200 mEq of Na^+ and 18,000 mEq of Cl^- each day (assuming GFR = 180 L/day), and more than 99% is reabsorbed by the nephrons, with less than 1% appearing in the urine. Although Na^+ and Cl^- uptake into cells across the apical membrane and NaCl reabsorption across the paracellular pathway are passive processes (i.e., they do not require the direct input of adenosine triphosphate [ATP]), they ultimately depend on the operation of the Na^+,K^+-ATPase. Accordingly, reabsorption of NaCl requires a considerable quantity of ATP, the synthesis of which by kidney cells requires large amounts of oxygen and, hence, high blood flow.

TABLE D-1			
Urine Flow Rate			
	0.5 L/DAY	1 L/DAY	2 L/DAY
Na^+, mEq/L	300	150	75
K^+, mEq/L	200	100	50
Cl^-, mEq/L	300	150	75
HCO_3^-, mEq/L	≈4	≈2	≈1
Ca^{++}, mg/dl	40	20	10
NH_4^+, mEq/L	100	50	25
Creatinine, mg/L	2,000	1,000	500
Glucose, mmol/L	1.0	0.5	0.25
Urea, mmol/L	600	300	150
Urea, mg/L	14,000	7,000	3,500
pH	5.0	to	7.0
Osmolality, mOsm/kg H_2O	1,600	800	400

TABLE D-2	
SOLUTE	SOLUTE EXCRETION/DAY
Na^+, mEq	150
K^+, mEq	100
Cl^-, mEq	150
HCO_3^-, mEq	≈2
Ca^{++}, mg	200
NH_4^+, mEq	50
Creatinine, mg	1000
Glucose, mmol	0.5
Urea, mmol	300
Urea, mg/L	7000
Osmolytes, mOsm	800

Modified from Valtin HV: *Renal function*, ed 2, Boston, 1983, Little, Brown. Lab values from DMS, 1989.

2. "Normal" or "average" urine composition does not actually exist because of the variability in the volume excreted, as well as variations in the intake of solutes in the diet. Consider Table D-1. Urine was collected on three different days from a subject who ate a consistent diet but ingested different amounts of water each day. Although the amount of each solute excreted was similar each day (Table D-2), the concentration of each solute in the urine was different because the volume of urine varied each day. This question demonstrates that the amount (or rate) of a solute excreted, not the concentration of the solute in the urine, is important in the clinical evaluation of urine.

3. Passive transport always occurs down an electrochemical gradient. Diffusion of a gas (e.g., O_2) through the lipid portion of the plasma membrane occurs passively. For coupled transporters (antiport and symport), the movement of one molecule down its electrochemical gradient can drive uphill movement of the coupled molecule. When this occurs, the uphill movement is termed secondary active transport because the transporter is not coupled directly to the hydrolysis of ATP. Active transport occurs against an electrochemical gradient and requires the direct input of energy (i.e., ATP). Some authors refer to such transport as primary active to emphasize the direct coupling to ATP.

4. Because the Na^+,K^+-ATPase is ultimately responsible for the reabsorption and secretion of all solutes (except H^+) and water by the nephron, complete inhibition of this transport protein would block all solute and water transport (both cellular and paracellular). Hence, in this hypothetical example, each day the kidneys would excrete 180 L of fluid (assuming GFR = 180 L/day) that would be similar in composition to the glomerular ultrafiltrate.

5. In the first phase of proximal reabsorption, Na^+ enters the cell across the apical membrane by several symport and antiport mechanisms (e.g., Na^+-glucose symporter, Na^+–amino acid symporter, and Na^+-H^+ antiporter). Na^+ exits from the cell into the blood through the Na^+,K^+-ATPase. Therefore, Na^+ is reabsorbed across the cell with glucose, amino acids, and HCO_3^-. When tubular fluid reaches the second half of the proximal tubule, the concentrations of glucose, amino acids, and HCO_3^- are greatly reduced. As a result, the tubular fluid at this point is primarily NaCl. In the second phase of proximal tubule reabsorption, NaCl uptake across the apical membrane occurs by the parallel operation of Na^+-H^+ and Cl^--anion antiporters. Na^+ efflux from the cell occurs through the Na^+,K^+-ATPase, and Cl^- exits through the K^+-Cl^- symporter. Paracellular NaCl reabsorption also occurs. Paracellular Cl^- reabsorption, in the second half of the proximal tubule, is driven by the Cl^- concentration gradient across the proximal tubule, which develops because relatively less Cl^- is reabsorbed in the first half of the proximal tubule compared with Na^+ (i.e., Na^+ is

reabsorbed with other solutes). Because the amount of water reabsorbed is proportionally more than the amount of Cl^- reabsorbed in the first half of the proximal tubule, the $[Cl^-]$ in tubular fluid increases, which provides the driving force for Cl^- diffusion across the tight junctions. Cl^- diffusion also renders the transepithelial voltage lumen positive, which in turn provides the driving force for the passive, paracellular diffusion of Na^+. The transport of solutes (NaCl) across the cellular and paracellular pathways lowers the osmolality of the tubular fluid and increases the osmolality of the interstitial fluid, which establishes a driving force for water reabsorption across the proximal tubule. Some solutes are reabsorbed with this water by the process of solvent drag. Starling forces across the wall of the peritubular capillary are important for the uptake of this interstitial fluid and can regulate the rate of solute and water back-flux across the tight junctions and thereby modulate net solute and water reabsorption.

6. NaCl is reabsorbed across the thick ascending limb by two mechanisms. First, transcellular transport involves Na^+ and Cl^- entry into the cell across the apical membrane by the $1Na^+$-$1K^+$-$2Cl^-$ symporter (some Na^+ is also reabsorbed by the apical membrane Na^+-H^+ antiporter) and exit across the basolateral membrane by the Na^+,K^+-ATPase (for Na^+) and a K^+-Cl^- symporter and Cl^- channel (for Cl^-, mechanism not shown in Figure 4-8). Second, Na^+ is also reabsorbed across the paracellular pathway, owing to the lumen-positive transepithelial voltage. Furosemide would have no effect on water reabsorption in the thick ascending limb because this segment of the nephron is relatively impermeable to water and water is not reabsorbed even when NaCl reabsorptive rates are high. Furosemide increases water excretion by reducing the osmolality of the medullary interstitial fluid, which in turn reduces water reabsorption from the descending thin limb of Henle's loop.

7. Glomerulotubular balance describes the phenomenon whereby an increase in the filtered load of water and NaCl is accompanied by a parallel increase in water and NaCl reabsorption by the proximal tubule. If a constant amount of NaCl and water was reabsorbed by the proximal tubule, increases in GFR and the filtered load of NaCl and water would result in an increased delivery to more distal segments. If these segments were not able to reabsorb the excess NaCl and water, large amounts could be lost in the urine. If such an increase in excretion were not accompanied by a corresponding rise in dietary intake, the organism would develop negative NaCl and water balance. Hence, glomerulotubular balance helps maintain NaCl and water homeostasis despite changes in GFR and the filtered load of water and NaCl.

8. See Table 4-6.

CHAPTER 5

1. This problem illustrates the importance of effective versus ineffective osmoles in regulating ADH secretion. Although plasma osmolality is elevated, the increased osmolality is due to urea. Because urea is an ineffective osmole with regard to ADH secretion, it is necessary to estimate the osmolality of plasma that is due to effective osmoles (Na^+ and its anions). The effective osmolality of the plasma is estimated by doubling the plasma $[Na^+]$, which yields a value of 270 mOsm/kg H_2O (see Chapter 1). Because the effective osmolality is reduced, ADH secretion is suppressed and plasma levels are reduced.

2. Osmolality of tubular fluid

Nephron Site	0-ADH	Max. ADH
Proximal tubule	300	300
Beginning of descending thin limb	300	300
Beginning of ascending thin limb	1200	1200
End of thick ascending limb	≈150	≈150
End of cortical collecting duct	<100	300
Urine	≈50	1200

Regardless of the presence or absence of ADH, tubular fluid osmolality is the same in all segments except the late portion of the distal tubule and collecting duct. When ADH is present, the tubular fluid within the lumen of these segments comes to osmotic equilibrium with the surrounding interstitial fluid (300 mOsm/kg H_2O in the cortex and 1200 mOsm/kg H_2O at the papilla). In the absence of ADH, solute reabsorption by these segments leads to further dilution of the tubular fluid.

3. a. *Decreased renal perfusion*: With a decrease in renal perfusion, as would occur with contraction of the extracellular fluid volume, delivery of solute and water to Henle's loop is reduced (GFR is decreased, and therefore filtered load is decreased and proximal tubule fractional reabsorption is enhanced [see Chapter 6]). As a result, there will be less separation of solute and water and a reduction in T^c_{H2O}. Urine osmolality will be maximal, but the total volume of solute-free water reabsorbed by the nephron (i.e., T^c_{H2O}) will be reduced.

   b. *Inhibition of thick ascending limb transport*: Inhibition of thick ascending limb NaCl transport decreases the separation of solute and water that occurs at this site. Because transport by the thick ascending limb is necessary for the generation of the medullary interstitial osmotic gradient, the osmolality of the interstitium falls. This impairs the reabsorption of water from the medullary collecting duct. As a result, T^c_{H2O} is reduced. The urine osmolality will approach 300 mOsm/kg H_2O, reflecting the fact that fluid entering Henle's loop from the proximal tubule has an osmolality of this value, and separation of solute and water is impaired.

   c. *Nephrogenic diabetes insipidus*: In nephrogenic diabetes insipidus, the collecting duct does not respond to ADH. As a result, water cannot be absorbed. This impairs the ability of the kidneys to concentrate the urine and reabsorb solute-free water (T^c_{H2O}). Dilute urine will be excreted.

   d. *Defect in the urea transporter in the vasa recta*: The urea transporter in the vasa recta (UT-B) helps to trap urea in the inner medulla by the process of countercurrent exchange. In the absence of this transporter, trapping of urea is impaired. As a result, the osmolality of the inner medullary interstitium is reduced and the urine cannot be maximally concentrated.

4. If daily solute excretion is 800 mOsm and the individual can produce concentrated urine that has an osmolality of only 400 mOsm/kg H_2O, the minimum volume of urine required for this solute excretion is:

$$\frac{800\,mOsm}{400\,mOsm/kg\,H_2O} = 2\,L$$

If insensible loss is 1 L, this individual must drink at least 3 L of water (or other dilute beverage) in that 24-hour period to prevent the development of hyperosmolality. This is slightly more than the average daily intake of most individuals. For the second individual, the daily water requirement is much less because of the ability to excrete a more concentrated urine. Minimum urine volume required in this individual:

$$\frac{800\,mOsm}{1200\,mOsm/kg\,H_2O} = 0.67\,L$$

With insensible loss of 1 L, daily water intake could be less than 2 L, and body fluid osmolality would be maintained. A corollary to these examples is that solute excretion also places constraints on the maximum volume of water that can be ingested. For example, if an individual who can dilute urine to 100 mOsm/kg H_2O excretes 800 mOsm of solute, this person could drink as much as 8 L of water without reducing body fluid osmolality. If, however, the individual excretes more solute (e.g., 1200 mOsm), 12 L of water could be ingested. Indeed, a decline in body fluid osmolality can be seen in individuals who drink large quantities of water without sufficient solute intake.

5. Osmolar clearance and free-water clearance are calculated as:

$$C_{osm} = \frac{200\,mOsm/kg\,H_2O \times 6\,L/day}{280\,mOsm/kg\,H_2O} = 4.3\,L$$

and

$$C_{H_2O} = 6\,L/day - 4.3\,L/day = 1.7\,L/day$$

CHAPTER 6

1. It is assumed that the 3-kg weight loss reflects only the loss of ECF. Because the plasma [Na^+] is unchanged, this represents a loss of isotonic fluid (3 L) from the ECF.

   Plasma osmolality: Because the plasma [Na^+] is unchanged, the plasma osmolality is unchanged.

   ECF volume: The ECF volume has been decreased by 3 L.

Effective circulating volume (ECV): The loss of fluid from the ECF will be detected by the vascular volume sensors as a decrease in the ECV.

Plasma ADH levels: The vascular volume sensors will detect the decreased ECV and cause increased ADH secretion (see Chapter 5).

Urine osmolality: The increased levels of ADH lead to water conservation by the kidneys and excretion of a concentrated urine (see Chapter 5).

Sensation of thirst: Again, the detection of a decrease in ECV by the vascular volume sensors leads to an enhanced sensation of thirst. The elevated levels of angiotensin II, which would also exist in this situation, will also stimulate the thirst center in the hypothalamus (see Chapter 5).

2. The individual is euvolemic. To maintain Na$^+$ balance, the amount of Na$^+$ ingested in the diet must equal the amount excreted from the body. Because the kidneys are the primary route for Na$^+$ excretion, the amount of Na$^+$ excreted daily is very nearly equal to the amount ingested in the diet (small amounts of Na$^+$ are lost in perspiration and feces). Therefore, the Na$^+$ excretion rate in this individual is approximately 100 mEq/day.

3.

	Volume Expansion	Volume Contraction
Renal sympathetic nerve activity	Decreased	Increased
ANP and BNP levels	Increased	Decreased
Angiotensin II levels	Decreased	Increased
Aldosterone levels	Decreased	Increased
Vasopressin levels	Decreased	Increased

4. Volume of accumulated edema fluid   4 L
   Amount of Na$^+$ retained by the kidneys   580 mEq

The man has gained 4 kg. This represents an increase in the volume of his ECF of 4 L of fluid (1 kg = 1 L). A portion of this will accumulate in the interstitial fluid compartment as edema because of the altered Starling forces across his capillary walls. The composition of this fluid is the same as that of serum and therefore has an [Na$^+$] of 145 mEq/L. Because the accumulation of the fluid requires NaCl and water retention by the kidneys, the amount of Na$^+$ retained by the kidneys must be equal to the amount contained in 4 L of fluid having an [Na$^+$] of 145 mEq/L or 580 mEq of Na$^+$.

5. Aldosterone stimulates Na$^+$ reabsorption primarily in the distal tubule and collecting duct, which explains the reduction in Na$^+$ excretion seen during the beginning of aldosterone treatment. As a result of the positive Na$^+$ balance, the ECF volume is increased. This in turn increases the GFR (i.e., increases the filtered load of Na$^+$), reduces proximal tubule reabsorption, and thereby enhances delivery of Na$^+$ to the distal tubule and collecting duct. In addition, natriuretic peptides (ANP and BNP) and urodilatin levels are increased, and their action on the collecting duct to inhibit Na$^+$ reabsorption, together with increased Na$^+$ delivery to this site, results in the return of Na$^+$ excretion to its previous level. A new steady state is reached (Na$^+$ intake = Na$^+$ excretion) but at an expanded ECF volume. Body weight is increased, reflecting the increased ECF volume. With cessation of aldosterone treatment, the Na$^+$ reabsorptive rate of the distal tubule and collecting duct decreases. Because of the increased ECF volume and, therefore, enhanced Na$^+$ delivery to the distal tubule, the reabsorptive capacity of the distal tubule and collecting duct is overwhelmed, and Na$^+$ excretion increases. After a period of negative Na$^+$ balance, the ECF volume decreases back to normal. A new steady state is reached (Na$^+$ intake = Na$^+$ excretion), and the body weight returns to its original value as the ECF volume decreases.

6. *ECF volume*: With decreased cardiac performance there is NaCl and water retention (see Figure 6-6). This will increase ECF volume, blood volume, and interstitial fluid volume. The increased interstitial fluid volume is manifested as edema.

ECV: Because of the poor cardiac performance (decreased blood pressure and cardiac output), the vascular volume receptors, especially those in the high-pressure side of the circulation, will detect a decreased ECV.

Plasma osmolality: Because the plasma [Na$^+$] is unchanged, the plasma osmolality is unchanged.

Fractional Na$^+$ excretion: Because the ECV is decreased, renal sympathetic nerve activity is increased, and the renin-angiotensin-aldosterone system is activated. This results in a decrease in the filtered load of Na$^+$ and also an increase in the reabsorption of Na$^+$ by the nephron. This increase in Na$^+$ reabsorption eliminates almost all the

Na⁺ from the urine. Therefore, the fractional Na⁺ excretion decreases.

Renal sympathetic nerve activity: The vascular volume sensors will detect the decreased ECV and increase the activity of the sympathetic fibers innervating the kidney.

ANP and BNP levels: Because of the increased blood and venous volumes, the heart will be dilated. This will stimulate ANP and BNP secretion, and their levels in the blood will be increased.

Angiotensin II levels: The vascular volume sensors will detect the decreased ECV and activate the renin-angiotensin-aldosterone system.

Aldosterone levels: The vascular volume sensors will detect the decreased ECV and activate the renin-angiotensin-aldosterone system.

Plasma ADH levels: The vascular volume sensors will detect the decreased ECV and cause increased ADH secretion (see Chapter 5).

CHAPTER 7

1. Intravenous infusion of K⁺ into a subject with a combination of sympathetic blockade (i.e., no catecholamine release) and insulin deficiency would result in significant hyperkalemia compared with a similar infusion of K⁺ in a normal subject. Although aldosterone secretion would be stimulated by the hyperkalemia, this hormone stimulates cell K⁺ uptake after a 1-hour lag period. In the first hour following K⁺ infusion, less than 50% of the infused K⁺ is excreted by the kidneys, and because sympathetic activity and insulin release are suppressed, most of the K⁺ remaining in the body is retained in the ECF.

2. Aldosterone deficiency would initially reduce urinary potassium excretion, and K⁺ would be retained in the body (i.e., dietary intake would exceed excretion). This would lead to hyperkalemia, which is a potent stimulus of K⁺ excretion. Because the individual is initially in positive K⁺ balance, plasma K⁺ rises until urinary K⁺ excretion becomes equal to dietary K⁺ intake. In the new steady state, K⁺ intake would equal K⁺ excretion; however, the subject has hyperkalemia. Thus, it is possible to match dietary K⁺ intake with excretion in the absence of aldosterone, although this occurs at an elevated plasma [K⁺].

3. In the first hour after a meal, the rise in plasma [K⁺] is blunted by the rapid (minutes) uptake of K⁺ into skeletal muscle, liver, bone, and red blood cells. Some K⁺ is excreted by the kidneys, but in the first hour after the meal, most K⁺ is sequestered in the intracellular fluid. In the ensuing hours, K⁺ slowly leaves the cells and is excreted by the kidneys, thereby maintaining K⁺ balance and plasma [K⁺].

4. Normally, K⁺ excretion is determined primarily by the rate of K⁺ secretion by the distal tubule and collecting duct and is largely independent of the GFR and the filtered load of K⁺. When 50% of the nephrons are lost, the distal tubules and collecting ducts in the remaining functioning nephrons secrete more K⁺ so that K⁺ excretion and plasma [K⁺] are maintained at normal levels. However, if 80% to 85% of the nephrons are lost and GFR falls below 15% to 20% of normal, K⁺ secretion by the distal tubule and collecting duct cannot increase enough to maintain constant urinary K⁺ excretion, and hyperkalemia ensues.

CHAPTER 8

1. If urinary buffers were not available, the 70 mEq of acid needed to be excreted by the kidneys to maintain acid-base balance (net acid excretion = nonvolatile acid production) would have to be excreted as free H⁺. If the minimum urine pH equals 4.0, this represents only 0.1 mEq/L of H⁺. Thus, for 70 mEq of H⁺ to be excreted, the daily urine output would need to be:

$$\frac{70 \text{ mEq/day}}{0.1 \text{ mEq/L}} = 700 \text{ L/day}$$

This exceeds the daily GFR (180 L/day). Thus, the urinary buffers are essential for the kidneys' ability to excrete sufficient quantities of H⁺ and maintain acid-base balance.

2.

pH	[HCO3-] (mEq/L)	Pco₂ mm Hg	Disorder
7.23	10	25	Metabolic acidosis
7.46	30	44	Metabolic alkalosis
7.37	28	50	Chronic respiratory acidosis
7.66	22	20	Acute respiratory alkalosis
7.34	26	50	Acute respiratory acidosis
7.54	18	22	Chronic respiratory alkalosis

3. The initial set of laboratory data indicates the presence of a metabolic alkalosis with appropriate respiratory compensation. Given the individual's history, the most likely cause of this simple acid-base disorder is the loss of gastric acid by vomiting. The second set of laboratory data continues to show the presence of metabolic alkalosis with respiratory compensation. In addition, there is evidence of fluid loss (decrease in body weight by 2 kg) and a resultant decrease in ECF volume (decrease in blood pressure). Given the worsening of this individual's metabolic alkalosis, it is somewhat surprising that the urine pH is so acidic. The appropriate renal response should be an increase in HCO_3^- excretion (i.e., decreased net acid excretion) to correct the alkalosis. However, the kidneys' response to the ECF volume contraction prevents this from occurring (see Chapter 6). Thus, the filtered load of HCO_3^- is decreased because of a reduction in GFR, and proximal tubule HCO_3^- reabsorption is enhanced because of the need to conserve Na^+ (i.e., H^+ secretion is stimulated because of the increased activity of the Na^+-H^+ antiporter). In addition, the ECF volume contraction stimulates aldosterone secretion, which increases H^+ secretion by the intercalated cells of the distal tubule and collecting duct. Therefore, the urine is more acidic than expected for the degree of alkalosis. The ECF volume must be restored to its normal value to correct this situation. Infusion of isotonic NaCl would accomplish this and also allow the kidneys to excrete the excess HCO_3^-, thereby restoring acid-base balance.

4. Carbonic anhydrase plays an important role in the secretion of H^+ (reabsorption of HCO_3^-) by the cells of the proximal tubule, thick ascending limb of Henle's loop, and intercalated cells of the distal tubule and collecting duct. Inhibition of this enzyme would therefore inhibit the secretion of H^+ by these nephron segments. Because the proximal tubule reabsorbs the largest fraction of the filtered load of HCO_3^- (80%), the effect of carbonic anhydrase inhibitors at this site is quantitatively the most important. With decreased reabsorption, more HCO_3^- would be excreted in the urine, and urine pH would become alkaline. This loss of HCO_3^- from the body would result in the development of metabolic acidosis.

5. This man has a metabolic acidosis with respiratory compensation. The plasma anion gap is calculated from the serum concentrations of Na^+, Cl^- and HCO_3^-, and is:

Anion gap = $[Na^+] - ([Cl^-] + [HCO_3^-])$
13 mEq/L = 137 mEq/L − (111 mEq/L + 13 mEq/L)

Thus, this is a normal anion gap metabolic acidosis, which may be seen either in patients who lose alkali in the feces secondary to diarrhea or in patients with renal tubular acidosis. Because his urine is more alkaline than expected for someone with his degree of acidosis (a urine pH of at least 5.5 would be expected), it is most probable that he has renal tubular acidosis. This would predispose him to the formation of kidney stones. Because of his acidosis, he will lose Ca^{++} from his bones (bones serve as a buffer source with chronic acidosis). This Ca^{++} will be excreted by the kidneys. However, the alkaline urine pH leads to Ca^{++} precipitation and thus stone formation.

CHAPTER 9

1. Approximately two thirds of Ca^{++} reabsorption across the proximal tubule occurs by solvent drag, a process that depends on Na^+ reabsorption. Mannitol would inhibit Ca^{++} reabsorption by blocking solvent drag in the proximal tubule and thereby increase urinary Ca^{++} excretion.

2. Furosemide would inhibit the $1Na^+$-$1K^+$-$2Cl^-$ symporter and reduce the lumen-positive transepithelial voltage to 0. This, in turn, would inhibit passive Ca^{++} reabsorption by the paracellular pathway.

3. A rise in plasma [Pi] increases the amount of Pi filtered by the glomeruli. Because the amount of Pi normally filtered is equal to the reabsorptive capacity of the kidneys, an increase in the amount of Pi filtered will increase urinary Pi excretion and reduce plasma [Pi].

CHAPTER 10

1. Nephrogenic diabetes insipidus is a condition in which the late portion of the distal tubule and collecting duct does not respond to ADH. As a

result, water reabsorption is impaired and a large volume of dilute urine is excreted. Long-term administration of thiazide diuretics provides symptomatic relief by reducing the volume of urine excreted. This occurs by two mechanisms. First, the diuretic-induced natriuresis reduces the volume of the ECF. This in turn reduces the GFR and enhances proximal tubule reabsorption (see Chapter 6 for details). As a result, less fluid is delivered to Henle's loop and ultimately to the distal tubule and collecting duct, where water reabsorption is impaired. The net effect is that urine volume is decreased. Second, thiazide diuretics increase the abundance of aquaporin-2 in the principal cells of the late portion of the distal tubule and collecting duct (at least in the form of nephrogenic diabetes insipidus associated with Li^+ ingestion). The increased expression of aquaporin-2 would thus allow increased water reabsorption and thereby reduce urine output.

2. **a.** The long-term effect of diuretic therapy is a reduction in the volume of the ECF. With such a decrease, the blood volume and thus cardiac output are reduced. Because blood pressure is equal to cardiac output multiplied by the total peripheral vascular resistance, a decrease in cardiac output therefore reduces blood pressure (cardiovascular reflexes activate sympathetic outflow so as to increase peripheral vascular resistance and thereby try to maintain blood pressure). In addition, diuretics may cause some degree of vascular smooth muscle vasodilatation, although the mechanism by which this occurs is not fully understood. This vasodilation reduces total peripheral vascular resistance, thereby decreasing blood pressure.

   b. Hypokalemia is a side effect of all diuretics acting proximal to the K^+ secretory site (late portion of the distal tubule and the cortical collecting duct). The most common diuretics given for the treatment of hypertension are thiazides. However, the loop diuretics, osmotic diuretics, and carbonic anhydrase inhibitors can also lead to hypokalemia. By their action, tubular fluid flow rate to the K^+ secretory site is enhanced, which stimulates K^+ secretion. In addition, the diuretic-induced decrease in ECF volume leads to stimulation of aldosterone and ADH, both of which stimulate K^+ secretion by the late portion of the distal tubule and cortical collecting duct.

   c. Treatment of the hypokalemia could involve supplementation of the diet with foods containing high levels of K^+ or with KCl tablets. Alternatively, a K^+-sparing diuretic could be given in combination with the thiazide diuretic.

3. Thiazide diuretics are secreted into the lumen of the proximal tubule by the same organic anion transport system that secretes penicillin. Competitive inhibition of secretion of the thiazide could decrease the effective concentration of the diuretic in the tubular field. Because thiazides act from the lumen, a reduction in their concentration at this site could reduce their effectiveness.

4. **a.** To maintain Na^+ balance, both individuals will excrete approximately 100 mEq/day of Na^+. Normally the kidneys excrete 90%+ of the daily ingested Na^+ load. The remainder is lost in the feces and in sweat. When individuals are treated chronically with a diuretic, they do not exhibit a sustained natriuresis. This is the diuretic braking phenomenon. After a relatively short period of negative Na^+ balance (i.e., intake < excretion), they again come into steady-state balance (i.e., intake = excretion). The ability to reestablish steady-state balance results from the diuretic-induced decrease in ECF volume and increased expression of Na^+ transporters. The decrease in ECF volume results in a decrease in the GFR and increased proximal tubule reabsorption. This in turn delivers less Na^+ to the portions of the nephron where the diuretic is acting. In addition, increased expression of Na^+ transporters in the segments where the diuretics act, as well as in other nephron segments, contributes to this response. Together, these modifications in renal Na^+ handling allow a new steady state to be reached where once again Na^+ excretion equals Na^+ ingestion.

   b. Individual A was treated with a loop diuretic. With inhibition of NaCl reabsorption by the thick ascending limb, less NaCl is deposited in the medullary interstitium. As a result, the osmolality of the interstitium declines, and water reabsorption from the collecting duct in the presence of ADH is reduced. Thus, the loop diuretic inhibits the reabsorption of solute-free water. Individual B was treated with a thiazide diuretic, which, in contrast, inhibits NaCl reabsorption in the early distal tubule. Because this segment is located in the cortex of the kidney, medullary interstitial osmolality is not affected. Thus, when ADH is present, the urine can be concentrated. Thus, thiazide diuretics do not impair solute-free water reabsorption.

c. Individual A is treated with a loop diuretic. Because the thick ascending limb has the highest rate of solute reabsorption of all the water-impermeable segments of the nephron (i.e., thin ascending limb, thick ascending limb, and early distal tubule), inhibition of solute transport at this site will greatly impair the kidneys' ability to dilute the urine. As a result, the urine osmolality will approach that of plasma (300 mOsm/kg H_2O), which is the osmolality of the glomerular filtrate as well as that of the tubular fluid exiting the proximal tubule. Individual B is treated with a thiazide diuretic, which acts only on cortical nephron segments (early distal tubule). This will impair urine dilution, but not as significantly because the thick ascending limb is still intact.

CASE 1

1a. The ECF volume of this man is increased above normal. The presence of edema, distention of the neck veins, and rales (sounds related to fluid in the lungs) is evidence of this increased volume. Additional evidence could be obtained by measuring weight gain because accumulation of each liter of extracellular fluid would increase body weight by 1 kg.

1b. The ECV in this man would be decreased from normal. With damage to the myocardium, cardiac output and therefore tissue perfusion would be reduced. This decreased cardiac performance will be sensed by the vascular baroreceptors as a decrease in the ECV.

1c. As noted previously, the reduced cardiac performance would be sensed by the vascular baroreceptors in the body as a decreased ECV. This will activate the sympathetic nervous system and the renin-angiotensin-aldosterone system and stimulate ADH secretion. Because ANP and BNP are secreted from the cardiac myocytes by stretch and because the heart is dilated (expanded ECF and vascular volume), ANP and BNP secretion will be stimulated.

1d. The kidneys would be avidly retaining Na^+. With a decrease in ECV, vascular volume sensors, especially in the high-pressure (juxtaglomerular apparatus, aortic arch, and carotid sinus) side of the circulation, would be activated and signals sent to the kidneys to retain Na^+.

- Sympathetic nerves innervating the afferent and efferent arterioles of the glomeruli would cause vasoconstriction. The net result would be to reduce the GFR. This in turn would reduce the filtered load of Na^+.

- Sympathetic innervation of the proximal tubule, thick ascending limb of Henle's loop, and collecting duct will also increase Na^+ reabsorption at these sites. This response is mediated by α_1-adrenoceptors on the cells.

- Increased sympathetic nerve activity, together with decreased perfusion pressure at the afferent arteriole, will result in the secretion of renin. This activation of the renin-angiotensin-aldosterone system will further stimulate Na^+ reabsorption because angiotensin II increases both proximal and distal tubule Na^+ reabsorption, and aldosterone increases Na^+ reabsorption in the distal tubule and collecting duct. Angiotensin II acts directly on the cells of the proximal tubule to stimulate Na^+ reabsorption.

- With the decreased ECV, the GFR decreases and the filtration fraction increases. This in turn decreases the hydrostatic pressure and increases the oncotic pressure in the peritubular capillaries and thereby enhances overall reabsorption of fluid by the proximal tubule.

- With the increases in the ECF and vascular volumes, the heart dilates and ANP and BNP levels are elevated. However, the effect of these natriuretic peptides (inhibition of renin secretion and natriuresis) appears to be blunted by the effect of the other factors, all of which act to reduce Na$^+$ excretion. The net effect of these responses is retention of Na$^+$ by the kidneys. As a result of this Na$^+$ retention (positive Na$^+$ balance), the ECF volume will increase, leading to the formation of edema as seen in the physical examination of this man.

1e. The development of hyponatremia indicates that this man is in positive water balance. In this case the ingestion of water has exceeded the capacity of the kidneys to excrete solute-free water. There are several reasons why solute-free water excretion is impaired in this man.

- ADH secretion is stimulated because of the decreased ECV. As a consequence, the collecting duct reabsorbs solute-free water.

- The decreased ECV results in a reduction in the filtered load of solute (NaCl) and water and an increase in fractional reabsorption by the proximal tubule (see earlier). As a result, there is decreased delivery of solute and water to the thick ascending limb, the primary site where solute-free water is generated.

1f. Hypokalemia in this man is the result of increased renal K$^+$ excretion. The major reason for increased K$^+$ excretion is related to the elevated levels of aldosterone in this man (secondary to decreased ECV). Aldosterone then acts on the distal tubule and collecting duct to stimulate K$^+$ secretion. The enhanced secretion of K$^+$ by the distal tubule and cortical collecting duct will result in increased K$^+$ excretion and the development of hypokalemia. Because delivery of Na$^+$ to the collecting duct is reduced in this man (see earlier), the hypokalemia will be mild. It is likely that extrarenal factors will also contribute to the development of hypokalemia because aldosterone causes K$^+$ to move into cells.

1g. In order to get an appropriate response to a loop diuretic, there needs to be adequate delivery of NaCl to the loop of Henle. As outlined before, GFR is reduced in congestive heart failure, which reduces the filtered load of NaCl. In addition, proximal tubule reabsorption is enhanced. The net result is a significant reduction in the delivery of NaCl to the thick ascending limb and thus a blunted response to the diuretic.

1h. As noted, the diuretic is given to prevent NaCl retention by the kidneys and thus reduce his edema. The additional NaCl lost from the ECF by the action of the diuretic will further reduce his ECV. As a result, the sympathetic nervous system will be further activated, as will the renin-angiotensin-aldosterone system. ADH secretion will also be stimulated.

1i. Loop diuretics increase the excretion K$^+$ and thus can lead to the development of hypokalemia. Two important effects contribute to this response. First, the thick ascending limb of Henle's loop reabsorbs approximately 20% of the filtered load of K$^+$. Loop diuretics inhibit this process. K$^+$ is reabsorbed by the Na$^+$-2Cl$^-$-K$^+$ symporter in the apical membrane and by the paracellular pathway driven by the lumen-positive transepithelial voltage (inhibition of the symporter results in a reduction in the lumen-positive voltage). Second, the loop diuretic will cause increased delivery of Na$^+$ and fluid to the distal tubule and cortical collecting duct and thereby stimulate K$^+$ secretion. Because aldosterone levels are also elevated (secondary to decreased ECV), K$^+$ secretion is further stimulated. Together, these effects will enhance K$^+$ secretion and thus renal K$^+$ excretion, leading to a worsening of the hypokalemia.

1j. Creatinine is excreted from the body primarily by glomerular filtration (10% is excreted as a result of secretion by the proximal tubule). Therefore, the amount of creatinine excreted is determined primarily by its filtered load. With a reduction in the ECV, the glomerular filtration rate is reduced. The reduced filtration rate will decrease the filtered load of creatinine and thus its excretion. As a result, the serum [creatinine] will increase. With the added decrement in the ECV caused by the loop diuretic, the glomerular filtration rate will fall further and thereby cause the serum [creatinine] to increase even more.

CASE 2

2a. This woman's symptoms and the electrolyte disturbances are most characteristic of decreased levels of adrenal cortical steroids and especially the mineralocorticoid hormone aldosterone. This is a patient with Addison's disease. The presence of hyperpigmentation suggests that the primary problem is at the level of the adrenal gland (i.e., nonresponsive to ACTH). ACTH levels are elevated in response to the decreased circulating levels of adrenal cortical steroids. (ACTH is synthesized as preproopiomelanocortin, and when this molecule is processed to ACTH several of the cleavage products have melanocyte-stimulating properties). These cleavage products act on the epidermal melanocytes leading to the hyperpigmentation of the gums and skin.

2b. Normally, the kidneys would respond to the decreased ECF volume present in this woman by dramatically reducing the excretion of Na$^+$. The urine [Na$^+$] is unexpectedly high in this woman because of the inability of her kidneys to reabsorb Na$^+$ in the thick ascending limb, distal tubule, and collecting duct (the distal tubule and collecting duct are especially important). This "Na$^+$ wasting" is a result of the low levels of aldosterone. Although the angiotensin II levels would be elevated in this woman, her adrenal glands are not secreting aldosterone in response to the angiotensin II. The hypotension is a result of the negative Na$^+$ balance present in this woman, which in turn reflects the decreased circulating levels of aldosterone. Because of the negative Na$^+$ balance, ECF volume will be decreased. Because plasma is a component of the ECF, vascular volume and hence blood pressure will be decreased.

2c. Hyponatremia indicates a problem in water balance. Thus, the ability of this woman's kidneys to excrete solute-free water is impaired, and she is in positive water balance (solute-free water ingestion > solute-free water excretion). There are several reasons for the decreased ability of this woman's kidneys to excrete solute-free water. Because of her decreased ECF and vascular volumes, her vascular baroreceptors are activated. As a result, the sympathetic nervous system and the renin-angiotensin-aldosterone system are activated. Nonosmotic release of ADH also occurs because of a fall in the ECF volume. As a consequence of the elevated ADH levels, solute-free water is reabsorbed by the late portion of the distal tubule and collecting duct. In addition, the decreased ECF volume results in a decrease in the filtered load of solute (NaCl) and water and an increase in fractional reabsorption by the proximal tubule. As a result, there is decreased delivery of solute and water to the thick ascending limb, the primary site where solute-free water is generated.

2d. Urinary K$^+$ excretion is determined in large part by the amount of K$^+$ secreted into tubular fluid by the distal tubule and cortical collecting duct. K$^+$ secretion at these nephron sites is reduced by the low levels of plasma aldosterone in this woman. In addition, aldosterone causes the uptake of K$^+$ into cells (e.g., skeletal muscle). In the absence of aldosterone, there will be less cellular uptake. This will also contribute to the development of hyperkalemia.

2e. This woman has a metabolic acidosis as evidenced by her low serum [HCO$_3^-$]. This is a result of the inability of her kidneys to excrete sufficient net acid to balance the nonvolatile acids produced each day through metabolism. The defect in her kidneys is reduced H$^+$ secretion by the intercalated cells of the late portion of the distal tubule and the collecting duct. H$^+$ secretion by these cells is dependent on aldosterone. This is both a direct and indirect effect. Aldosterone directly stimulates the intercalated cells to secrete H$^+$. It is also responsible for stimulating Na$^+$ reabsorption by the principal cells in these segments. This reabsorption of Na$^+$ generates a lumen-negative transepithelial voltage that facilitates H$^+$ secretion by the intercalated cell. Therefore, in the absence of aldosterone, H$^+$ secretion is impaired. This will reduce HCO$_3^-$ reabsorption, the excretion of H$^+$ with urinary buffers, and the excretion of NH$_4^+$. Thus, net acid excretion is reduced.

CASE 3

3a. Na$^+$ excretion is determined by diet and ECF volume status. In a euvolemic individual, the amount of Na$^+$ excreted in the urine each day is approximately equal to the amount ingested in the diet. Because the man appears to be euvolemic, his daily Na^+ intake would be approximately 80 mEq/day. The hyponatremia in this man reflects a disorder of water balance. Specifically, the unregulated secretion of ADH prevents his kidneys from excreting solute-free water. As a result, his water intake exceeds the ability of his kidneys to excrete solute-free water and he is in positive water balance.

3b. Infusion of 1 L of isotonic saline will add 300 mOsm of NaCl (150 mmoles of NaCl = 300 mOsm) to his ECF together with 1 L of water. This will transiently increase the ECF volume and raise the plasma osmolality and $[Na^+]$. However, over time the entire amount of NaCl will be excreted because he is in steady-state Na^+ balance (excretion = intake). However, because of the inappropriate secretion of ADH, he will not be able to excrete the water. With a U_{osm} of 600 mOsm/kg H_2O, he will excrete the infused NaCl (300 mOsm) in 0.5 L of urine. Thus, 0.5 L of solute-free water will remain in the body, and the plasma $[Na^+]$ will decrease. For this man, the addition of 0.5 L of solute-free water to his body fluid will reduce the plasma $[Na^+]$ to 119 mEq/L.

Total body osmoles (unchanged) = 240 mOsm/L × 42 L
$$= 10,080 \text{ mOsm}$$

New total body water   = 42 L + 0.5 L = 42.5 L

New plasma osmolality $= \dfrac{10,080 \text{ mOsmoles}}{42.5 \text{ L}}$

$$= 237 \text{ mOsm/kg } H_2O$$

New plasma $[Na^+]$ $= \dfrac{237 \text{ mOsm/kg } H_2O}{2}$

$$= 119 \text{ mEq/L}$$

3c. A 3% saline solution contains 513 mmol/L of NaCl (MW = 58.5 g/mole), which is 1026 mOsm/L. Thus, 1 L of fluid and 1026 mOsm of solute are added to the body fluids. With the establishment of a new steady state, the infused NaCl will be excreted with 1.7 L of urine.

$$\frac{1,026 \text{ mOsmole}}{600 \text{ mOsm/kg } H_2O} = 1.7 \text{ L}$$

(U_{osm} = 600 mOsm/kg H_2O because of the unregulated secretion of ADH. Therefore, 1 L of infused water is excreted together with an additional

0.7 L of solute-free water. This will result in a new plasma $[Na^+]$ of 122 mEq/L.

Total body osmoles (unchanged) = 240 mOsm/L × 42 L
$$= 10,080 \text{ mOsm}$$

New total body water   = 42 L − 0.7 L = 41.3 L

New plasma osmolality $= \dfrac{10,080 \text{ mOsmoles}}{41.3 \text{ L}}$

$$= 244 \text{ mOsm/kg } H_2O$$

New plasma $[Na^+]$ $= \dfrac{244 \text{ mOsm/kg } H_2O}{2}$

$$= 122 \text{ mEq/L}$$

3d. The simplest treatment option would be to restrict his intake of fluids so that intake does not exceed the ability of his kidneys to excrete solute-free water (i.e., he should drink only in response to thirst). Another treatment option would be to block the effect of ADH on the collecting duct. Currently, ADH receptor antagonists (aquaretics) are available for this purpose.

CASE 4

4a. The acid-base disorder of this man is a metabolic acidosis. In the absence of insulin, the metabolism of fats and carbohydrates is altered such that nonvolatile acids (keto acids) are produced. The nonvolatile acids are rapidly buffered by cellular and extracellular buffers. Buffering in the extracellular fluid results in a decrease in the plasma $[HCO_3^-]$, which lowers the pH. The deep rapid breathing reflects the respiratory compensation (P_{CO_2} is lowered). The plasma anion gap is calculated using the following formula (normal value is 8 to 16 mEq/L):

Anion gap = $[Na^+] - ([Cl^-] + [HCO_3^-])$ or $130 - (95 + 7)$
$$= 28 \text{ mEq/L}$$

The plasma anion gap is elevated because of the presence of unmeasured anions; in this case the anions would be the keto acids such as acetoacetate and β-hydroxybutyrate.

4b. Despite the hyperkalemia in this man, he is probably K^+ depleted. The K^+ depletion is a result of K^+ shift out of the cells (see later) and enhanced K^+ excretion by the kidneys because of the glucose-induced osmotic diuresis (i.e., increased urinary flow rate increases K^+ secretion in the collecting duct). Hyperkalemia is a result of a shift of K^+ out of cells (e.g., skeletal muscle) into the extracellular fluid. This shift occurs because of the lack of insulin and the hypertonicity of the ECF secondary to the elevated [glucose]. The acidosis is probably not a major contributing factor to the development of hyperkalemia in this situation. When acidosis is induced by mineral acids (e.g., HCl), movement of H^+ into cells during the process of intracellular buffering results in a shift of K^+ out of the cells into the ECF. However, with organic acidosis, as occurs in this situation, the cellular buffering of the organic acids does not result in a significant shift of K^+ out of the cell. The polyuria is a result of an osmotic diuresis induced by glucose (also the keto acids). Normally, all of the filtered load of glucose is reabsorbed by the proximal tubule. However, in this man the filtered load of glucose exceeds the reabsorptive capacity of the proximal tubule. Consequently, the nonreabsorbed glucose will remain in the lumen of the proximal tubule, where it will act as an osmotically active particle. This will establish an osmotic gradient opposite to that generated by the NaCl reabsorptive processes. This glucose-induced osmotic diuresis will increase the delivery of NaCl and water to the distal tubule and cortical collecting duct, which stimulates K^+ secretion at these sites. As a result, K^+ excretion from the body will be increased. In addition, keto acids (anions) are excreted with a cation (Na^+ and K^+). Thus, some additional K^+ will be excreted because of the high excretion rate of the keto acids. Increased K^+ excretion together with the shift of K^+ from the ICF to the ECF noted previously (secondary to the insulin deficiency and hyperosmolality) will lead to progressive whole-body K^+ depletion. Accordingly, an increase in serum [K^+] is not always indicative of positive K^+ balance. This man is in negative K^+ balance and is at risk for the development of hypokalemia when insulin is administered and the metabolic abnormalities are corrected.

4c. The serum [K^+] fell for several reasons. Insulin causes K^+ to move into cells. The mechanism responsible for this effect of insulin is related to

stimulation of the Na^+,K^+-ATPase. With increased activity of the Na^+,K^+-ATPase, K^+ uptake into the cell is enhanced. In addition, insulin's effect on glucose metabolism will lower the serum [glucose]. As a consequence, the osmolality of the ECF will decrease and cause additional K^+ to move into cells. Finally, administration of fluids will reexpand the ECF and dilute the K^+ in this compartment. For all of these reasons, K^+ is usually administered during the course of treatment so as not to induce hypokalemia.

CASE 5

5a. This is a metabolic acidosis with a normal anion gap (anion gap = 13 mEq/L). The two most frequent causes of nonanion gap acidosis are defects in renal acid excretion (renal tubular acidosis) and loss of HCO_3^- from the body (e.g., diarrhea). In this case, the relatively alkaline urine pH in the presence of systemic acidosis suggests a defect in renal acid excretion. Normally, the urine should be maximally acidic with this degree of systemic acidosis. The most likely diagnosis is distal renal tubular acidosis (i.e., a defect in H^+ secretion or H^+ permeability of the distal tubule and collecting duct). The renal stone that brought this man to the physician is probably a calcium-containing stone because the solubility of calcium is reduced in alkaline urine. His filtered load of Ca^{++} is also elevated, reflecting the loss of Ca^{++} from his bones because of buffering of the acidosis.

5b. Normally, the kidneys respond to a metabolic acidosis by increasing net acid excretion. This typically occurs with a urine pH of less than 5.5. Thus, the urine pH of 6.4 indicates some defect in renal acid excretion. As noted, this is a case of distal renal tubular acidosis, where the defect is an inability of the distal nephron to acidify the urine maximally. Because of this defect, there is impaired HCO_3^- reabsorption, decreased excretion of titratable acid, and decreased excretion of NH_4^+. Therefore, net acid excretion is less than nonvolatile acid production, and metabolic acidosis (nonanion gap) develops.

5c. Urinary net charge should be negative under normal conditions, reflecting the excretion of

NH_4^+ in the urine. The positive value confirms the fact that the kidney is the cause of the acidosis because insufficient amounts of NH_4^+ are being excreted.

CASE 6

6a. This is a mixed acid-base disorder because the P_{CO_2} is elevated and the serum $[HCO_3^-]$ is decreased. There is a component related to respiratory acidosis caused by poor gas exchange in the lungs. In addition, her hypoxia (low P_{O_2}) has resulted in anaerobic metabolism by her tissues with the generation of lactic acid. Buffering of the lactic acid has resulted in a decrease in her serum $[HCO_3^-]$.

6b. This girl was given an injection of epinephrine by the paramedics in order to dilate her airways. Epinephrine is a β-selective agonist that not only acts to relax her constricted airways but also stimulates the Na^+,K^+-ATPase, causing enhanced K^+ uptake into cells (e.g., skeletal muscle).

REVIEW EXAMINATION

1. The daily excretion rate of total osmoles for an individual is 900 mOsm. If this individual has a urine-concentrating defect and can produce urine having a maximum osmolality of only 300 mOsm/kg H$_2$O, what is the minimum volume of water that must be ingested in order to prevent a rise in the osmolality of the body fluids? (Assume that insensible water loss is 1.5 L/day.)
   a. 1.5 L/day
   b. 3.0 L/day
   c. 4.5 L/day
   d. 6.0 L/day
   e. 7.5 L/day

   $U_{oSM} = 300$
   $E = 0 \cdot V$
   $V = 3 \, kg \, H_2O$
   $ +1.5$
   $ \overline{4.5}$

2. Three individuals, each weighing 55 kg and each having a plasma [Na$^+$] of 145 mEq/L, are infused with different solutions. Individual A is infused with 1 L of isotonic NaCl (290 mOsm/kg H$_2$O), individual B is infused with 1 L of a mannitol solution (290 mOsm/kg H$_2$O), and individual C is infused with 1 L of a D5W (5% dextrose) solution (290 mOsm/kg H$_2$O). Assuming that there is no urine output, and after complete equilibration of the ECF and ICF, which of these individuals has a lower plasma [Na$^+$]?
   a. Individual A (NaCl infusion)
   b. Individual B (mannitol infusion)
   c. Individual C (D5W infusion)
   d. Individuals A, B, and C have the same plasma [Na$^+$]

3. Intravenous infusion of 2 L of which of the following solutions leads to the largest increase in ICF volume?
   a. D5W $\frac{1}{3} ECF + \frac{2}{3} ICF$
   b. Isotonic NaCl
   c. Hypotonic NaCl
   d. Hypertonic NaCl

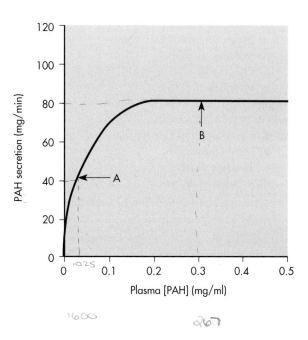

	A	B	C
TBW	33	33	33
ECF			
ICF			

For questions 4 through 6, consider the graph on p. 205. PAH (p-aminohippuric acid) is freely filtered at the glomerulus and secreted into the urine by the organic anion secretory process in the proximal tubule. At low plasma concentrations of PAH (i.e., less than the tubular transport maximum for secretion), virtually all PAH is excreted in the urine in a single pass through the kidneys. The graph depicts the rate of proximal tubule PAH secretion (y-axis) as a function of plasma PAH concentration (x-axis).

4. The amount of PAH <u>filtered</u> at the glomerulus is:
   a. Greater at point A than at point B.
   b. Less at point A than at point B.
   c. The same at points A and B. ×

5. The amount of PAH excreted in the urine is:
   a. Greater at point A than at point B.
   b. Less at point A than at point B.
   c. The same at points A and B.

6. The clearance of PAH is: C= excrete
   a. Greater at point A than at point B.   Px
   b. Less at point A than at point B.
   c. The same at points A and B.

7. Proximal tubule <u>HCO$_3^-$ reabsorption</u> is inhibited by which of the following?
   a. Increased P$_{CO_2}$ ×
   b. Expansion of the ECF volume
   c. Systemic acidosis ×
   d. Endothelin
   e. Hypokalemia ×

For questions 8 through 11, match the appropriate diuretic with the statement.
   a. Carbonic anhydrase inhibitor
   b. Loop diuretic ✓
   c. Thiazide diuretic ✓
   d. K$^+$-sparing diuretic ✓

8. Administration of this diuretic leads to an <u>increase</u> in the kidneys' ability to excrete solute-free water (C$_{H_2O}$). A

9. Administration of this diuretic may lead to the development of hyperkalemia. D

10. Administration of this diuretic impairs the kidneys' ability to reabsorb solute-free water (T$^c_{H_2O}$). B

11. Administration of this diuretic results in a decrease in renal Ca^{++} excretion. C

↓ ECF

12. An individual is stricken with an illness characterized by nausea, vomiting, and diarrhea. Over a 2-day period, this individual experiences a <u>3-kg loss</u> in weight without a change in the plasma [Na$^+$]. What can be concluded about body fluid volumes and composition in this individual?
   a. The volume of ICF is increased.
   b. The volume of the ECF is reduced. ✓
   c. The total body osmoles increased. ∨
   d. The plasma osmolality is reduced. ×

13. An individual weighs 60 kg and ingests a diet containing 100 mEq/day of Na$^+$. This individual is placed on a <u>thiazide diuretic.</u> After 2 weeks of taking this diuretic and with no change in diet, what can be concluded about Na$^+$ balance in the individual?
   a. Total body Na$^+$ content is increased.
   b. Urine Na$^+$ excretion is greater than 100 mEq/day. ×
   c. Na$^+$ content of the ECF is reduced.
   d. The plasma [Na$^+$] is increased. ×
   e. The Na$^+$ content of the ICF is increased. ×

Match the acid-base disturbance with the clinical scenario and arterial blood gases described in questions 14 through 18.
   a. Metabolic acidosis with respiratory compensation
   b. Metabolic alkalosis with respiratory compensation
   c. Respiratory acidosis with renal compensation (chronic respiratory acidosis)
   d. Respiratory acidosis without renal compensation (acute respiratory acidosis)
   e. Metabolic acidosis and respiratory acidosis

14. An individual with an asthma attack   D
    ↓pH = 7.32; ↑[HCO$_3^-$] = 25 mEq/L; ↑P$_{CO_2}$ = 50 mm Hg
    Resp Acid w/ comp.

15. An individual with diabetes mellitus, who forgets to take insulin   A
    ↓pH = 7.29; ↓[HCO$_3^-$] = 12 mEq/L; ↓P$_{CO_2}$ = 26 mm Hg
    Metabolic acidosis w/ comp

16. An individual with cardiopulmonary arrest
    ↓pH = 6.85; ↑[HCO$_3^-$] = 10 mEq/L; ↑P$_{CO_2}$ = 60 mm Hg E
    Acidosis

17. An individual with a gastric ulcer who ingests large quantities of antacids   B
    ↑pH = 7.45; ↑[HCO$_3^-$] = 30 mEq/L; ↑P$_{CO_2}$ = 45 mm Hg

    Alkalosis Metabolic

18. An individual with a 20-year history of smoking 3 packs/day who has emphysema: C

$\downarrow$pH = 7.37; $\uparrow$[HCO$_3^-$] = 28 mEq/L; $\uparrow$Pco$_2$ = 50 mm Hg

Acidosis Respiratory

19. An individual is treated with a thiazide diuretic for mild hypertension. After 3 months of therapy, the plasma [Na$^+$] has decreased from 143 to 135 mEq/L. Which of the following factors plays a role in the development of hyponatremia in this individual?
    a. Enhanced reabsorption of solute-free water by the early distal tubule ✗
    b. Reduced excretion of solute-free water
    c. Shift of water from the ICF to the ECF
    d. Diuretic-induced stimulation of the thirst center ✗
    e. Reduced effect of antidiuretic hormone (ADH) on the collecting duct ✗

20. An individual has a tumor of the adrenal gland that secretes aldosterone. What effect would the high levels of aldosterone have on renal electrolyte handling in this individual?
    a. Stimulation of Na$^+$ reabsorption by the principal cells of the distal tubule and collecting duct
    b. Reduced K$^+$ secretion by the principal cells of the distal tubule and collecting duct
    c. Stimulation of proximal tubule Na$^+$ reabsorption ✗
    d. Reduced secretion of H$^+$ by the intercalated cells of the distal tubule and collecting duct ✗
    e. Reduced reabsorption of Ca^{++} by the early distal tubule ✗

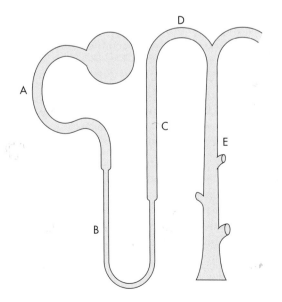

D

A

C

E

B

Match the portion of the nephron to the function described in questions 21 through 24.

21. Major site of NH$_4^+$ production

22. Site where calcitriol is synthesized

23. Site where parathyroid hormone (PTH) stimulates Ca^{++} reabsorption   D

24. Site where natriuretic peptides and urodilatin inhibit NaCl reabsorption   E

25. Which of the following maneuvers would be expected to stimulate ADH secretion?   ↓ECV
    a. Infusion of 1 L of hypertonic NaCl ✓
    b. Infusion of 1 L of an isosmotic urea solution
    c. Expansion of the ECV ✗
    d. Infusion of 1 L of D5W (assume no dextrose metabolism)
    e. An acute increase in blood pressure ✗

26. A portion of Na$^+$ reabsorption in the late portion of the proximal tubule is passive through the paracellular pathway. What is the primary driving force for this passive reabsorption of Na$^+$?
    a. A lower luminal than peritubular hydrostatic pressure ✗
    b. A higher luminal than peritubular [Na$^+$]
    c. A lumen-positive transepithelial voltage
    d. A lower interstitial fluid than luminal fluid oncotic pressure

27. During a 24-hour period, an individual excretes in the urine 60 mmol of NH$_4^+$, 40 mmol of titratable acid, and 10 mmol of HCO$_3^-$. If this individual is in acid-base balance, how much nonvolatile acid was produced from metabolism?
    a. 80 mmol/day $(60+40)-10 = 90$
    b. 90 mmol/day ✓
    c. 100 mmol/day
    d. 110 mmol/day
    e. 120 mmol/day

28. According to the tubuloglomerular feedback theory, an increase in tubular fluid NaCl delivery to the macula densa results in which of the following?   ↓[ADH]
    a. A decrease in the glomerular filtration rate of the same nephron
    b. An increase in renal blood flow to the glomerulus of the same nephron
    c. Activation of the renal sympathetic nerves ✗
    d. An increase in proximal tubule solute and water reabsorption ✗
    e. An increase in renin secretion ✗

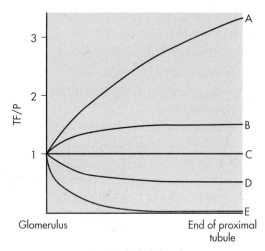

Glomerulus

End of proximal tubule

Proximal tubule length

Questions 29 through 31: The graph above depicts the change in tubular fluid concentration of various substances along the length of the proximal tubule plotted as the tubular fluid-to-plasma concentration ratio (TF/P). Thus, the TF/P = 1 for a substance that is at the same concentration in the tubular fluid and plasma (all substances that are freely filtered have a TF/P equal to 1 at the glomerulus).

Match the following substances to the appropriate TF/P curve.

29. Na$^+$ C

30. Creatinine

31. Glucose E

32. An individual has no urine output over a 2-day period. During this time, the body weight increases by 2 kg. Plasma [Na$^+$] is unchanged. What can be concluded about the volumes and composition of the body fluids?
    a. The volume of the ICF is decreased. x
    b. The volume of the ECF is increased. ✓
    c. The total body water is normal.
    d. The plasma osmolality is decreased. x

33. Na$^+$ reabsorption by the thick ascending limb of Henle's loop is
    a. Inhibited by a decrease in peritubular capillary hydrostatic pressure. x
    b. Inhibited by angiotensin II. x
    c. Increased with increased delivered load of Na$^+$.
    d. Inhibited by K$^+$-sparing diuretics. x
    e. Increased by natriuretic peptides. ✓

34. A reduction in dietary K$^+$ intake would be expected to alter K$^+$ transport in which segment of the nephron?
    a. Proximal convoluted tubule
    b. Descending limb of Henle's loop
    c. Proximal straight tubule
    d. Collecting duct
    e. Thick ascending limb of Henle's loop

35. Infusion of 1 L of which of the following solutions leads to the largest increase in the volume of the ECF?
    a. Isotonic D5W
    b. Isotonic NaCl ✓
    c. Hypotonic NaCl
    d. Hypertonic NaCl

36. Which of the following structures is a barrier to the filtration of proteins across the glomerulus?
    a. Capillary endothelial cells ✓
    b. Basement membrane x
    c. Lacis cells
    d. Parietal epithelial cells x
    e. Mesangial cells x

37. Starling forces regulate sodium and water reabsorption by the proximal tubule. Which of the following changes in Starling forces would increase reabsorption?
    a. Increase in capillary hydrostatic pressure ✓
    b. Increase in capillary oncotic pressure
    c. Decrease in capillary oncotic pressure
    d. Decrease in the permeability of the peritubular capillary to sodium and water

38. Which of the following occurs with a decrease in the ECF volume?
    a. Increase in GFR x
    b. Increase in angiotensin II levels ✓
    c. Increase in natriuretic peptide levels x
    d. Increase in free water clearance x
    e. Increase in fractional excretion of Na$^+$ x

39. Which of the following increases the reabsorption of sodium and chloride in the distal tubule and collecting duct?
    a. Uroguanylin x
    b. Peritubular Starling forces
    c. Natriuretic peptides x
    d. Aldosterone ✓
    e. Urodilatin x

40. Which of the following enhances urinary potassium excretion?
  a. An osmotic diuresis
  b. Acute metabolic acidosis
  c. Hypoaldosteronism
  d. Decreased tubular flow rate
  e. A water diuresis

41. Which of the following hormones plays an important role in keeping the plasma concentration of potassium within normal limits?
  a. Calcitriol
  b. Vasopressin
  c. PTH
  d. Insulin
  e. Glucagon

42. The use of a thiazide diuretic that inhibits NaCl reabsorption in the distal tubule does which of the following?
  a. Decreases the ability of the kidneys to excrete solute-free water
  b. Decreases the urinary excretion of NaCl
  c. Decreases the urinary excretion of K^+
  d. Increases the ability of the kidneys to excrete a concentrated urine
  e. Increases plasma $[K^+]$

43. Diuretics that inhibit NaCl reabsorption by the thick ascending limb of Henle's loop do which of the following?
  a. Stimulate calcium reabsorption by the thick ascending limb
  b. Decrease urine flow rate
  c. Stimulate urinary excretion of K^+
  d. Stimulate countercurrent multiplication
  e. Increase the osmolality of the medullary interstitial fluid

44. A 56-year-old woman has congestive heart failure with generalized edema. Which of the following plays an important role in the formation of edema in this woman?
  a. Increased interstitial hydrostatic pressure
  b. Decreased interstitial oncotic pressure
  c. Increased plasma oncotic pressure
  d. Decreased renal excretion of Na^+
  e. Decreased venous pressure

45. Vasopressin has which of the following actions?
  a. Increases the water permeability of the thick ascending limb of Henle's loop
  b. Increases the urea permeability of the cortical portion of the collecting duct
  c. Increases the water permeability of the collecting duct
  d. Decreases the GFR
  e. Increases the water permeability of the proximal tubule

46. A patient has polyuria and polydipsia, and the urine osmolality is 100 mOsm/kg H_2O. After an intravenous injection of ADH, urine volume decreases and urine osmolality increases. What is the most likely disorder in this patient?
  a. SIADH (syndrome of inappropriate ADH secretion)
  b. Osmotic diuresis
  c. Central diabetes insipidus
  d. Nephrogenic diabetes insipidus
  e. Nephrolithiasis (renal stone)

47. A healthy individual, weighing 60 kg, is infused with 1 L of isotonic saline to which 20 mEq of K^+ has been added. Following the infusion, the plasma $[K^+]$ of this individual has increased from 3.5 to 7.8 mEq/L. What is the most likely explanation for the development of hyperkalemia in this individual?
  a. Shift of K^+ from the ICF into the ECF
  b. Impaired renal excretion of K^+
  c. The increase in plasma $[K^+]$ of 4.3 mEq/L is what is expected from the addition of 20 mEq/L of K^+ to the ECF.
  d. Contraction of the ECF volume
  e. Development of hyperosmolality

48. An individual with polyuria resulting from nephrogenic diabetes insipidus is treated with a thiazide diuretic. After several weeks of therapy, daily urine output has decreased. What is the most likely explanation for the ability of the thiazide diuretic to reduce urine output in this individual?
   a. Stimulation of ADH secretion
   b. Decrease in ECF volume
   c. Decreased water permeability of the collecting duct
   d. Increased expression of V_2 receptors by collecting duct cells
   e. Stimulation of NaCl reabsorption by the thick ascending limb of Henle's loop

49. Two individuals ingest a diet containing 100 mEq/day of Na^+. One has a GFR of 180 L/day, and the other has a GFR of 90 L/day. Assuming both individuals are in steady-state Na^+ balance, what would be the expected Na^+ excretion of the individual with the reduced GFR?
   a. 0 mEq/day
   b. 50 mEq/day
   c. 100 mEq/day
   d. 150 mEq/day
   e. 200 mEq/day

50. In response to a metabolic acidosis, the kidneys increase the excretion of net acid. Which of the following is the most important component of this compensatory response?
   a. Increased filtered load of HCO_3^-
   b. Enhanced reabsorption of HCO_3^- by the proximal tubule
   c. Increased synthesis and excretion of NH_4^+
   d. Reduced H^+ secretion by the distal tubule and collecting duct
   e. Reduced secretion of HCO_3^- by the collecting duct

51. A patient receives an infusion of hypertonic saline. What will be the effect of this infusion on plasma osmolality and the Starling forces across capillary walls?

	Plasma Osmolality	Capillary Starling Forces
a.	↑	No change
b.	↑	↑Filtration
c.	No change	↑Filtration
d.	No change	No change
e.	↓	↓Filtration

52. The kidneys maintain a constant plasma osmolality by regulating the excretion of which of the following?
   a. Glucose
   b. Na^+
   c. Creatinine
   d. Water
   e. K^+

53. A 25-year-old woman has a decreased ECF volume as a result of several days of diarrhea. She has orthostatic changes in blood pressure and pulse as well as poor skin turgor. Which set of parameters would you predict for this woman? (*Note*: The arrows indicate changes from the euvolemic state.)

	GFR	Filtration Fraction	Proximal Tubule Reabsorption
a.	↑	↑	↑
b.	↓	↓	↓
c.	↓	↑	↑
d.	↓	↓	↑
e.	↑	↓	↓

54. Urinary K^+ excretion is increased by which of the following?
   a. Hypokalemia
   b. Hyperaldosteronism
   c. Antidiuretic hormone (ADH)
   d. A decrease in GFR
   e. Administration of amiloride

55. A 56-year-old man was admitted to the hospital with a myocardial infarction. At admission, his serum creatinine was 1.2 mg/dl, and his creatinine clearance was 100 ml/min. Over the next 3 days, he had several periods of hypotension, and his serum creatinine is now increased to 3.6 mg/dl. Assuming that he is in steady-state balance for creatinine (i.e., amount excreted = amount produced), what is his predicted creatinine clearance?
   a. 10 ml/min
   b. 33 ml/min
   c. 50 ml/min
   d. 66 ml/min
   e. 100 ml/min

56. A patient receives a 1-L infusion of isotonic saline. What effect will this infusion have on serum [Na$^+$] and urinary Na$^+$ excretion?

	Serum [Na$^+$]	Urinary Na$^+$ excretion
a.	No change	No change
b.	No change	↓
c.	No change	↑
d.	↑	↑
e.	↓	↓

57. A 21-year-old man with insulin-dependent (type 1) diabetes mellitus, who forgot to inject his insulin, is seen in the emergency department. The following laboratory data are obtained:

Serum [Na$^+$]	=	140 mEq/L (normal: 135 to 147 mEq/L)
Serum [K$^+$]	=	6.5 mEq/L (normal: 3.5 to 5.0 mEq/L)
Serum [HCO$_3^-$]	=	10 mEq/L (normal: 22 to 28 mEq/L)
Blood pH	=	7.0 (normal: 7.35 to 7.45)
Arterial P$_{CO_2}$	=	25 mm Hg (normal: 33 to 44 mm Hg)
Serum [glucose]	=	1000 mg/dl (normal: 70 to 110 mg/dl)

Which of the following plays the most important role in the generation of hyperkalemia in this man?

a. A low plasma osmolality
b. Low arterial P$_{CO_2}$
c. Hyponatremia
d. Metabolic acidosis
e. Low plasma insulin concentration

58. The man described in question 57 reported having polyuria and polydipsia before coming to the emergency department. What is the most likely cause of his polyuria?

a. Increased filtered load of glucose
b. Hyperkalemia
c. Reduced ADH levels
d. Kidneys not responding to ADH
e. Increased water ingestion

59. A 78-year-old woman with congestive heart failure develops pitting edema of her legs. Compared with a healthy (i.e., euvolemic) individual, what set of parameters would be expected in this woman?

	Plasma Volume	ECF Volume	ECV
a.	↓	↓	↓
b.	↓	↑	↓
c.	↑	↑	↓
d.	↑	↑	↑
e.	↑	↓	↓

60. The macula densa is part of which of the following structures in the kidney?

a. Extraglomerular matrix
b. Vasa recta
c. Afferent arteriole
d. Juxtamedullary nephron
e. Juxtaglomerular apparatus

61. Hyponatremia can sometimes be seen in individuals whose ECF volume is decreased by more than 10%. Which of the following factors contributes to the development of hyponatremia in this situation?

a. Decreased levels of ADH
b. Elevated levels of natriuretic peptides
c. Increased excretion of Na$^+$ by the kidneys
d. Reduced excretion of solute-free water by the kidneys
e. Development of positive Na$^+$ balance

62. A 45-year-old woman has a blood pressure of 140/90 mm Hg. Her doctor recommends a low-salt diet. What would you predict her serum [Na$^+$] and ECF volume would be compared with their values on her previous diet? (*Note*: Assume she has reached a new steady state on her new diet.)

	Serum [Na$^+$]	ECF Volume
a.	No change	↓
b.	No change	No change
c.	No change	↑
d.	↓	No change
e.	↓	↓

63. A 55-year-old woman has acute renal failure following a surgical procedure. Urine output is essentially zero. Over the course of 2 days, she gains 3 kg of weight and her serum [Na⁺] is unchanged. What would you conclude about the volume and composition of her body fluids?
    a. Intracellular fluid (ICF) volume is decreased.
    b. Hematocrit is increased.
    c. Today body water is unchanged.
    d. Effective plasma osmolality is increased.
    e. ECF volume is increased.

64. A 35-year-old man is diagnosed with an aldosterone-secreting adrenal tumor. What effect would the elevated levels of aldosterone have on his serum [K⁺] and plasma renin levels? (*Note*: Changes are indicated compared with a state of normal aldosterone levels.)

	Serum [K⁺]	Plasma Renin Levels
a.	↑	↑
b.	↑	↓
c.	↓	No change
d.	↓	↑
e.	↓	↓

65. A 20-year-old woman runs a marathon in 90° F weather. If she replaces all volume lost in sweat by drinking distilled water, what would happen to the volume and composition of her body fluids? (*Note*: Sweat is a hypotonic NaCl solution.)
    a. Total body water would be decreased.
    b. Hematocrit would be decreased.
    c. ICF volume would be decreased.
    d. ECF volume would be increased.
    e. Plasma osmolality would be decreased.

66. The efferent arteriole of some juxtamedullary nephrons enters the renal medulla and becomes which of the following vessels?
    a. Interlobular artery
    b. Arcuate artery
    c. Vasa recta
    d. Glomerular capillary
    e. Interlobar artery

67. A 6-year-old boy presents to the emergency department with fever, abdominal cramps, and diarrhea. Arterial blood gases are as follows:

pH: 7.28 (normal: 7.35 to 7.45)
P_{CO_2}:   24 mm Hg (normal: 33 to 44 mm Hg)
HCO_3^-:   11 mEq/L (normal: 22 to 28 mEq/L)

What is the acid-base disorder?
    a. Metabolic acidosis with respiratory compensation
    b. Metabolic acidosis with respiratory acidosis
    c. Acute respiratory acidosis
    d. Chronic respiratory acidosis

68. A patient has polyuria and polydipsia, and the urine osmolality is 100 mOsm/kg H₂O. The polyuria and polydipsia are not corrected by intravenous injection of ADH, nor does the exogenous ADH alter urine osmolality. What is the most like disorder in this patient?
    a. SIADH (syndrome of inappropriate ADH secretion)
    b. Osmotic diuresis
    c. Central diabetes insipidus
    d. Nephrogenic diabetes insipidus
    e. Nephrolithiasis (renal stone)

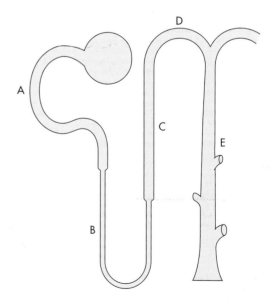

Match the portion of the nephron to the function described in questions 69 through 72.

69. Tubular fluid is hyperosmotic at this site when a dilute urine is being excreted.

70. The largest percentage of the filtered load of Na^+ is reabsorbed at this site.

71. Urine pH is the most acidic at this site.

72. NH_4^+ is reabsorbed from the tubular fluid at this site.

73. Which of the following situations would be expected to cause an increase in ADH secretion by the posterior pituitary?
    a. 5% decrease in arterial blood pressure
    b. 5% increase in arterial blood pressure
    c. 1% decrease in plasma osmolality
    d. 1% increase in plasma osmolality

74. Low-pressure volume receptors (baroreceptors) are located in which of the following vascular structures?
    a. Aortic arch
    b. Cardiac atria
    c. Carotid sinus
    d. Juxtaglomerular apparatus of the kidney
    e. Renal veins

75. What would be the expected neural and hormonal profile in a person whose ECF volume was decreased? (*Note*: Changes are in comparison with the euvolemic state.)

	Sympathetic Nerve Activity	Aldosterone Levels	ANP Levels
a.	No change	↑	↑
b.	↑	↑	↓
c.	↑	↑	No change
d.	No change	↑	↓
e.	↓	↓	↑

76. Which of the following statements regarding the GFR is true?
    a. Plasma oncotic pressure is constant along the length of the glomerular capillary.
    b. Net filtration pressure decreases from the afferent to the efferent end of the capillary.
    c. Net filtration pressure increases from the afferent to the efferent end of the capillary.
    d. Filtration occurs at the afferent end and reabsorption at the efferent end of the capillary.
    e. Plasma oncotic pressure decreases along the length of the glomerular capillary.

77. Which of the following responses to a fall in arterial pressure accounts for the ability of the kidneys to autoregulate GFR?
    a. Decreased resistance of the efferent arteriole
    b. Increased delivery of fluid to the end of the proximal tubule
    c. Increase resistance of the afferent arteriole
    d. Increased [NaCl] in tubular fluid at the macula densa
    e. Decreased in resistance of the afferent arteriole

78. GFR decreases in which of the following conditions?
    a. Dilation of the afferent arteriole
    b. Decrease in renal nerve activity
    c. Decrease in plasma oncotic pressure
    d. Increase in hydrostatic pressure in Bowman's space
    e. Increase in renal blood flow

79. A healthy 25-year-old woman donates a kidney to her identical twin, who has chronic renal failure. Her serum [creatinine] before removal of the kidney is 1.0 mg/dl. After donating her kidney, her serum [creatinine] increases to 2.0 mg/dL. One month later her serum [creatinine] has decreased to 1.5 mg/dL. Which of the following accounts for the fact that her serum [creatinine] fell from 2.0 to 1.5 mg/dL.
    a. Decreased production of creatinine by skeletal muscle
    b. Enhanced secretion of creatinine by the proximal tubule
    c. Increase in the GFR of each of the remaining nephrons
    d. Expansion of her ECF volume

80. The woman described in question 79 has not modified her diet since removal of her kidney. What is the change in renal handling of Na^+ now that she has only one kidney?

	Urinary Na^+ Excretion/24 hr	Fractional Excretion of Na^+
a.	No change	No change
b.	No change	↑
c.	↑	↑
d.	↓	↓
e.	↓	↑

81. A 45-year-old man is prescribed an angiotensin-converting enzyme inhibitor as part of his therapy for hypertension. If he does not change his diet, what changes in his serum [Na⁺] and serum [K⁺] would you expect?

	Serum [Na⁺]	Serum [K⁺]
a.	No change	↓
b.	No change	↑
c.	↓	No change
d.	↑	↑
e.	↓	↓

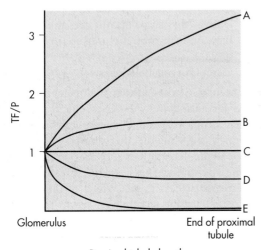

Glomerulus   End of proximal tubule

Proximal tubule length

Questions 82 through 85: The above graph depicts the change in tubular fluid concentration of various substances along the length of the proximal tubule plotted as the tubular fluid to plasma concentration ratio (TF/P). Thus, the TF/P = 1 for a substance that is the same concentration in the tubular fluid and plasma (all substances that are freely filtered have a TF/P = 1 at the glomerulus). Match the following to the appropriate TF/P curve.

82. Cimetidine (organic cation)

83. Amino acids

84. Cl⁻

85. Tubular fluid osmolality

86. A substance (Y) is found in the plasma at a concentration of 2 mg/dL. A 24-hour urine collection is done to determine the renal clearance of Y. The following data are obtained.
Urine volume: 1.44 L
Urine [Y]:   500 mg/L

What is the renal clearance of Y?
a. 5 ml/min
b. 25 ml/min
c. 50 ml/min
d. 100 ml/min
e. 250 ml/min

87. Starling forces are measured across a capillary wall, and the following values are obtained:
Capillary hydrostatic pressure: 30 mm Hg
Capillary oncotic pressure: 25 mm Hg
Interstitial hydrostatic pressure: 0 mm Hg
Interstitial oncotic pressure: 15 mm Hg
If the reflection coefficient for protein across this capillary wall is 0.5, what are the pressure and direction of fluid flow across the capillary wall?

	Net Pressure	Direction of Fluid Flow
a.	5 mm Hg	Into capillary
b.	10 mm Hg	Out of capillary
c.	15 mm Hg	Out of capillary
d.	20 mm Hg	Out of capillary
e.	25 mm Hg	Out of capillary

88. A 65-year-old man has chronic renal failure. What are the expected changes in his serum Ca⁺⁺, Pi, and calcitriol levels? (*Note:* Changes are those expected compared with an individual with normal renal function.)

	Serum [Ca⁺⁺]	Serum [Pi]	Calcitriol Level
a.	↓	↑	↓
b.	↑	↑	↑
c.	↑	↓	↓
d.	↓	↓	↓
e.	↑	↑	↓

89. Hyperkalemia will most likely be seen under which of the following conditions?
a. Metabolic alkalosis
b. Exercise
c. Insulin injection
d. Decreased plasma osmolality
e. Administration of a β-adrenergic agonist

90. A 60-year-old woman comes to the emergency department with shortness of breath. An arterial blood sample is obtained.

PO_2:   75 mm Hg (normal: 75 to 100 mm Hg)
PCO_2:   58 mm Hg (normal: 33 to 44 mm Hg)
HCO_3^-: 24 mEq/L (normal: 22 to 28 mEq/L)
pH: 7.24 (normal: 7.35 to 7.45)

What is this woman's acid-base disorder?
  a. Metabolic acidosis
  b. Metabolic alkalosis
  c. Acute respiratory acidosis
  d. Acute respiratory alkalosis
  e. Chronic respiratory acidosis

91. Which of the following conditions would be expected to reduce the free (i.e., ionized) $[Ca^{++}]$ in the plasma?
  a. Metabolic acidosis
  b. Reduced dietary intake of phosphate
  c. A tumor secreting parathyroid hormone–like peptide
  d. Ingestion of calcitriol
  e. Acute respiratory alkalosis

92. A 42-year-old woman is recovering in the hospital after removal of a benign brain tumor. She develops SIADH, and her serum $[Na^+]$ falls from 142 to 128 mEq/L. Urine osmolality is 600 mOsm/kg H_2O. Administration of 1 L of isotonic saline to this woman would result in which of the following changes in her plasma $[Na^+]$ and urinary Na^+ excretion?

	Serum $[Na^+]$	Urinary Na^+ Excretion/24 hr
a.	No change	↑
b.	↑	↑
c.	↓	↑
d.	↑	No change
e.	↓	↓

93. A 35-year-old man is prescribed a thiazide diuretic for hypertension. If you measured his urine within the first 24 hours after starting the diuretic, what would you expect to happen to his excretion of Na^+, K^+, and Ca^{++}?

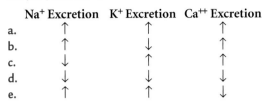

	Na^+ Excretion	K^+ Excretion	Ca^{++} Excretion
a.	↑	↑	↑
b.	↑	↓	↑
c.	↓	↑	↑
d.	↓	↓	↓
e.	↑	↑	↓

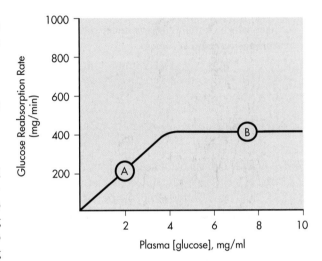

Questions 94 through 96: The above graph depicts proximal tubule glucose reabsorption as a function of the plasma concentration of glucose.

94. The amount of glucose filtered at the glomerulus is:
  a. Greater at point B than at point A.
  b. Less at point B than at point A.
  c. The same at points A and B.

95. The amount of glucose excreted in the urine is:
  a. Greater at point B than at point A.
  b. Less at point B than at point A.
  c. The same at points A and B.

96. The clearance of glucose is:
  a. Greater at point B than at point A.
  b. Less at point B than at point A.
  c. The same at points A and B.

97. An individual drinks 2 L of distilled water. The kidneys respond to the ingestion of this water load by:
   a. Increasing the GFR.
   b. Decreasing proximal tubule reabsorption of water.
   c. Increasing tubular fluid dilution by the thick ascending limb of Henle's loop.
   d. Decreasing water reabsorption by the collecting duct.
   e. Decreasing solute excretion.

98. Administration of a loop diuretic to a healthy individual for several weeks would be expected to have which of the following effects on body fluid composition and volume?

	P_{osm}	ECF Volume	ICF Volume
a.	↑	↓	↓
b.	No change	↓	No change
c.	↓	No change	↑
d.	↓	↑	↓
e.	No change	No change	No change

99. A healthy 21-year-old man participates in a clinical trial of a new loop diuretic. Before administration of this new diuretic, his urine osmolality is 600 mOsm/kg H_2O and his urine output is 1.5 L/day. Which of the following values for urine osmolality and urine output would you predict as a result of the diuretic's action on his thick ascending limb of Henle's loop?

	Urine Osmolality (mOsm/kg H_2O)	Urine Output (L/day)
a.	1200	0.75
b.	1000	0.9
c.	600	1.5
d.	300	3.0
e.	200	4.5

100. A 65-year-old woman cannot dilute her urine below 200 mOsm/kg H_2O. Her daily intake of food requires the excretion of 600 mmol/day of solute in the urine. What is the maximum volume of water she can ingest each day that will not result in a decrease in her body fluid osmolality? (*Note*: Assume water loss by nonrenal routes is 0.5 L/day.)
   a. 2.0 L/day
   b. 2.5 L/day
   c. 3.0 L/day
   d. 3.5 L/day
   e. 4.0 L/day

A N S W E R S

1. c	21. a	41. d	61. d	81. b
2. b	22. a	42. a	62. a	82. a
3. a	23. d	43. c	63. e	83. e
4. b	24. e	44. d	64. e	84. b
5. b	25. a	45. c	65. e	85. c
6. a	26. c	46. c	66. c	86. b
7. b	27. b	47. a	67. a	87. e
8. a	28. a	48. b	68. d	88. a
9. d	29. c	49. c	69. b	89. b
10. b	30. a	50. c	70. a	90. c
11. c	31. e	51. a	71. e	91. e
12. b	32. b	52. d	72. c	92. c
13. c	33. c	53. c	73. d	93. e
14. d	34. d	54. b	74. b	94. a
15. a	35. d	55. b	75. b	95. a
16. e	36. b	56. c	76. b	96. a
17. b	37. b	57. e	77. e	97. d
18. c	38. b	58. a	78. d	98. b
19. b	39. d	59. c	79. c	99. d
20. a	40. a	60. e	80. b	100. d

INDEX

Page numbers followed by f indicate figures; t, tables, b, boxes.

A

ACE. *See* Angiotensin-converting enzyme (ACE)
Acetazolamide, 167
Acid, definition of, 129
Acid-base balance, 129-148
　ammonium synthesis and excretion, 132
　HCO_3^- buffer system, 130
　HCO_3^- formation in, 137-141, 137f
　HCO_3^- reabsorption in, 132-135
　net acid excretion by kidneys, 131-132
　overview of, 130-131
　plasma $[K^+]$ alterations and, 117, 117t
　potassium excretion and, 125, 126f, 127
　regulation of, 2
　regulation of H^+ secretion, 135-137, 135t
Acid-base disorders
　analysis of, 145-146, 146f
　metabolic acidosis, 117, 125, 126f, 127, 143-144
　metabolic alkalosis, 143b, 144
　metabolic vs. respiratory, 141
　mixed, 146
　respiratory acidosis, 144-145
　respiratory alkalosis, 145
　response to, 141-143
　simple, 143-145, 144t
Acidosis, 130
　metabolic. *See* Metabolic acidosis
　renal tubular, 140b-141b
　respiratory, 144-145
α-actinin 4 *(ACTN4)*, 27
Active transport, 50
Addison's disease, 158b
Adenosine, 38, 44
Adenosine monophosphate, cyclic (cAMP), 77
Adenosine triphosphate (ATP), 38, 44
Adrenomedullin, 67, 99
Afferent arteriole, 20
Albumin, plasma, 152
Aldosterone, 97
　antagonists, 168b
　in NaCl/water reabsorption regulation, 65, 65t

Aldosterone—cont'd
　plasma K^+ regulation, 117, 117t
　potassium secretion regulation, 122-123, 122f
　secretion of, 28
Alkali, definition of, 129
Alkalosis, 130
　metabolic, 143b, 144
　respiratory, 145
Alport's syndrome, 28b
Amiloride, 168
Ammoniagenesis, 138, 139f, 140
Ammonium (NH_4^+)
　excretion assessment of, 140b
　production of, 137-141, 139f
　regulation by acid-base balance, 140
　synthesis and excretion of, 132
Amphotericin B, 140b
Angiotensin-converting enzyme (ACE), 97
　in RBF/GFR regulation, 45
　inhibitors of, 45b, 66b
Angiotensin I, 97
Angiotensin II, 97
　in NaCl/water reabsorption regulation, 65, 65t
　in RBF/GFR regulation, 42, 43f
　receptor antagonists, 45b
　renin and formation of, 28
Angiotensinogen, 97
Anion gap, 143b
ANP. *See* Atrial natriuretic peptide (ANP)
Antidiuresis
　ADH levels and, 73, 84-85
　mechanisms of, 82f, 83-85, 83t
Antidiuretic hormone (ADH)
　body fluid osmolality and, 73-78, 73f
　extracellular fluid volume and, 97
　hemodynamic control of secretion, 75-76, 75f, 77f
　in antidiuresis, 73, 84-85
　NaCl/water reabsorption regulation by, 67
　plasma osmolality and, 74-75, 75f
　potassium secretion regulation by, 123-124, 123f

Antidiuretic hormone—cont'd
　renal actions of, 76-79
　secretion of, 73-74, 74f
　thirst and secretion of, 79-80
Antiport mechanisms, 50
Aquaporins (AQPs), 13, 13b
　ADH and, 77
　in water reabsorption, 56b
　membrane permeability and, 85b
　nephrogenic diabetes insipidus and, 79b
　thiazide diuretics and, 166b
Aquaretics, 163, 164, 164f, 169
Arcuate artery, 20
Arcuate vein, 20
Arterial blood gases, normal values, 183
Arterioles, 20, 41, 42f
Ascites, 93b
ATP (adenosine triphosphate), 38, 44
Atrial natriuretic peptide (ANP)
　as volume pressure sensor, 94
　extracellular fluid volume and, 99
　in RBF/GFR regulation, 44
　NaCl/water reabsorption regulation by, 66
Autoregulation, 35, 38-41, 38f, 39f
Autosomal dominant hypocalcemia, 155b

B

Baroreceptors, 76, 94-95, 96t
Bartter's syndrome, 49t, 62b
Basement membrane, 24, 26
Bicarbonate (HCO_3^-)
　as buffer system, 130
　diuretics and excretion of, 169t, 170-171
　extracellular fluid osmolality and, 10
　formation of, 137-141, 137f
　production of, 130-131
　reabsorption of, 132-135, 132f-134f
Blood-brain barrier, 14b
BNP. *See* Brain natriuretic peptide (BNP)
Body fluid osmolality, 1, 71-90.
　　See also Water balance
　antidiuretic hormone and, 73-78, 73f
　medullary interstitium and, 85-86

Body fluid osmolality—cont'd
  renal diluting and concentrating ability, assessment of, 87b-88b
  thirst and, 79-80
  urine dilution and concentration mechanisms, 80-87, 82f, 83t
  water balance disorders and, 72
Body fluids, 3-17. *See also* Electrolyte solutions
  capillary exchange of, 11-14, 12f
  cellular exchange of, 13-14, 13b
  composition of compartments, 10-11
  exchange between compartments, 11-14
  total body water, 9
  volume regulation in, 1
  volumes of compartments, 9-10, 10f
Body water. *See* Water *terms*
Bone, as extracellular buffer, 142
Bowman's capsule, 21, 21f, 22f, 24
Bowman's space, 24
Bradykinin, 44
Brain natriuretic peptide (BNP)
  as volume pressure sensor, 94
  extracellular fluid volume and, 99
  in RBF/GFR regulation, 44
  NaCl/water reabsorption regulation by, 66
Brush border, 22
Buffers, 130, 131, 141-142
Bumetanide, 167
BUN (urea nitrogen), normal values of, 183

C

Calcitonin
  Ca^{++} excretion and, 155
  in Ca^{++} and Pi homeostasis, 151, 151f, 159, 160f
Calcitriol, 150-151, 151f
  Ca^{++} excretion and, 155
  in Ca^{++} and Pi homeostasis, 159, 160f
  secretion of, 2
Calcium (Ca^{++})
  body content of, 150, 150t
  plasma forms of, 151-152, 152t
  reabsorption of, 2, 151-154, 153f
Calcium balance, 149-155
  Ca^{++} excretion regulation in, 154-155, 154t
  Ca^{++} transport, 152-154, 152f
  calcium-sensing receptor and, 151, 155
  homeostasis in, 150-152, 150f
Calcium-sensing receptor (CaSR), 151, 155
Calyces, 19, 20f
cAMP (cyclic adenosine monophosphate), 77
CAP1 (channel activating protease), 122
Capillary filtration coefficient (K_f), 11, 37, 37b
Capillary fluid exchange, 11-13, 12f
Capillary hydrostatic pressure, 106
Capillary permeability, 107
Carbon dioxide (CO_2), 130
Carbonic anhydrase inhibitors, 167, 171

Carbonic anhydrases, 133
Cardiac arrhythmias, 114b
Case studies, 179-181, 203-208
Catecholamines, 67
CD2-AP, 26f, 27
Cell lysis, 117t, 118
Cell membrane permeability
  ADH and, 76-79
  membrane transport principles in, 48, 50
  tonicity and, 7-8
Cellular fluid exchange, 13-14, 13b
Channel activating protease (CAP1), 122
Chemoreceptors, 142
Chloride (Cl^-), 10
Chlorothiazide, 168
Cilia, primary, 22, 23f
Cirrhosis, hepatic, 93b
Cl^--HCO_3^- antiporter, 135
Claudin-16, 154b
CO_2 (carbon dioxide), 130
Collecting duct system, 21-22
  ADH and water permeability in, 76-77
  HCO_3^- reabsorption by, 133
  NaCl and water reabsorption by, 63-64, 64f
Congestive heart failure
  aldosterone antagonists for, 168b
  edema in, 107-108, 108f
  extracellular fluid volume in, 93, 93b
Corpuscle, renal, 21, 24-28, 24f-26f
Cortex (kidney), 19, 20f
Cortical collecting duct, 21-22
Cortisol, 136
Countercurrent multiplication, 83-84
Coupled transport, 50
Creatinine clearance, 33-34
  normal values of, 183
Cubilin, 56b
Cyclic adenosine monophosphate (cAMP), 77
Cystinosis, 140b

D

Dextrans, 35, 35f
Diabetes insipidus, 76b, 79b
Diabetes mellitus
  carbohydrate metabolism in, 131b
  metabolic acidosis in, 142b
  nitric oxide production in, 44b
Diabetic ketoacidosis, 143b
Diffusion, 50, 138
Diffusion trapping, 138
1,25-Dihydroxyvitamin D_3. *See* Calcitriol
Diluting segment of kidney, 83
Distal renal tubular acidosis, 140b-141b
Distal tubule, 21, 22f
  delivery of sodium to, 101
  disorders of, 140b-141b
  HCO_3^- reabsorption by, 133
  in urinary excretion, 170
  NaCl and water reabsorption by, 63-64

Diuresis
  ADH levels and, 73
  diuretics vs., 163
  mechanisms of, 81, 82f, 83
Diuretic braking phenomenon, 165-166, 165f
Diuretics, 163-173
  adequate delivery of, 164-165
  aquaretics, 163, 164, 164f, 169
  braking phenomenon of, 165-166, 165f
  Ca^{++} and Pi excretion and, 169t, 171-172
  carbonic anhydrase inhibitors, 167
  diuresis vs., 163
  excretion of water and solutes and, 169-172
  general principles of action, 163-165
  HCO_3^- excretion, 169t, 170-171
  K^+ excretion, 169t, 170
  K^+-sparing diuretics, 168-169, 170-171
  loop diuretics, 165b, 167-168
  osmotic diuretics, 166-167
  sites of action of, 164, 164f
  solute-free water excretion and, 169-170, 169t
  thiazide diuretics, 154, 165b-166b, 168
Donnan effect, 10
Dopamine, 44, 67

E

ECF. *See* Extracellular fluid (ECF)
ECV (effective circulating volume), 92-93
Edema, 106-108
  congestive heart failure and, 93b
  localized vs. generalized, 107b
Effective circulating volume (ECV), 92-93
Effective osmoles, 8, 88b
Efferent arteriole, 20
Electrolyte balance, regulation of, 1-2
Electrolyte solutions
  for fluid replacement therapy, 14b
  molarity and equivalence of, 5-6
  oncotic pressure in, 8
  osmolarity and osmolality of, 7
  physicochemical properties of, 5-9
  plasma protein concentration and osmotic pressure in, 9f
  specific gravity of, 8, 8b
  tonicity of, 7-8
  units of measurement of, 7t
Electrolytes, serum, normal values of, 183
Endocytosis, 50
Endothelial cells, 44, 45f
Endothelin, 44, 136
Epinephrine, 116, 117t
Eplerenone, 168
Equivalence, of electrolyte solutions, 5-6
Erythropoietin, 2
ESRD (end-stage renal disease), 3
Estrogens, 159b
Ethacrynic acid, 167
Euvolemia, 96, 99-102
Exercise, 118

Extracellular buffers, 141-142
Extracellular fluid (ECF), 91-111
    composition of, 9-10
    diuretic action and volume of, 165-166
    edema and, 106-108
    effective circulating volume of, 92-93
    NaCl excretion control of, 99-102
    osmolality of, 91
    tubular flow rate and potassium
        excretion, 124-125, 124f
    volume contraction and NaCl excretion
        control, 104-106, 107f
    volume expansion and NaCl excretion
        control, 102-104, 103f
    volume-sensing systems of, 93-99, 93t
Extraglomerular mesangial cells, 28

F
Facilitated diffusion, 50
Familial hypocalciuric hypercalcemia, 155b
Familial hypomagnesemic
    hypercalcemia, 154b
Fanconi's syndrome, 54b, 140b
Fibroblast growth factor 23 (FGF-23), 158
Fick principle, 31
Filtration barrier, 24, 24f-27f, 26
    negative charges and, 35b, 36f
Filtration slit diaphragm, 25f, 27
Filtration slits, 27
Free-water clearance, 87
Frizzled-related protein 4 (FRP-4), 158
Furosemide, 167

G
G-T (glomerulotubular) balance, 69, 101
Generalized edema. See Edema
GFR. See Glomerular filtration rate (GFR)
Gitelman's syndrome, 114
Glomerular capillaries, 20
    hydrostatic pressure in, 12
    ultrastructure of, 24, 24f-25f, 26, 27f
Glomerular disease, immune
    complex-mediated, 28b
Glomerular filtration, 34-37, 36f
Glomerular filtration rate (GFR), 32-34
    autoregulation of, 38-41, 38f, 39f, 101
    extracellular fluid volume expansion
        and, 102
    formula for, 37
    hormones influencing, 41t
    in end-stage renal disease, 3
    measurement of, 33-34, 34f
    mesangial cells and, 28
    regulation of, 41-45
Glomerulotubular (G-T) balance,
    69, 101
Glomerulus. See Glomerular capillaries
Glucocorticoids, 44, 127, 127t
Glucose, normal values of, 183
Glutamine, 137-138
Granular cells, 28
Growth hormone, 158b
Guanylin, 67, 92b

H
H+. See Hydrogen ion (H+)
H+, K+-ATPase, 134
HCO3− buffer system, 130, 141-142.
        See also Bicarbonate (HCO3−)
Hemorrhage, 42b
Henderson-Hasselbalch equation, 130, 142
Henle's loop, 21
    antidiuresis and, 83-84
    diuresis and, 81, 82f, 83, 83t
    HCO3− reabsorption by, 133
    in urinary excretion, 170
    reabsorption of Ca++, 153, 153f, 154b
    reabsorption of NaCl and water,
        61-62, 61f
Hepatic baroreceptors, 95
Hepatic cirrhosis, 93b
Hepatic sensors, 95
HHS (hypomagnesemia-hypercalciuria
        syndrome), 154b
High-pressure volume sensors,
        vascular, 94
Histamine, 44
Hormones
    potassium secretion and, 127, 127t
    regulatory effects of, 41t, 64, 65t
    renal secretion of, 2-3
Hydrogen ion (H+)
    NH4+ excretion and, 138
    secretion, regulation of,
        135-137, 135t
Hydrostatic pressure
    capillary, 11-12, 106
    in body fluid exchange, 11
    in ultrafiltration, 36, 36f
Hyperaldosteronism, 98b
Hypercalcemia, 150, 151, 151b
    Ca++ excretion and, 154, 154t
    familial hypocalciuric, 155b
    familial hypomagnesemic, 154b
Hyperkalemia, 113, 114, 115f
    chronic, 121b
    exercise and, 118b
    in kidney disease, 119b
Hyperosmolality, 72b-73b
Hyperparathyroidism, 151b, 157b
Hypertension, 44b
Hypertonic solutions, 7
Hypo-osmolality, 72b-73b, 80b
Hypocalcemia, 150, 151
    autosomal dominant, 155b
    parathyroid hormone secretion and, 159
Hypocalcemic tetany, 150, 151b, 152
Hypokalemia, 113-114, 115f
    chronic, 121b
    in kidney disease, 120b
Hypomagnesemia-hypercalciuria
        syndrome (HHS), 154b
Hyponatremia, 80b
Hypoparathyroidism, 151b
Hypothalamus, 73, 74f
Hypotonic solutions, 7-8
Hypoxia, 131b

I
ICF (intracellular fluid), 9, 10, 11
Ineffective osmoles, 8, 77
Inner medullary collecting duct, 21f, 22,
        22f, 78
Insensible water loss, 71
Insulin, 116-117, 117t
Intercalated cells
    in H+ secretion, 133
    in potassium secretion, 120
    NaCl and water reabsorption by,
        63-64, 64f
    of collecting duct, 22
Intercellular spaces, lateral, 50, 51f
Interlobar artery, 20
Interlobar vein, 20
Interlobular artery, 20
Interlobular vein, 20
Interstitial fluid, 9
    hydrostatic pressure in, 12
    medullary, 85-86
Intracellular buffers, 141, 142
Intracellular fluid (ICF), 9, 10, 11
Isosmotic solutions, 7-8
Isotonic solutions, 7

J
Juxtaglomerular apparatus
    as volume pressure sensor, 94
    in tubuloglomerular feedback, 38, 39f
    ultrastructure of, 24f, 28
Juxtamedullary nephron, 23

K
K+. See Potassium (K+)
K+-sparing diuretics, 168-169, 170-171
Ketoacidosis, diabetic, 143b
Kf (capillary filtration coefficient),
        11, 37, 37b
Kidney. See also Juxtaglomerular
        apparatus; Nephrons; Renal terms
    diluting segment of, 83
    excretory function of, 2
    gross anatomy of, 19-20, 20f
    innervation of, 28
    mass balance relationships of, 31-32, 32f
    overview of, 1-3
    renal corpuscle, 21, 24-28,
        24f-26f
    vascular system of, 19-20,
        20f, 21f
Kidney diseases
    glomerular filtration rate decline in,
        34b, 34f
    medullary sponge kidney, 140b
    polycystic, 23b
    potassium disorders in,
        119b-120b
    prevalence of, 2b
    renal replacement therapies for, 3
    transport proteins in, 49t
Kidney failure, chronic, 157b
Kussmaul's respiration, 142b

L

Laboratory values, normal, 183
Lacis cells (extraglomerular mesangial
    cells), 28
Liddle's syndrome, 66b
Liver cirrhosis, 93b
Localized edema, 107b
Loop diuretics, 165b, 167-168, 171
Loop of Henle. See Henle's loop
Low-pressure volume sensors, vascular, 94
Lymphatic obstruction, 106-107

M

Macula densa
    in autoregulation, 38-39, 39f
    of juxtaglomerular apparatus, 28
    in renin secretion, 96
Major calyx, 19, 20f
Mannitol, 14b, 166
Mass balance relationship, 31-32, 32f
Medulla, 19, 20f
Medullary collecting duct, 21f, 22, 22f, 86
Medullary interstitium, 85-86
Medullary sponge kidney, 140b
Megalin, 56b
Mesangial cells, 28
Mesangial matrix, 28
Mesangium, 27f, 28
Metabolic acid-base disorders, 141
Metabolic acidosis, 143-144
    plasma K^+ alterations and, 117
    potassium excretion and,
        125, 126f, 127
Metabolic alkalosis, 143b, 144
Metolazone, 168
Minor calyx, 19, 20f
Mixed acid-base disorders, 146
Molarity, 5-6
Multiligand endocytic receptors, 56b
Myogenic mechanism, 38

N

Na^+. See Sodium (Na^+)
Na^+, K^+-ATPase (sodium-potassium
        adenosine triphosphatase)
        pump
    aldosterone activation of, 122-123
    distal tube and collecting duct and,
        63-64, 64f
    in intracellular fluid, 11
    in potassium balance, 114, 120, 121f
    in reabsorption by Henle's loop,
        61-62
    in sodium reabsorption, 51, 51f
Na^+-H^+ antiporter (NHE3), 132
Na^+-Pi symporters, 157, 158f
NaCl. See Sodium chloride (NaCl)
NAE (net acid excretion), 132
Natriuresis, 93, 163
    diuretic braking phenomenon and,
        165-166, 165f
    loop diuretics and, 167

Natriuretic peptides
    as volume pressure sensors, 94
    extracellular fluid volume and, 99
    in RBF/GFR regulation, 44
    NaCl/water reabsorption regulation by, 66
Negative Na^+ balance, 92
Negative water balance, 72
NEPH-1, 27
Nephrin (NPHS1), 27
Nephrons, 19, 20f
    function by segment, 188
    function by transport process, 185-187
    HCO_3^- reabsorption by, 132-135,
        132f-134f
    in urine concentration and dilution, 83t
    NaCl transport along, 57t
    sodium handling in euvolemia,
        99-101, 101f
    superficial vs. juxtamedullary, 23
    ultrastructure of, 20-24, 21f, 22f
    water reabsorption by, 52
    water transport along, 60t
Nephrotic syndrome, 27b, 107b
Net acid excretion (NAE), 132
Neurohypophysis, 73
NH_4^+. See Ammonium (NH_4^+)
NHE3 (Na^+-H^+ antiporter), 132
Nitric oxide, 43-44, 44b
Nonionic diffusion, 138
Nonvolatile acid, 130-131

O

Oncotic pressure, 8, 12-13, 106
Organic anions, 57-61, 58f, 59b, 59f, 165
Organic cations, 60-61, 60f, 165
Osmolality, 7. See also Body fluid
        osmolality; Plasma osmolality (P_{OSM})
    of extracellular fluid, 10, 91
    of medullary interstitial fluid, 85
    serum, normal values, 183
Osmolar clearance (C_{OSM}), 87
Osmolarity, 7
Osmoles, 8, 88b
Osmoreceptors, 75
Osmosis, 5-6, 6f, 48
Osmotic coefficient, 8
Osmotic diuretics, 166-167
Osmotic pressure, 5-6, 6f
    in body fluid exchange, 11
    cell membrane permeability and, 8
Osteitis fibrosa cystica, 157b

P

P_{OSM}. See Plasma osmolality (P_{OSM})
Papilla, 19
Paracellin 1 (PCLN-1), 154b
Paracellular pathway, 50, 51f, 54
Parathyroid hormone (PTH)
    Ca^{++} excretion and, 154-155, 154t
    calcium homeostasis and, 151, 151f
    H^+ secretion and, 136-137
    in Ca^{++} and Pi homeostasis, 159, 159f

Pi excretion and, 157, 158t
Parathyroid hormone-related peptide
        (PTHRP), 151b
Paraventricular nuclei (hypothalamus), 73
Parietal layer (Bowman's capsule), 24
Passive transport, 48
PCLN-1 (paracellin 1), 154b
Pelvis (kidney), 19, 20f
Peripheral edema, 107b
Peritubular capillaries, 20
Phosphate (Pi)
    diuretics and excretion of, 169t, 172
    homeostasis, 149, 156, 156f
    in bone, 155
    nephron transport of, 157, 157f, 158f
    plasma forms of, 151, 152f
    urinary excretion of, 157-158, 158t
Phosphatonins, 158
Pituitary gland, 73-74, 74f
PKA (protein kinase A), 77
Plasma, 9
    composition of, 10
    oncotic pressure of, 12, 106
    osmotic pressure of, 9f
Plasma [K^+]
    alterations of, 117-118, 117t,
        120-121, 122f
    hormone regulation of, 115-117
Plasma osmolality (P_{OSM}), 10, 11b
    ADH secretion and, 74-75, 75f
    extracellular fluid volume expansion
        and, 103-104
    set point in, 75
    water balance disorders and,
        72, 72b-73b
Plasma proteins
    as extracellular buffers, 142
    oncotic pressure of, 12
    osmotic pressure of, 9f
Podocin (NPHS2), 27
Podocytes, 24-27
Polycystic kidney disease, 23b
Polycystins, 23b
Polydipsia, 76b
Polyuria, 76b
Positive Na^+ balance, 92
Positive water balance, 72
Potassium (K^+). See also Plasma [K^+]
    cellular mechanisms of secretion,
        120, 121f
    diuretics and excretion of, 169t, 170
    secretion of, 120-124
Potassium balance regulation, 113-127
    factors affecting excretion of, 124-127
    function of, 114, 114f
    H^+ secretion and, 137
    homeostasis, overview of, 113-115,
        115f, 116f
    hormones and, 115-117
    in intracellular fluid, 11
    K^+ excretion by kidneys, 118-119,
        119f, 121t

Potassium balance regulation—cont'd
    K⁺-sparing diuretics and, 168-169, 170-171
    transport of, 63-64, 64f
Principal cells (collecting duct),
        22, 63-64, 64f
Prostatin, 122
Protein kinase A (PKA), 77
Protein reabsorption, 56-57
Proteins, serum, normal values of, 183
Proteinuria, 27b, 57, 107b
Proximal renal tubular acidosis, 140b
Proximal tubule, 21, 22f
    Ca⁺⁺ reabsorption by, 152-154, 153f
    Na⁺ reabsorption by, 51-55
    organic anion secretion by, 58b, 58-61,
        59b, 59f
    protein reabsorption by, 56-57
    solute reabsorption routes in, 58f
    water reabsorption by, 54-56, 58f
Pseudohyperkalemia, 114
Pseudohypoaldosteronism (PHA), 66b
PTH. See Parathyroid hormone (PTH)
PTHRP (parathyroid hormone-related
        peptide), 151b
Pulmonary edema, 93b, 107b
Pyramid (kidney), 19, 20f

R
Reflection coefficient, 8
Renal artery, 20, 20f
Renal artery stenosis, 41b
Renal blood flow, 37-41
    autoregulation of, 38-41, 38f, 39f
    hormones influencing, 41t
    regulation of, 41-45
Renal clearance, 31-34
    equations for, 32
    glomerular filtration rate and, 32-34
    mass balance relationship in, 31-32, 32f
Renal compensation, 142-143
Renal corpuscle, 21, 24-28, 24f-26f
Renal disease. See Kidney diseases
Renal plasma flow (RPF), 31
Renal replacement therapies, 3
Renal transport mechanisms, 47-70
    distal tube and collecting duct, 63-64
    in urine formation, 47-48
    membrane transport, 48, 50
    Na⁺, K⁺-ATPase pump, 51, 51f
    Na⁺ reabsorption, 52-54, 53f-55f
    organic anion secretion, 58b, 57-61, 59b
    transepithelial solute and water transport,
        general principles of, 50-52, 51f
Renal tubular acidosis (RTA), 140b
Renal vein, 20, 20f
Renalase, 2, 42
Renin, 2, 28, 96-97b
Renin-angiotensin-aldosterone system
    diuretics and, 166b
    H⁺ secretion and, 136
    in extracellular fluid volume regulation,
        96-98, 98f

Respiratory acid-base disorders, 141
    acidosis, 144-145
    alkalosis, 145
    buffering in, 142
Respiratory compensation, 142
Review examination, 209-221
Rhabdomyolysis, 118
RhBG (protein), 138b
RhCG (protein), 138b
Rhesus glycoproteins, 138b
ROMK channel (KCNJ1), 125b
RPF (renal plasma flow), 31
RTA (renal tubular acidosis), 140b

S
Secondary active transport, 50
Secretion, in urine formation, 47
Self-study problems, 189-201. See also
        problems at end of each chapter.
Serum electrolytes, normal values of, 183
Serum glucocorticoid-stimulated kinase
        (Sgk), 65b-66b
Serum proteins, normal values of, 183
Set point, 75
SIADH (syndrome of inappropriate ADH
        secretion), 76b
Single effect, in antidiuresis, 84
Sjögren's syndrome, 140b
Small cell carcinoma, 76b
Sodium (Na⁺)
    alterations in balance and
        H⁺ secretion, 136
    central nervous system sensors of, 95
    diuretic action and excretion of, 163
    excretion control with ECF volume
        contraction, 104-106, 107f
    excretion control with ECF volume
        expansion, 102-104, 103f
    filtered load of, 100, 101f
    in extracellular fluid, 10
    in intracellular fluid, 11
    reabsorption of, 51-55, 53f-55f, 101-102,
        102-103, 104
Sodium chloride (NaCl)
    cellular fluid exchange and, 13-14
    dietary intake and excretion of, 99-100, 100f
    excretion of, 91-92, 99-102
    extracellular fluid volume and, 91-92
    Henle's loop and reabsorption of, 61-62
    in autoregulation, 38, 39f
    osmotic diuretics and, 166-167
    reabsorption of, 52, 64-69, 65t
    transport along nephron, 57t
Solute-free water, 87, 169-170, 169t
Solvent drag, 48, 51
Specific gravity, 8, 8b
Spironolactone, 168
Starling forces, 11, 12f, 13
    in edema, 106-107
    in ultrafiltration, 34-35, 36-37, 36f
    peritubular, 67-69, 68f
Steady state, 91-92, 166

Supraoptic nuclei (hypothalamus), 73
Sweating, 71
Sympathetic nerves, 41-42, 95-96
Symport mechanisms, 50
Syndrome of inappropriate ADH secretion
        (SIADH), 76b

T
Tamm-Horsfall glycoprotein, 57
Tetany, 150, 151b, 152
Thiazide diuretics, 154, 165b-166b, 168
    Ca⁺⁺ excretion and, 171-172
    Na⁺ excretion and, 170
Thick ascending limb (Henle's loop), 170
Thirst, 79-80
Tight junctions, 52b, 62b
Titratable acids, 131
Tonicity, 7-8
Torsemide, 167
Total body water, 9
Transcellular pathway, 50-52, 51f, 54-55
Transcellular pathway, 50-52, 51f, 54-55
Triamterene, 168
Tubular conservation of water, 87
Tubules, renal, 21, 22f
Tubuloglomerular feedback, 38, 39b,
        39f-40f, 96
Tumor lysis syndrome, 118

U
Ultrafiltration
    dynamics of, 36-37, 36f
    in urine formation, 24, 34-35, 47
    ultrafiltrate composition,
        determinants of, 35, 35f
Uniport, 50
Urea, 77, 85-86
Urea nitrogen (BUN), normal
        values of, 183
Ureter, 19, 20f
Urinalysis, 57
Urinary bladder, 19, 20f
Urinary buffers, 131
Urine. See also Antidiuresis; Diuresis
    composition of, 48t
    dilution and concentration mechanisms,
        80-87, 82f, 83t
    formation of, 47-48, 48t
    renal diluting and concentrating ability,
        assessment of, 87b-88b
    specific gravity of, 8b
    ultrafiltration and formation of,
        24, 34-35
Urine anion gap, 140b
Urodilatin, 66-67, 98
Uroguanylin, 67, 92b, 99

V
V₂ (vasopressin 2) receptor
    ADH binding and membrane
        permeability, 76-77b, 78f
van't Hoff's law, 7
Vasa recta, 23-24, 86b-87b

Vascular baroreceptors, 94-95
Vascular resistance, renal, 38, 38f, 41, 42f
Vascular volume sensors, 94-95
Vasopressin. *See* Antidiuretic hormone
    (ADH)
Visceral layer (Bowman's capsule), 24
Vitamin D_3, 151, 160f
Volatile acid, 130
Volume contraction (extracellular fluid),
    92, 104-106, 107f
Volume expansion (extracellular fluid), 92,
    102-104, 103f
Volume sensors. *See* Baroreceptors

W

Water balance. *See also* Antidiuresis; Body
    fluid osmolality; Diuresis
    environmental factors in, 71, 72t
    excessive intake and, 80b
    osmotic diuretics and, 166-167
    plasma ADH levels and, 73, 73f
    positive vs. negative, 72
    regulation of, 71-73
    thirst and, 79-80
    water loss, routes of, 71, 72t
Water channels. *See* Aquaporins
Water intake, social/cultural aspects of, 80b

Water reabsorption, 54-56
    aquaporins in, 56b
    by nephron, 52
    Henle's loop and, 61-62, 78
    in extracellular fluid volume
        contraction, 104
    in urine formation, 47
    regulation of, 64-69, 65t
    urine dilution or concentration and, 85

Z

Zonula occludens (tight junction),
    52b, 62b